Renal Cell Cancer

Guest Editor

TONI K. CHOUEIRI, MD

HEMATOLOGY/ONCOLOGY CLINICS OF NORTH AMERICA

www.hemonc.theclinics.com

Consulting Editors
GEORGE P. CANELLOS, MD
NANCY BERLINER, MD

August 2011 • Volume 25 • Number 4

SAUNDERS an imprint of ELSEVIER, Inc.

W.B. SAUNDERS COMPANY
A Division of Elsevier Inc.

1600 John F. Kennedy Blvd. ● Suite 1800 ● Philadelphia, PA 19103-2899

http://www.theclinics.com

HEMATOLOGY/ONCOLOGY CLINICS OF NORTH AMERICA Volume 25, Number 4
August 2011 ISSN 0889-8588, ISBN 13: 978-1-4557-1103-1

Editor: Patrick Manley

Photocopying
Single photocopies of single articles may be made for personal use as allowed by national copyright laws. Permission of the Publisher and payment of a fee is required for all other photocopying, including multiple or systematic copying, copying for advertising or promotional purposes, resale, and all forms of document delivery. Special rates are available for educational institutions that wish to make photocopies for non-profit educational classroom use. For information on how to seek permission visit www.elsevier.com/permissions or call: (+44) 1865 843830 (UK)/(+1) 215 239 3804 (USA).

Derivative Works
Subscribers may reproduce tables of contents or prepare lists of articles including abstracts for internal circulation within their institutions. Permission of the Publisher is required for resale or distribution outside the institution. Permission of the Publisher is required for all other derivative works, including compilations and translations (please consult www.elsevier.com/permissions).

Electronic Storage or Usage
Permission of the Publisher is required to store or use electronically any material contained in this journal, including any article or part of an article (please consult www.elsevier.com/permissions). Except as outlined above, no part of this publication may be reproduced, stored in a retrieval system or transmitted in any form or by any means, electronic, mechanical, photocopying, recording or otherwise, without prior written permission of the Publisher.

Notice
No responsibility is assumed by the Publisher for any injury and/or damage to persons or property as a matter of products liability, negligence or otherwise, or from any use or operation of any methods, products, instructions or ideas contained in the material herein. Because of rapid advances in the medical sciences, in particular, independent verification of diagnoses and drug dosages should be made.

Although all advertising material is expected to conform to ethical (medical) standards, inclusion in this publication does not constitute a guarantee or endorsement of the quality or value of such product or of the claims made of it by its manufacturer.

Hematology/Oncology Clinics (ISSN 0889-8588) is published bimonthly by Elsevier Inc., 360 Park Avenue South, New York, NY 10010-1710. Months of issue are February, April, June, August, October, and December. Business and Editorial Offices: 1600 John F. Kennedy Blvd., Ste. 1800, Philadelphia, PA 19103–2899. Customer Service Office: 3251 Riverport Lane, Maryland Heights, MO 63043. Periodicals postage paid at New York, NY and at additional mailing offices. Subscription prices are $327.00 per year (domestic individuals), $541.00 per year (domestic institutions), $160.00 per year (domestic students/residents), $371.00 per year (Canadian individuals), $662.00 per year (Canadian institutions) $442.00 per year (international individuals), $662.00 per year (international institutions), and $216.00 per year (international and Canadian students/residents). International air speed delivery is included in all *Clinics* subscription prices. All prices are subject to change without notice. **POSTMASTER:** Send address changes to *Hematology/Oncology Clinics of North America*, Elsevier Health Sciences Division, Subscription Customer Service, 3251 Riverport Lane, Maryland Heights, MO 63043. Customer Service (orders, claims, online, change of address): Elsevier Health Sciences Division, Subscription Customer Service, 3251 Riverport Lane, Maryland Heights, MO 63043. Tel: 1-800-654-2452 (U.S. and Canada); 314-447-8871 (outside U.S. and Canada). Fax: 314-447-8029. E-mail: journalscustomerservice-usa@elsevier.com (for print support); journalsonlinesupport-usa@elsevier.com (for online support).

Reprints. For copies of 100 or more, of articles in this publication, please contact the Commercial Reprints Department, Elsevier Inc., 360 Park Avenue South, New York, New York 10010-1710; Tel.: 212-633-3813, Fax: 212-462-1935, E-mail: reprints@elsevier.com.

Hematology/Oncology Clinics of North America is covered in *MEDLINE/PubMed (Index Medicus), EMBASE/ Excerpta Medica, and BIOSIS.*

Printed and bound by CPI Group (UK) Ltd, Croydon, CR0 4YY

Transferred to Digital Print 2011

Contributors

CONSULTING EDITORS

GEORGE P. CANELLOS, MD
William Rosenberg Professor of Medicine, Department of Medical Oncology, Dana-Farber Cancer Institute, Boston, Massachusetts

NANCY BERLINER, MD
Chief, Division of Hematology, Brigham and Women's Hospital; Professor of Medicine, Harvard Medical School, Boston, Massachusetts

GUEST EDITOR

TONI K. CHOUEIRI, MD
Director, Kidney Cancer Center, Dana-Farber Cancer Institute/Brigham and Women's Hospital and Harvard Medical School, Boston, Massachusetts

AUTHORS

HANS-OLOV ADAMI, MD
Department of Epidemiology, Harvard School of Public Health, Boston, Massachusetts; Department of Medical Epidemiology and Biostatistics, Karolinska Institutet, Stockholm, Sweden

LAURENCE ALBIGES, MD
Medical Oncology Department, Institut Gustave Roussy, Villejuif, France

LAURIE APPLEBY, APRN, MS
The Lank Center for Genitourinary Oncology, Dana-Farber Cancer Institute, Harvard Medical School, Boston, Massachusetts

MICHAEL B. ATKINS, MD
Professor of Medicine, Harvard Medical School; Deputy Chief, Division of Hematology/Oncology, Beth Israel Deaconess Medical Center; Leader, Kidney Cancer Program, Dana-Farber/Harvard Cancer Center, Boston, Massachusetts

BRADLEY ATKINSON, PharmD
Clinical Pharmacist, Department of Genitourinary Medical Oncology, The University of Texas MD Anderson Cancer Center, Houston, Texas

JOAQUIM BELLMUNT, MD, PhD
Hospital del Mar, Barcelona, Spain

STEVEN C. CAMPBELL, MD, PhD
Center for Urologic Oncology, Cleveland Clinic, Glickman Urological and Kidney Institute, Cleveland, Ohio

DANIEL C. CHO, MD
Assistant Professor of Medicine, Harvard Medical School; Director, Experimental Therapeutics Program, Division of Hematology/Oncology, Beth Israel Deaconess Medical Center; Member, Kidney Cancer Program, Dana-Farber/Harvard Cancer Center, Boston, Massachusetts

EUNYOUNG CHO, ScD
Channing Laboratory, Department of Medicine, Harvard Medical School, Brigham and Women's Hospital; Department of Nutrition, Harvard School of Public Health, Boston, Massachusetts

TONI K. CHOUEIRI, MD
Director, Kidney Cancer Center, Dana-Farber Cancer Institute/Brigham and Women's Hospital and Harvard Medical School, Boston, Massachusetts

SIMON CHOWDHURY, MA, MRCP, PhD
Department of Medical Oncology, Guy's Hospital, London, United Kingdom

BERNARD ESCUDIER, MD
Medical Oncology Department, Institut Gustave Roussy, Villejuif, France

CHUNKIT FUNG, MD
Oncology Fellow, Division of Hematology/Oncology, Department of Medicine, Abramson Cancer Center, University of Pennsylvania, Philadelphia, Pennsylvania

ANGELA A. GIARDINO, MD
Department of Imaging, Dana-Farber Cancer Institute; Department of Radiology, Brigham and Women's Hospital; Assistant Professor of Radiology, Harvard Medical School, Boston, Massachusetts

NAOMI B. HAAS, MD
Associate Professor, Division of Hematology/Oncology, Department of Medicine, Abramson Cancer Center, University of Pennsylvania, Philadelphia, Pennsylvania

DANIEL Y.C. HENG, MD, MPH, FRCPC
Clinical Assistant Professor, Department of Oncology, Tom Baker Cancer Center, University of Calgary, Calgary, Alberta, Canada

WILLIAM G. KAELIN Jr, MD
Investigator, Department of Medical Oncology, Howard Hughes Medical Institute (HHMI), Chevy Chase, Maryland; Professor, Dana-Farber Cancer Institute, Brigham and Women's Hospital, Boston, Massachusetts

JOSE A. KARAM, MD
Urologic Oncology Fellow, Department of Urology, The University of Texas MD Anderson Cancer Center, Houston, Texas

KATHERINE M. KRAJEWSKI, MD
Department of Imaging, Dana-Farber Cancer Institute; Department of Radiology, Brigham and Women's Hospital; Instructor in Radiology, Harvard Medical School, Boston, Massachusetts

LIANJIE LI, PhD
Research Associate, Howard Hughes Medical Institute (HHMI), Chevy Chase, Maryland; Research Fellow, Department of Medical Oncology, Dana-Farber Cancer Institute, Brigham and Women's Hospital, Boston, Massachusetts

PER LINDBLAD, MD, PhD
Department of Urology, Örebro University Hospital, Örebro, Sweden

MARC R. MATRANA, MD, MS
Hematology and Medical Oncology Fellow, Department of Genitourinary Medical Oncology, The University of Texas MD Anderson Cancer Center, Houston, Texas

DAVID F. MCDERMOTT, MD
Assistant Professor of Medicine, Clinical Director, Biologic Therapy Program, Department of Medicine, Beth Israel Deaconess Medical Center, Harvard Medical School; Chair, Clinical Research Sub-Committee, Dana-Farber/Harvard Cancer Center Renal Cancer Program, Boston, Massachusetts

ANA M. MOLINA, MD
Genitourinary Oncology Service, Department of Medicine, Memorial Sloan-Kettering Cancer Center, New York, New York

STEPHANIE MORRISSEY, RN, BSN
The Lank Center for Genitourinary Oncology, Dana-Farber Cancer Institute, Harvard Medical School, Boston, Massachusetts

ROBERT J. MOTZER, MD
Genitourinary Oncology Service, Department of Medicine, Memorial Sloan-Kettering Cancer Center, New York, New York

IVAN PEDROSA, MD
Director, Body MRI, Department of Radiology, Beth Israel Deaconess Medical Center; Associate Professor of Radiology, Harvard Medical School, Boston, Massachusetts

BRIAN RINI, MD
Department of Solid Tumor Oncology, Cleveland Clinic Taussig Cancer Institute, Cleveland, Ohio

JONATHAN ROSENBERG, MD
The Lank Center for Genitourinary Oncology, Dana-Farber Cancer Institute, Harvard Medical School, Boston, Massachusetts

JACALYN ROSENBLATT, MD
Instructor in Medicine, Department of Medicine, Beth Israel Deaconess Medical Center, Harvard Medical School, Boston, Massachusetts

PAUL RUSSO, MD, FACS
Attending Surgeon; Professor of Urology, Urology Service, Department of Surgery, Memorial Sloan Kettering Cancer Center, Weill Medical College, Cornell University, New York, New York

MOHAMED SALEM, MD
Department of Solid Tumor Oncology, Cleveland Clinic Taussig Cancer Institute, Cleveland, Ohio

MATTHEW N. SIMMONS, MD, PhD
Center for Urologic Oncology, Cleveland Clinic, Glickman Urological and Kidney Institute, Cleveland, Ohio

MARC C. SMALDONE, MD
Urologic Oncology Fellow, Division of Urologic Oncology, Department of Surgery, Fox Chase Cancer Center, Philadelphia, Pennsylvania

PATRICIA A. TANG, MD, FRCPC
Clinical Assistant Professor, Department of Oncology, Tom Baker Cancer Center, University of Calgary, Calgary, Alberta, Canada

NIZAR M. TANNIR, MD, FACP
Associate Professor, Department of Genitourinary Medical Oncology, The University of Texas MD Anderson Cancer Center, Houston, Texas

CHRISTOPHER TSANG, BA
Department of Medical Oncology, Guy's Hospital, London, United Kingdom

ROBERT G. UZZO, MD, FACS
Professor and Chairman, Division of Urologic Oncology, Department of Surgery, Fox Chase Cancer Center, Philadelphia, Pennsylvania

ANNICK D. VAN DEN ABBEELE, MD
Chief, Department of Imaging, Dana-Farber Cancer Institute; Department of Radiology, Brigham and Women's Hospital; Associate Professor of Radiology, Harvard Medical School, Boston, Massachusetts

MICHAEL M. VICKERS, MD, FRCPC
Clinical Assistant Professor, Department of Oncology, Tom Baker Cancer Center, University of Calgary, Calgary, Alberta, Canada

MARTIN H. VOSS, MD
Genitourinary Oncology Service, Department of Medicine, Memorial Sloan-Kettering Cancer Center, New York, New York

CHRISTOPHER G. WOOD, MD, FACS
Professor, Department of Urology, The University of Texas MD Anderson Cancer Center, Houston, Texas

YUKA YAMAGUCHI, MD
Department of Urology, Cleveland Clinic, Glickman Urological and Kidney Institute, Cleveland, Ohio

KATHERINE ZUKOTYNSKI, MD
Department of Imaging, Dana-Farber Cancer Institute; Department of Radiology, Brigham and Women's Hospital; Instructor in Radiology, Harvard Medical School, Boston, Massachusetts

Contents

The majority of kidney cancer tumors are small renal masses (SRMs). Partial nephrectomy is now established as the preferred treatment modality. In some patients the potential morbidity may outweigh the oncologic risk. Based on active surveillance studies, restriction of radical therapy to patients with aggressive tumors has been proposed. This has spurred renewed interest in development of radiologic and biopsy-based diagnostic techniques that can identify high-risk disease. This article discusses the natural history and pathologic features of SRMs, the evolving role of biopsy, and provides an overview of outcomes of various treatment approaches and current recommendations for management.

There were an estimated 58,240 new cases and 13,040 deaths from kidney cancer in the United States in 2010. The increased treatment and cure of small, incidentally discovered renal tumors, most of which are nonlethal in nature, has not offset the increased mortality caused by advanced and metastatic tumors. In this article, the optimum approach to the surgical management of localized renal tumors and its impact on renal function are discussed.

Renal cell carcinoma (RCC) is considered a relatively rare malignancy worldwide. Around a third of patients with RCC present with metastatic disease, and among those patients treated with nephrectomy with curative intent, more than one-third develop metastases during postoperative follow-up. Due to the absence of curative medical treatments for metastatic RCC, surgery remains the mainstay of therapy. Surgery plays a key role in two aspects: cytoreductive nephrectomy to remove the primary renal tumor in the presence of known metastatic disease, and metastasectomy to remove distant metastatic foci in patients with metastatic RCC.

The standard of care for renal cell carcinoma (RCC) is surgical resection as a monotherapy or as part of a multimodal approach. A significant number of patients undergoing surgery for localized RCC experience recurrence, suggesting that there are some individuals in whom surgical excision is necessary but insufficient because of the presence of micrometastatic disease at diagnosis. This review summarizes current algorithms used to identify patients at high risk for disease recurrence following the surgical resection of RCC, the outcomes of contemporary adjuvant systemic therapy trials, and the rationale supporting the use of neoadjuvant therapy.

Although several cytokines have shown antitumor activity in renal cell carcinoma (RCC), the most consistent results have been reported with interleukin-2 (IL-2) and interferon (IFN). Recent insights into how the immune response to a tumor is regulated hold the promise of allowing patients to obtain a durable response to immunotherapy, perhaps without the significant toxicity associated with conventional approaches. This review describes how improvements in patient selection, combination therapy, and investigational agents might expand and better define the role of immunotherapy in metastatic RCC.

Vascular endothelial growth factor (VEGF) is, to date, the key element in the pathogenesis of renal cell carcinoma (RCC). VEGF pathway activation is responsible for the recruitment, migration, and expansion of endothelial cells, with this angiogenesis tumor model being characteristic of RCC. Different strategies have been developed for almost a decade to block the VEGF pathway in this setting. Four different compounds were approved for metastatic RCC (mRCC) in the past 6 years: bevacizumab, sunitinib, sorafenib, and pazopanib. Axitinib and tivozanib are also promising compounds under evaluation. The revolution in the management and prognosis of patients with mRCC is ongoing.

Better understanding of the molecular biology of renal cell carcinoma (RCC) has led to the development of several targeted anti-cancer agents, several of which have since received approval for treatment of advanced disease. Two of these, the intravenous agent temsirolimus and the oral everolimus, exhibit antitumor effects through inhibition of the mammalian target of rapamycin (mTOR) pathway. This article reviews their mechanisms of action in the context of the current understanding of RCC pathophysiology, the clinical data leading to their approval, class-specific toxicities, potential molecular mechanisms behind treatment resistance and novel treatment approaches for RCC that incorporate mTOR blockade.

Insights into the biology of clear-cell renal cell carcinoma (CCRCC) have identified multiple pathways associated with the pathogenesis and progression of this cancer. This progress has led to the development of multiple agents targeting these pathways, including the tyrosine kinase inhibitors sorafenib, sunitinib, and pazopanib, the monoclonal antibody bevacizumab, and the mTOR inhibitors temsirolimus and everolimus. With the exception of temsirolimus, phase 3 trials tested these agents in patients with clear-cell histology; therefore, their efficacy in non-CCRCC is unclear. To date, there is no established effective therapy for patients with advanced non-CCRCC. This article focuses on treatment options for metastatic non-CCRCC.

The current treatment paradigm for metastatic renal cell carcinoma (RCC) includes agents that target the vascular endothelial growth factor (VEGF) and mammalian target of rapamycin (mTOR) pathways. Because these agents have revolutionized RCC over the past five years, new clinical and molecular predictive and prognostic tools are required. These are potentially important for therapy selection, patient counseling, and clinical trial stratification. This review examines clinical prognostic models and molecular biomarkers in RCC.

The advent of targeted agents for the treatment of advanced renal cell carcinoma has led to dramatic improvements in therapy. However, the chronic use of these medications has also led to the identification of new toxicities that require long-term management. Effective management of toxicity is needed to maximize the benefits of treatment and improve patients' quality of life. In addition, toxicity from these agents may affect treatment compliance, particularly with daily oral agents. This review delineates the toxicities that require monitoring, the underlying pathophysiology (when known), and treatments that may have benefits in relieving symptoms and side effects.

Emerging from a largely cytokine-based era, the last several years have witnessed a dramatic change in the therapeutic landscape of renal cancer. Molecularly targeted and antiangiogenic agents now form the backbone of most therapeutic strategies for patients with advanced renal cell carcinoma (RCC). Although the next few years may not see such broad paradigm shifts, there remains significant room for improvement in the care of patients with RCC. This review discusses challenges that face physicians and researchers as well as innovations that may contribute to improving the therapeutic outcomes for patients with RCC.

THE CLINICS ARE NOW AVAILABLE ONLINE!

Access your subscription at:
www.theclinics.com

Preface

Renal Cell Carcinoma

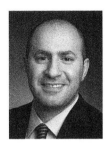

Toni K. Choueiri, MD
Guest Editor

Since December 2005 and as of August 2011, the date of this issue, six "targeted" drugs have been approved in metastatic renal cell carcinoma (RCC). Several others are expected to be approved in the near future.

With the elucidation of von Hippel Lindau gene dysregulation, scientists have enabled clinical investigators to approach clear-cell RCC—the most common type of RCC—at the molecular level. The discovery that this tumor is driven by angiogenesis (see Li and Kaelin) has led to establishing the vascular endothelial growth factor (VEGF) and the mammalian target of rapamycin as the cornerstone of therapy for RCC (see Voss and Albiges). Overall, patients with advanced RCC now live longer and have options.

The success of these therapies in the advanced setting makes them attractive options to be tested in the adjuvant and neoadjuvant settings (see Smaldone and colleagues), and in non-clear-cell histologies (see Chowdhury and colleagues). These agents can cause "class-effect" toxicities such as hypertension, diarrhea, wound healing, cardiovascular events, metabolic derangements, and others. It is therefore essential that health care providers be familiar with the management of side effects from these novel agents (see Appleby and colleagues) to maximize therapeutic benefit.

Immunotherapy is considered an old standard in advanced RCC; nevertheless, high-dose interleukin-2 remains the only therapy with durable (albeit quite rare), complete remissions and insights into patient selection for such a toxic therapy is key (see Rosenblatt and McDermott).

RCC accounts for ~2% of all malignant diseases and incidence rates in the US have been rising steadily for over three decades. However, the increasing incidence of RCC cannot fully be explained by increasing availability and use of novel sensitive imaging (see Krajewski and colleagues) and may indicate an increase in the prevalence of etiologic risk factors. While smoking, hypertension, and obesity are established risk factors, several other occupational and lifestyle factors may also affect the risk of RCC (see Cho and colleagues).

Hematol Oncol Clin N Am 25 (2011) xiii–xiv
doi:10.1016/j.hoc.2011.06.001
0889-8588/11/$ – see front matter © 2011 Elsevier Inc. All rights reserved.
hemonc.theclinics.com

Surgery remains the mainstay of curative therapy for nonmetastatic RCC. Surgical techniques are evolving. We understand now more than ever that partial nephrectomy, when feasible, will lead to an equivalent long-term oncologic control to radical nephrectomy with the advantage of saving nephrons (see Russo).

Small renal masses (SRMs) are increasingly encountered in clinical practice and represent a challenging scenario with risk of overtreatment, particularly in the elderly and patients with limited life expectancy. Studies are now emerging with pathologic data suggesting that a large number of these SRMs are benign lesions or indolent cancers. Active surveillance or ablative therapies may therefore be appropriate in selected cases (see Yamaguchi and colleagues).

Surgery also plays a role in advanced RCC. In appropriately selected patients, cytoreductive nephrectomy as well as metastectomy can prolong survival. Whether this is applicable to the new era of targeted therapy remains unclear (see Karam and Wood).

While significant strides have been made in RCC biology and treatment in the last several years, many challenges will continue to face researchers and clinicians. Why do patients eventually progress; what are the mechanisms underlying VEGF-targeted therapy resistance, and is the strategy of combining "active" drugs better than sequencing them? How should we think beyond 2011? (see Cho and Atkins). Patient selection/stratification remains essential in the targeted era and biomarkers of efficacy are more than ever needed in the complicated therapeutic landscape in RCC (see Tang and colleagues).

In this issue of *Hematology/Oncology Clinics of North America*, I have assembled a panel of thought leaders in the field, many of whom played pivotal roles in the development of our current treatment paradigms. Together, their contributions provide a comprehensive and up-to-date review of the management of this disease, and what we can anticipate on the horizon for the treatment of RCC.

Toni K. Choueiri, MD
Kidney Cancer Center
Dana-Farber Cancer Institute/Brigham and Women's Hospital
and Harvard Medical School
450 Brookline Avenue
Boston, MA 02215, USA

E-mail address:
Toni_Choueiri@dfci.harvard.edu

Epidemiology of Renal Cell Cancer

Eunyoung Cho, ScD[a,b,*], Hans-Olov Adami, MD[c,d],
Per Lindblad, MD, PhD[e]

KEYWORDS

- Renal cell cancer • Epidemiology • Risk factors • Incidence
- Mortality • Smoking • Obesity • Hypertension

More than 90% of kidney cancers arise in the renal parenchyma, and the remainder in the renal pelvis.[1] Most cancers in the parenchyma are renal cell carcinomas (RCC), a heterogeneous class of tumors arising from different cell types within the nephron with a clinical course ranging from indolent to highly aggressive. Advances in our understanding of the genetics underlying the pathogenesis of renal cell neoplasms have led to a histopathologic classification into several subgroups, of which "clear-cell" histology is the most common (75%–80%). As the increasing incidence of RCC observed for the past several decades in most parts of the world cannot fully be explained by the increasing availability of medical services and the use of novel sensitive imaging procedures, an increase in the prevalence of etiologic risk factors must also play a role.

DESCRIPTIVE EPIDEMIOLOGY

It is difficult to obtain clear population-based patterns of incidence and mortality from RCC because population data from different regions are presented for RCC and renal pelvis cancer combined. Hence, kidney cancer in this section, unless otherwise specified, includes cancers of the renal parenchyma and renal pelvis.

The authors have nothing to disclose.
[a] Channing Laboratory, Department of Medicine, Harvard Medical School and Brigham and Women's Hospital, 181 Longwood Avenue, Boston, MA 02115, USA
[b] Department of Nutrition, Harvard School of Public Health, 665 Huntington Avenue, Boston, MA 02115, USA
[c] Department of Epidemiology, Harvard School of Public Health, 677 Huntington Avenue, Boston, MA 02215, USA
[d] Department of Medical Epidemiology and Biostatistics, Karolinska Institutet, SE-171 77 Stockholm, Sweden
[e] Department of Urology, Örebro University Hospital, SE-701 85 Örebro, Sweden
* Corresponding author. Channing Laboratory, 181 Longwood Avenue, Boston, MA 02115.
E-mail address: eunyoung.cho@channing.harvard.edu

Hematol Oncol Clin N Am 25 (2011) 651–665
doi:10.1016/j.hoc.2011.04.002
0889-8588/11/$ – see front matter © 2011 Elsevier Inc. All rights reserved.

Incidence

The global incidence of kidney cancer increased from the 1970s until the mid 1990s, then leveled out or decreased in many countries.[2,3] In 2008, kidney cancer was estimated to afflict about 270,000 individuals worldwide, accounting for more than 2% of all malignant diseases.[4] In the United States annual incidence rose by 2.6% per year between 1997 and 2007, and it was estimated that more than 58,000 men and women would be diagnosed in 2010.[5] Kidney cancer was the seventh (4% of total cancer) leading malignant condition among men and the eighth (3%) among women in the United States in 2010.[6] In the United States incidence rates are somewhat higher among the black than among the white population. RCC is more common in men than in women; male to female ratios are generally between 1.5:1 and 2.5:1. The incidence rates are highest in the sixth and seventh decades.

Globally, the incidence of kidney cancer varies more than 10-fold between populations and geographic areas (**Fig. 1**),[1] suggesting that lifestyle factors may play major role in the difference in incidence across the continents. The highest rates are found in North America, Europe, and Australia, and the lowest in Asia. Moreover, genetic variations among populations may play a role. The increasing incidence observed for past decades in almost all areas and the geographic differences in incidences may also be explained in part by increased use of novel diagnostic imaging methods such as ultrasonography and computed tomography (CT). The widespread use of these imaging procedures has led to an increase in diagnosis of incidentally detected RCCs, which tend to be at a lower stage and more likely localized than symptomatic.[7]

Incidence rates for RCC in the United States have been rising steadily for more than 3 decades, more rapidly among African Americans than Caucasians. In the United States also, RCC incidence differs among racial and ethnic populations (see **Fig. 1**). A recent study reported overall increased incidence rates (2.39%), mainly due to a remarkable increase in the incidence of localized RCC (4.29%) from 1988 to 2006.[8] The incidence of distant stage decreased over time but those of regional spread remained unchanged. This finding strongly indicates changes in the diagnosis of RCC compared with earlier diagnoses in recent years.[8]

In Europe there have been regional differences in rates and trends over time, with high rates remaining in several countries in central and eastern Europe, whereas in Sweden over the last decades there have been decreases in rates, with stable rates in Denmark. In other northern European countries, except for the United Kingdom, incidence rates have tended to decrease or stabilize.[3]

Mortality

Trends in mortality from kidney cancer have reflected trends in incidence, but with a smaller increase over time in the past decades. The worldwide mortality rates of kidney cancer were estimated to be 116,000 in 2008, which is 1.5% of all cancer deaths. Similar to incidence, mortality varies considerably between regions.[4] Among women, mortality rates were in general about half those of men.

In Europe, death rates increased until the early 1990s and thereafter declined or stabilized. In general, the decreases were larger in men of middle age in western European countries. Nevertheless, in the early 2000s there was a greater than threefold difference in kidney cancer mortality within Europe, with high rates remaining especially in the Czech Republic and Baltic countries and the lowest rates in Greece, Spain, Portugal, and Romania.[3,9]

In the United States it was estimated that 13,000 deaths from kidney cancer occurred in 2010,[6] making it the tenth most common death in malignancy among

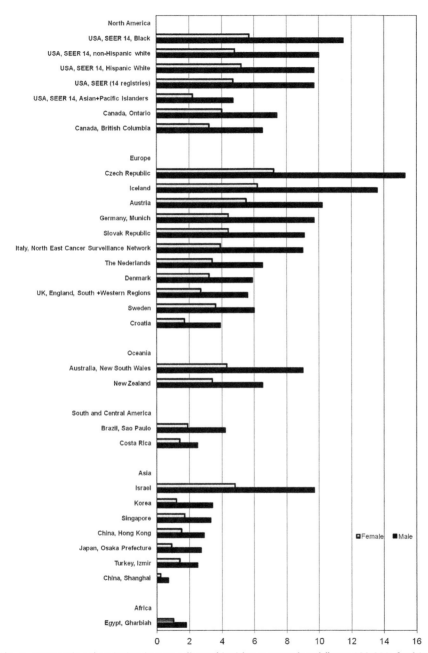

Fig. 1. International variation in age-adjusted incidence rates (world) per 100,000, for histologic verified renal cell cancer in selected countries. (*From* Curado MP, Edwards B, Shin HR, et al. Cancer incidence in five continents, vol. 9. Lyon (France): IARC; 2007; with permission.)

men. Death rates were highest among American Indians and Alaska Natives. Between the mid-1970s and mid-1990s, kidney cancer mortality increased despite the increasing proportion of localized, incidentally detected tumors; this could in part be the result of increase in all stages including advanced disease.[10] The diagnosis of

RCC with smaller tumors and at an earlier stage probably has contributed to the recent plateauing in mortality seen in the United States and also in many European countries.[3]

However, in a recent analysis of RCC cases diagnosed from 1988 to 2006 based on 17 registries from the Surveillance Epidemiology and End Results (SEER) database, the overall estimated age-adjusted rates increased annually by 0.78% where mortality rates for localized RCC increased by 3.16%, but those with regional and distant RCC decreased by 0.46% and 0.53%, respectively, over time.[8] Together this could imply that thus far it has not been shown that early treatment is efficacious. Moreover, the decreased mortality in advanced RCC could in part be due to improvement in the treatment for advanced stages.

Survival

Relative survival rates for kidney cancer are higher in the United States than in Europe.[11] From 2000 to 2002, for data from 47 European cancer registries (EUROCARE-4), the mean 5-year relative survival for kidney cancer was 55.7% compared with 62.6% from 13 United States SEER registries.[11] In the Nordic region relative survival has been increasing in all countries from 1964 to 2003.[12]

In the United States, the 5-year relative survival rates increased from 1983 to 2002 across all stages.[13] In a new report reevaluating SEER data including RCCs diagnosed from 1988 to 2006, 5-year relative survival for RCC of all stages increased from 63.7% in 1988 to 73.9% in 2002. For localized disease, survival rates increased from 91.7% in 1988 to 92.8% in 2002 whereas the rates remained unchanged for regional (63.7% to 64.2%) and metastatic disease (12.1% to 11.9%) over time.[8] This improvement in survival confined to localized disease may reflect the effect of lead-time bias, due to earlier diagnosis than in the past and also detection of indolent, nonlethal tumors with new imaging techniques.

RISK FACTORS
Tobacco Use

Cigarette smoke, containing a wide range of carcinogenic compounds including poly-cyclic aromatic hydrocarbons, aromatic amines, heterocyclic amines, and N-nitrosa-mines, can both initiate and promote tumor development in animals. Cigarette smoking is also one of the well-established risk factors for RCC. According to The International Agency for Research on Cancer (IARC) there is sufficient evidence to define tobacco smoking as a cause of RCC.[14] A meta-analysis of 24 (19 case-control and 5 cohort) studies reported a relative risk of 1.38 (95% confidence interval 1.27–1.50) for ever-smokers compared with lifetime never-smokers. Men had a 54% and women had a 22% increased risk for RCC. There was also a dose-dependent increase in risk related to the number of cigarettes smoked per day.[15] Smoking cessation for more than 10 years may reduce the elevated risk attributable to smoking.

Anthropometric Measures

Overweight, especially obesity, is another well-established risk factor for RCC in both women and men. According to a meta-analysis of 17 epidemiologic studies, a 5-unit increase in body mass index increases risk for RCC by 24% in men and 34% in women.[16] Later studies also supported the positive association in both genders.[17] Most studies found a dose-response relationship with increasing body mass index. Waist circumference and waist-hip ratio provide an estimate of abdominal or central obesity, a powerful contributor to metabolic abnormalities such as insulin resistance and hyperinsulinemia. In a few studies, waist circumference or waist-hip ratio was positively associated with RCC risk,[17–19] as was weight gain[17,20] or loss.[21] The proportion of all cases of RCC attributable to overweight and obesity has been estimated to be about 40% in the United States and up to about 30% in European countries.[22,23] There is still an unexplained stronger association in women than in men.

The mechanisms by which obesity influences renal carcinogenesis are not clear, but several plausible although speculative explanations exist. For example, sex steroid hormones may affect renal cell proliferation and growth by direct endocrine receptor-mediated effects, by regulation of receptor concentrations, or through paracrine growth factors such as epidermal growth factor. Further, obesity is related to several endocrine disorders such as decreased levels of sex hormone-binding globulin and progesterone, anovulation, insulin resistance, and increased levels of growth factors such as insulin-like growth factor 1 and high circulating levels of leptin. Lower adiponectin levels have also been observed among RCC patients than in healthy controls. There is also some evidence that link obesity, inflammation, and development of insulin resistance.[24]

Adult height is a complex variable because of its multiple determinants, including genetic, nutritional, and health-related factors. Most,[17,25–27] but not all[19,28] studies have found a positive association between height and risk of RCC.

Physical Activity

Because energy expenditure is an important determinant of adult weight and obesity, a role of physical activity in renal carcinogenesis is plausible. The impact of occupational and/or recreational physical activity on the risk of RCC has been reported in several case-control and cohort studies.[29] Some of the studies found that either occupational[30,31] or recreational[29,32–34] physical activity was associated with reduced risk of RCC. It remains unclear whether the association is independent of obesity.

Foods

Meat intake has been hypothesized to elevate risk for RCC, presumably because of its fat and protein content. Besides these nutrients, products in cooked meat such as heterocyclic amines, polycyclic aromatic hydrocarbons, and in cured meat nitrites and nitrates may mediate the renal carcinogenic process.[35,36] Studies suggest an association between fried,[37] processed,[38,39] or barbecued meat[36] and RCC risk. A meta-analysis of 13 case-control studies found a positive association between consumption of poultry, processed meat, red meat, and all meat and RCC risk, with 20% to 30% elevated risk among those in the highest compared with the lowest intake category for each of the meat groups.[40] Later case-control studies also supported the positive association between red meat intake and RCC risk.[39,41,42] By contrast, a recent pooled analysis of 13 prospective studies from North America and Europe found no association between intakes of red meat, processed meat, poultry, or seafood and RCC risk,[43] nor did a large prospective European study.[44]

Fruits and vegetables contain antioxidant nutrients and other dietary factors that may reduce RCC risk. Several case-control studies found a protective effect of vegetables and/or fruits, often strong for vegetables, especially the dark green and cruciferous varieties.[37,38,41,42,45] A pooled analysis of 13 prospective studies also found an inverse association between fruit and vegetable consumption and RCC risk.[46] However, in the large prospective European study, no associations between consumption of fruits and vegetables, except root vegetables, and RCC risk were observed.[47]

Neither coffee nor tea drinking has been conclusively associated with RCC risk,[48] although a pooled analysis of 13 prospective studies found an inverse association with both coffee and tea.[49]

Two studies have examined dietary pattern and RCC; one study found an inverse association with "drinker pattern" (wine, hard liquor, beer, and snacks)[50] and the other found a positive association with high-fat and high-protein diets.[51]

Nutrients

Fat and protein intake and RCC risk has been examined in several case-control studies, some of which found a positive association.[39] However, a recent pooled analysis of 13 prospective studies from North America and Europe found no association between intakes of fat and protein or their subtypes and RCC risk.[43] On the other hand, antioxidant nutrients including carotenoids,[45,52] vitamin C,[37,53] and vitamin E[18,38,53] have been associated with reduced risk of RCC. A pooled analysis of 13 prospective studies found an inverse association between β-carotene intake and RCC risk.[46]

Alcohol

Although alcohol intake is related to elevated risk of several cancer sites such as oral cavity, esophagus, and breast, several case-control[37,38,54,55] studies, a pooled analysis of 13 prospective studies, and a large European study consistently found an inverse association between alcohol consumption and RCC risk.[44,56] Overall, evidence is convincing that alcohol intake does not increase but most likely reduces risk of RCC, perhaps through enhancement of insulin sensitivity and risk of diabetes.[57,58]

Hypertension and Antihypertensive Medications

History of hypertension has been consistently associated with an elevated risk of RCC.[59] There is indeed sufficient evidence that hypertension is an independent risk factor for RCC. Use of antihypertensive medications including diuretics and nondiuretic antihypertensive medications[60–63] has also been associated with elevated risk of RCC. However, these data likely reflect confounding by indication rather than a causal association.[64–67] As suspected, some studies reported that the association with hypertensive medications disappeared once hypertension was accounted for[59,61,63,68] and high blood pressure was associated with an increased risk also among men and women who never took antihypertensive medications.[62] The association between risk of RCC and hypertension has also been shown to be independent of obesity. The biological mechanism for the association between risk for RCC and hypertension is not known.

Other Medical Conditions

End-stage renal disease

The incidence of RCC in patients with end-stage renal disease developing acquired cystic kidney disease has been reported to be elevated compared with the general population.[69–73] An increased risk has also been seen in native kidneys after renal transplantation.[74–77] While proliferation of proximal tubular epithelial cells has been identified as the major pathogenic mechanism of cyst formation, hormones (eg, estrogens), growth factors, and their receptors may stimulate cell proliferation and promote carcinogenesis. This mechanism may also explain, in part, the onset of multiple renal adenomas and bilateral carcinomas that develop in patients with acquired cystic kidney disease.[78]

Diabetes mellitus

Most case-control studies found either no increased risk with diabetes[60,63,79–82] or an excess risk confined to women.[54,83–86] Few cohort studies exist, but some reported a significantly increased incidence of RCC among diabetic patients.[87–89] However, diabetes may not be an independent risk factor because of its strong relation to obesity and hypertension. Elevated levels of growth factors and growth factor receptors may mediate the possible relationship between diabetes and RCC.[89]

Chronic hepatitis C infection

One recent prospective study found that chronic infection with hepatitis C virus was associated with a significantly increased risk of RCC (hazard ratio 1.77), after adjusting for age, gender, ethnicity, and the presence of chronic kidney disease.[90]

Analgesics

Phenacetin-containing analgesics have been implicated chiefly in the etiology of renal pelvic cancer,[91] but their role in RCC risk is less clear. Several studies have found a moderately elevated RCC risk with regular or long-term use of phenacetin.[80,83,85,92–95] More recent studies had limited power to evaluate phenacetin because the drug has been unavailable for many years. Among other analgesics, a few studies have found a positive association between acetaminophen, a metabolite of phenacetin, and RCC risk.[20,96,97] A meta-analysis of 5 case-control studies and 3 cohort studies found some suggestion of positive association between use of aspirin and RCC risk.[98] More recently, prospective data from more than 140,000 individuals found that the risk for RCC was increased among subjects who used nonaspirin, nonsteroidal anti-inflammatory drugs.[99] Aspirin use was not associated with RCC risk.

Reproductive Factors and Hormones

The reason for the consistent gender difference in RCC incidence is unknown, but hormone-related factors may play a role. Several studies found no associations with use of oral contraceptives or hormone replacement therapy,[100] but in some studies risk of RCC was significantly reduced following oral contraceptive use among nonsmokers.[100–102] Hysterectomy has been associated with increased risk of RCC in case-control studies and one recent cohort study, but not in all.[100,101,103] At least 8 studies have consistently found a positive association with number of births.[18,85,100,104] The possible role of reproductive factors in RCC etiology remains poorly understood, but there is some evidence that certain hormone-related factors are associated with the risk, although these associations seem unlikely to explain the lower incidence among women than in men.

Occupation

In contrast to bladder cancer, RCC is generally not considered an occupation-related cancer, although associations have been reported with asbestos,[105,106] gasoline and other petroleum products,[107–109] hydrocarbons,[110–112] lead,[106,113] cadmium,[106] and trichloroethylene (TCE).[114] The IARC has considered TCE, used mainly in metal degreasing and dry cleaning, as carcinogenic in animals and probably also in humans. A possible association between TCE and RCC has been reported in numerous studies[114,115] but is not yet proven as causal. It is interesting that RCC patients with high exposure of TCE have been shown to have more frequent somatic von Hippel-Lindau (VHL) mutations.[116]

GENETIC FACTORS

Although most RCCs are sporadic, 2% to 4% have a hereditary cause. Several genetic diseases are associated with RCC, including VHL syndrome, hereditary papillary renal carcinoma (HPRCC), hereditary leiomyomatosis RCC, Birt-Hogg-Dube (BHD) syndrome, chromosome 3 translocation, and tuberous sclerosis (TCS1, TCS2).[117]

VHL syndrome is a dominantly inherited multisystemic disorder including tumors in several organs: kidneys (often multiple, and bilateral tumors), pancreas, adrenal glands, epididymis, eyes, spine, and cerebellum.[118] The cumulative risk of RCC is more than 70% by the age of 60 years, and renal cell cancer is the most common cause of death.[119] Located on chromosome 3p, the VHL tumor-suppressor gene is involved in both spontaneous and hereditary RCC and is inactivated via several mechanisms, including mutation and silencing by DNA methylation.[120] This gene is exclusively involved in the conventional (clear cell) carcinoma. Somatic mutation of the VHL gene explains at least 50% of sporadic clear cell RCC while methylation of the gene explains another 10% to 20%.[120] Loss of VHL gene function correlates with increased expression of angiogenetic factors such as vascular endothelial growth factor. Overexpression of endothelial growth factor in vascularized tumors such as RCC may promote growth and progression.[121] The VHL tumor suppressor protein (pVHL) plays a central role also in the mammalian oxygen-sensing pathway through hypoxia-inducible factor (HIF).[120] In the absence of pVHL, HIF induces the expression of several genes that are related to regulation of angiogenesis, cell growth, or cell survival.

HPRCC is characterized by multifocal, bilateral tumor. This syndrome has an autosomal dominant inheritance pattern, distinct from that of other hereditary RCCs. It is caused by a germline mutation of the c-MET proto-oncogene on chromosome 7q (type 1 papillary RCC) or loss-of-function mutations of Fumarate Hydratase gene (type 2 papillary RCC). Apart from this, there is no loss of alleles of the short arm of chromosome 3 in papillary renal cell carcinoma; trisomies mainly of chromosomes 7, 16, and 17 and, in men, loss of chromosome Y are found.

BHD syndrome, caused by germline loss of function mutations of the BHD gene, is characterized by fibrofolliculomas, lung cysts, and a spectrum of renal carcinomas of varying histologic subtypes (chromophobe, oncocytoma, clear cell, or papillary).[120,122] Families with RCC have also been characterized by constitutionally balanced translocations between chromosomes 3 and 6 or 8 and between chromosomes 2 and 3.[122]

Few epidemiologic studies have analyzed family history of RCC and risk of RCC. Two studies found about 50% to 60% increased risk, and another a 2.5-fold increased

Table 1
Summary of risk factors for RCC

Convincing	Probable	Possible
Smoking	Alcohol—inverse	Fruits and vegetables—inverse
Obesity	Physical activity—inverse	Protein and/or fat
Hypertension	Height	Analgesics
Acquired cystic kidney disease	Parity	Other reproductive factors (eg, oral contraceptives)
Inherited susceptibility (eg, von Hippel-Lindau)	—	Occupational exposures (eg, asbestos, cadmium, hydrocarbons, gasoline, trichloroethylene)
—	—	Diabetes

risk of RCC if a first-degree relative was affected with the disease,[123-125] whereas no association was found in a smaller study.[85]

Several genes have been studied in relation to RCC risk and certain exposures, for example, GST, NAT2 and cigarette smoking, VHL and trichloroethylene.[116,126,127]

SUMMARY

The increasing incidence of RCC in most populations may be due in part to incidental detection of indolent, nonlethal tumors with new sensitive imaging modalities, which would entail a spuriously improved survival for localized disease. However, the increasing incidence is not restricted to small local tumors but also includes more advanced tumors, which explains the still high mortality rates in some countries. RCC is increasingly diagnosed at an early stage in many countries, which likely contributes to the recent leveling of RCC mortality in the United States and many European countries. However, over all stages nearly 50% of the patients die within 5 years after diagnosis.

Cigarette smoking and obesity may account for approximately 40% of all incidental cases in high-risk countries. Besides obesity, rising prevalence of hypertension may also play a growing role. Several other occupational and lifestyle factors may also affect the risk of RCC (**Table 1**). In terms of dietary factors, there are several leads but no association has been accepted as causal, as an expert panel organized by World Cancer Research Fund and American Institute for Cancer Research has concluded.[128] Genetic variations may also be important as a cause of the difference among populations. Continued research in RCC etiology is needed alongside better treatment options for nonlocalized disease. With the aim of prevention, the continued search for environmental causes should take into account the fact that RCC consists of different types with specific genetic molecular characteristics. In some cases, these genetic alterations have been purportedly associated with specific exposures. Furthermore, genetic polymorphisms may have a modulating effect on metabolic activation and detoxification enzymes. Therefore, better understanding of the genetic and molecular processes involved in RCC will, it is hoped, provide a better knowledge of how to analyze and interpret exposure associations that have importance for both initiation and progression of RCC.

REFERENCES

1. Curado MP, Edwards B, Shin HR, et al. Cancer incidence in five continent, vol. 9. Lyon (France): IARC; 2007.
2. Mathew A, Devesa SS, Fraumeni JF Jr, et al. Global increases in kidney cancer incidence, 1973–1992. Eur J Cancer Prev 2002;11(2):171–8.
3. Levi F, Ferlay J, Galeone C, et al. The changing pattern of kidney cancer incidence and mortality in Europe. BJU Int 2008;101(8):949–58.
4. Ferlay J, Shin HR, Bray F, et al. GLOBOCAN 2008: cancer incidence and mortality worldwide. Lyon (France): International Agency for Research on Cancer; 2010.
5. SEER cancer statistics review, 1975–2007. National Cancer Institute. 2010. Available at: http://seer.cancer.gov/csr/1975_2007/. Accessed May 20, 2011.
6. Jemal A, Siegel R, Xu J, et al. Cancer statistics, 2010. CA Cancer J Clin 2010; 60(5):277–300.
7. Bensalah K, Pantuck AJ, Crepel M, et al. Prognostic variables to predict cancer-related death in incidental renal tumours. BJU Int 2008;102(10):1376–80.

8. Sun M, Thuret R, Abdollah F, et al. Age-adjusted incidence, mortality, and survival rates of stage-specific renal cell carcinoma in North America: a trend analysis. Eur Urol 2011;59(1):135–41.

9. Levi F, Lucchini F, Negri E, et al. Declining mortality from kidney cancer in Europe. Ann Oncol 2004;15(7):1130–5.

10. Chow WH, Devesa SS, Warren JL, et al. Rising incidence of renal cell cancer in the United States. JAMA 1999;281(17):1628–31.

11. Verdecchia A, Francisci S, Brenner H, et al. Recent cancer survival in Europe: a 2000–02 period analysis of EUROCARE-4 data. Lancet Oncol 2007;8(9): 784–96.

12. Engholm G, Gislum M, Bray F, et al. Trends in the survival of patients diagnosed with cancer in the Nordic countries 1964–2003 followed up to the end of 2006. Material and methods. Acta Oncol 2010;49(5):545–60.

13. Chow WH, Linehan WM, Devesa SS. Re: Rising incidence of small renal masses: a need to reassess treatment effect. J Natl Cancer Inst 2007;99(7): 569–70 [author reply: 570–1].

14. IARC. IARC monographs on the evaluation of carcinogenic risks to humans: tobacco smoke and involuntary smoking, vol. 83. Lyon (France): IARC Press; 2004.

15. Hunt JD, van der Hel OL, McMillan GP, et al. Renal cell carcinoma in relation to cigarette smoking: meta-analysis of 24 studies. Int J Cancer 2005;114(1):101–8.

16. Renehan AG, Tyson M, Egger M, et al. Body-mass index and incidence of cancer: a systematic review and meta-analysis of prospective observational studies. Lancet 2008;371(9612):569–78.

17. Adams KF, Leitzmann MF, Albanes D, et al. Body size and renal cell cancer incidence in a large US Cohort Study. Am J Epidemiol 2008;168(3):268–77.

18. Nicodemus KK, Sweeney C, Folsom AR. Evaluation of dietary, medical and lifestyle risk factors for incident kidney cancer in postmenopausal women. Int J Cancer 2004;108(1):115–21.

19. Pischon T, Lahmann PH, Boeing H, et al. Body size and risk of renal cell carcinoma in the European Prospective Investigation into Cancer and Nutrition (EPIC). Int J Cancer 2006;118(3):728–38.

20. Mellemgaard A, Lindblad P, Schlehofer B, et al. International renal-cell cancer study. III. Role of weight, height, physical activity, and use of amphetamines. Int J Cancer 1995;60(3):350–4.

21. Lindblad P, Wolk A, Bergstrom R, et al. The role of obesity and weight fluctuations in the etiology of renal cell cancer: a population-based case-control study. Cancer Epidemiol Biomarkers Prev 1994;3(8):631–9.

22. Bergstrom A, Hsieh CC, Lindblad P, et al. Obesity and renal cell cancer—a quantitative review. Br J Cancer 2001;85(7):984–90.

23. Calle EE, Kaaks R. Overweight, obesity and cancer: epidemiological evidence and proposed mechanisms. Nat Rev Cancer 2004;4(8):579–91.

24. Osorio-Costa F, Rocha GZ, Dias MM, et al. Epidemiological and molecular mechanisms aspects linking obesity and cancer. Arq Bras Endocrinol Metabol 2009;53(2):213–26.

25. Tulinius H, Sigfusson N, Sigvaldason H, et al. Risk factors for malignant diseases: a cohort study on a population of 22,946 Icelanders. Cancer Epidemiol Biomarkers Prev 1997;6(11):863–73.

26. Bjorge T, Tretli S, Engeland A. Relation of height and body mass index to renal cell carcinoma in two million Norwegian men and women. Am J Epidemiol 2004; 160(12):1168–76.

27. van Dijk BA, Schouten LJ, Kiemeney LA, et al. Relation of height, body mass, energy intake, and physical activity to risk of renal cell carcinoma: results from the Netherlands Cohort Study. Am J Epidemiol 2004;160(12):1159–67.
28. Chow WH, Gridley G, Fraumeni JF Jr, et al. Obesity, hypertension, and the risk of kidney cancer in men. N Engl J Med 2000;343(18):1305–11.
29. Moore SC, Chow WH, Schatzkin A, et al. Physical activity during adulthood and adolescence in relation to renal cell cancer. Am J Epidemiol 2008;168(2):149–57.
30. Bergstrom A, Moradi T, Lindblad P, et al. Occupational physical activity and renal cell cancer: a nationwide cohort study in Sweden. Int J Cancer 1999; 83(2):186–91.
31. Tavani A, Zucchetto A, Dal Maso L, et al. Lifetime physical activity and the risk of renal cell cancer. Int J Cancer 2007;120(9):1977–80.
32. Bergstrom A, Terry P, Lindblad P, et al. Physical activity and risk of renal cell cancer. Int J Cancer 2001;92(1):155–7.
33. Menezes RJ, Tomlinson G, Kreiger N. Physical activity and risk of renal cell carcinoma. Int J Cancer 2003;107(4):642–6.
34. Chiu BC, Gapstur SM, Chow WH, et al. Body mass index, physical activity, and risk of renal cell carcinoma. Int J Obes (Lond) 2006;30(6):940–7.
35. Augustsson K, Skog K, Jagerstad M, et al. Dietary heterocyclic amines and cancer of the colon, rectum, bladder, and kidney: a population-based study. Lancet 1999;353(9154):703–7.
36. De Stefani E, Fierro L, Mendilaharsu M, et al. Meat intake, 'mate' drinking and renal cell cancer in Uruguay: a case-control study. Br J Cancer 1998;78(9): 1239–43.
37. Wolk A, Gridley G, Niwa S, et al. International renal cell cancer study. VII. Role of diet. Int J Cancer 1996;65(1):67–73.
38. Hu J, Mao Y, White K. Diet and vitamin or mineral supplements and risk of renal cell carcinoma in Canada. Cancer Causes Control 2003;14(8):705–14.
39. Brock KE, Gridley G, Chiu BC, et al. Dietary fat and risk of renal cell carcinoma in the USA: a case-control study. Br J Nutr 2009;101(8):1228–38.
40. Faramawi MF, Johnson E, Fry MW, et al. Consumption of different types of meat and the risk of renal cancer: meta-analysis of case-control studies. Cancer Causes Control 2007;18(2):125–33.
41. Hsu CC, Chow WH, Boffetta P, et al. Dietary risk factors for kidney cancer in eastern and central Europe. Am J Epidemiol 2007;166(1):62–70.
42. Grieb SM, Theis RP, Burr D, et al. Food groups and renal cell carcinoma: results from a case-control study. J Am Diet Assoc 2009;109(4):656–67.
43. Lee JE, Spiegelman D, Hunter DJ, et al. Fat, protein, and meat consumption and renal cell cancer risk: a pooled analysis of 13 prospective studies. J Natl Cancer Inst 2008;100(23):1695–706.
44. Allen NE, Roddam AW, Sieri S, et al. A prospective analysis of the association between macronutrient intake and renal cell carcinoma in the European Prospective Investigation into Cancer and Nutrition. Int J Cancer 2009;125(4):982–7.
45. Yuan JM, Gago-Dominguez M, Castelao JE, et al. Cruciferous vegetables in relation to renal cell carcinoma. Int J Cancer 1998;77(2):211–6.
46. Lee JE, Giovannucci E, Smith-Warner SA, et al. Intakes of fruits, vegetables, vitamins A, C, and E, and carotenoids and risk of renal cell cancer. Cancer Epidemiol Biomarkers Prev 2006;15(12):2445–52.
47. Weikert S, Boeing H, Pischon T, et al. Fruits and vegetables and renal cell carcinoma: findings from the European prospective investigation into cancer and nutrition (EPIC). Int J Cancer 2006;118(12):3133–9.

48. Montella M, Tramacere I, Tavani A, et al. Coffee, decaffeinated coffee, tea intake, and risk of renal cell cancer. Nutr Cancer 2009;61(1):76–80.

49. Lee JE, Hunter DJ, Spiegelman D, et al. Intakes of coffee, tea, milk, soda and juice and renal cell cancer in a pooled analysis of 13 prospective studies. Int J Cancer 2007;121(10):2246–53.

50. Rashidkhani B, Akesson A, Lindblad P, et al. Major dietary patterns and risk of renal cell carcinoma in a prospective cohort of Swedish women. J Nutr 2005; 135(7):1757–62.

51. Handa K, Kreiger N. Diet patterns and the risk of renal cell carcinoma. Public Health Nutr 2002;5(6):757–67.

52. Hu J, La Vecchia C, Negri E, et al. Dietary vitamin C, E, and carotenoid intake and risk of renal cell carcinoma. Cancer Causes Control 2009;20(8):1451–8.

53. Lindblad P, Wolk A, Bergstrom R, et al. Diet and risk of renal cell cancer: a population-based case-control study. Cancer Epidemiol Biomarkers Prev 1997;6(4): 215–23.

54. Goodman MT, Morgenstern H, Wynder EL. A case-control study of factors affecting the development of renal cell cancer. Am J Epidemiol 1986;124: 926–41.

55. Parker AS, Cerhan JR, Lynch CF, et al. Gender, alcohol consumption, and renal cell carcinoma. Am J Epidemiol 2002;155(5):455–62.

56. Lee JE, Hunter DJ, Spiegelman D, et al. Alcohol intake and renal cell cancer in a pooled analysis of 12 prospective studies. J Natl Cancer Inst 2007;99(10): 801–10.

57. Davies MJ, Baer DJ, Judd JT, et al. Effects of moderate alcohol intake on fasting insulin and glucose concentrations and insulin sensitivity in postmenopausal women: a randomized controlled trial. JAMA 2002;287(19):2559–62.

58. Facchini F, Chen YD, Reaven GM. Light-to-moderate alcohol intake is associated with enhanced insulin sensitivity. Diabetes Care 1994;17(2):115–9.

59. Flaherty KT, Fuchs CS, Colditz GA, et al. A prospective study of body mass index, hypertension, and smoking and the risk of renal cell carcinoma (United States). Cancer Causes Control 2005;16:1099–106.

60. McCredie M, Stewart JH. Risk factors for kidney cancer in New South Wales, Australia. II. Urologic disease, hypertension, obesity, and hormonal factors. Cancer Causes Control 1992;3(4):323–31.

61. McLaughlin JK, Chow WH, Mandel JS, et al. International renal-cell cancer study. VIII. Role of diuretics, other anti-hypertensive medications and hypertension. Int J Cancer 1995;63(2):216–21.

62. Shapiro JA, Williams MA, Weiss NS, et al. Hypertension, antihypertensive medication use, and risk of renal cell carcinoma. Am J Epidemiol 1999;149(6): 521–30.

63. Yuan JM, Castelao JE, Gago-Dominguez M, et al. Hypertension, obesity and their medications in relation to renal cell carcinoma. Br J Cancer 1998;77(9): 1508–13.

64. Heath CW Jr, Lally CA, Calle EE, et al. Hypertension, diuretics, and antihypertensive medications as possible risk factors for renal cell cancer. Am J Epidemiol 1997;145(7):607–13.

65. Prineas RJ, Folsom AR, Zhang ZM, et al. Nutrition and other risk factors for renal cell carcinoma in postmenopausal women. Epidemiology 1997;8(1): 31–6.

66. Fryzek JP, Poulsen AH, Johnsen SP, et al. A cohort study of antihypertensive treatments and risk of renal cell cancer. Br J Cancer 2005;92(7):1302–6.

67. Weikert S, Boeing H, Pischon T, et al. Blood pressure and risk of renal cell carcinoma in the European prospective investigation into cancer and nutrition. Am J Epidemiol 2008;167(4):438–46.
68. Shapiro JA, Williams MA, Weiss NS. Body mass index and risk of renal cell carcinoma. Epidemiology 1999;10(2):188–91.
69. Denton MD, Magee CC, Ovuworie C, et al. Prevalence of renal cell carcinoma in patients with ESRD pre-transplantation: a pathologic analysis. Kidney Int 2002; 61(6):2201–9.
70. Ishikawa I. Uremic acquired renal cystic disease. Natural history and complications. Nephron 1991;58(3):257–67.
71. Maisonneuve P, Agodoa L, Gellert R, et al. Cancer in patients on dialysis for end-stage renal disease: an international collaborative study. Lancet 1999; 354(9173):93–9.
72. Marple JT, MacDougall M, Chonko AM. Renal cancer complicating acquired cystic kidney disease. J Am Soc Nephrol 1994;4(12):1951–6.
73. Stewart JH, Buccianti G, Agodoa L, et al. Cancers of the kidney and urinary tract in patients on dialysis for end-stage renal disease: analysis of data from the United States, Europe, and Australia and New Zealand. J Am Soc Nephrol 2003;14(1):197–207.
74. Doublet JD, Peraldi MN, Gattegno B, et al. Renal cell carcinoma of native kidneys: prospective study of 129 renal transplant patients. J Urol 1997; 158(1):42–4.
75. Kliem V, Kolditz M, Behrend M, et al. Risk of renal cell carcinoma after kidney transplantation. Clin Transplant 1997;11(4):255–8.
76. Adami J, Gabel H, Lindelof B, et al. Cancer risk following organ transplantation: a nationwide cohort study in Sweden. Br J Cancer 2003;89(7):1221–7.
77. Neuzillet Y, Lay F, Luccioni A, et al. De novo renal cell carcinoma of native kidney in renal transplant recipients. Cancer 2005;103(2):251–7.
78. Concolino G, Lubrano C, Ombres M, et al. Acquired cystic kidney disease: the hormonal hypothesis. Urology 1993;41(2):170–5.
79. La Vecchia C, Negri E, Franceschi S, et al. A case-control study of diabetes mellitus and cancer risk. Br J Cancer 1994;70:950–3.
80. McLaughlin JK, Gao YT, Gao RN, et al. Risk factors for renal-cell cancer in Shanghai, China. Int J Cancer 1992;52(4):562–5.
81. Wynder EL, Mabuchi K, Whitmore WF Jr. Epidemiology of adenocarcinoma of the kidney. J Natl Cancer Inst 1974;53(6):1619–34.
82. Asal NR, Geyer JR, Risser DR, et al. Risk factors in renal cell carcinoma. II. Medical history, occupation, multivariate analysis, and conclusions. Cancer Detect Prev 1988;13(3–4):263–79.
83. McLaughlin JK, Mandel JS, Blot WJ, et al. A population-based case-control study of renal cell carcinoma. J Natl Cancer Inst 1984;72(2):275–84.
84. O'Mara BA, Byers T, Schoenfeld E. Diabetes mellitus and cancer risk: a multisite case-control study. J Chronic Dis 1985;38:435–41.
85. Kreiger N, Marrett LD, Dodds L, et al. Risk factors for renal cell carcinoma: results of a population-based case-control study. Cancer Causes Control 1993;4(2):101–10.
86. Mellemgaard A, Niwa S, Mehl ES, et al. Risk factors for renal cell carcinoma in Denmark: role of medication and medical history. Int J Epidemiol 1994;23(5): 923–30.
87. Adami HO, McLaughlin J, Ekbom A, et al. Cancer risk in patients with diabetes mellitus. Cancer Causes Control 1991;2:307–14.

88. Wideroff L, Gridley G, Mellemkjaer L, et al. Cancer incidence in a population-based cohort of patients hospitalized with diabetes mellitus in Denmark. J Natl Cancer Inst 1997;89(18):1360–5.

89. Lindblad P, Chow WH, Chan J, et al. The role of diabetes mellitus in the aetiology of renal cell cancer. Diabetologia 1999;42(1):107–12.

90. Gordon SC, Moonka D, Brown KA, et al. Risk for renal cell carcinoma in chronic hepatitis C infection. Cancer Epidemiol Biomarkers Prev 2010;19(4): 1066–73.

91. IARC. Phenacetin and analgesic mixtures containing phenacetin; monographs on the evaluation of carcinogenic risks of chemicals to humans: an updating of IARC monographs. Lyon (France): IARC Press; 1987.

92. Maclure M, MacMahon B. Phenacetin and cancer of urinary tract. N Engl J Med 1985;(313):1479.

93. McLaughlin JK, Blot WJ, Mehl ES, et al. Relation of analgesic use to renal cancer: population-based findings. Natl Cancer Inst Monogr 1985;69:217–22.

94. McCredie M, Ford JM, Stewart JH. Risk factors for cancer of the renal parenchyma. Int J Cancer 1988;42(1):13–6.

95. McCredie M, Stewart JH, Day NE. Different roles for phenacetin and paracetamol in cancer of the kidney and renal pelvis. Int J Cancer 1993;53(2):245–9.

96. Derby LE, Jick H. Acetaminophen and renal and bladder cancer. Epidemiology 1996;7(4):358–62.

97. Gago-Dominguez M, Yuan JM, Castelao JE, et al. Regular use of analgesics is a risk factor for renal cell carcinoma. Br J Cancer 1999;81(3):542–8.

98. Bosetti C, Gallus S, La Vecchia C. Aspirin and cancer risk: an updated quantitative review to 2005. Cancer Causes Control 2006;17(7):871–88.

99. Cho E, Hankinson SE, Curhan GC, et al. Prospective study of use of analgesics in relation to the risk of renal cell cancer: The Nurses' Health Study and Health Professionals Follow-up Study. AACR Meeting. April 18–22, 2009 [abstract: 4864].

100. Lee JE, Hankinson SE, Cho E. Reproductive factors and risk of renal cell cancer: the Nurses' Health Study. Am J Epidemiol 2009;169(10):1243–50.

101. Lindblad P, Mellemgaard A, Schlehofer B, et al. International renal-cell cancer study. V. Reproductive factors, gynecologic operations and exogenous hormones. Int J Cancer 1995;61(2):192–8.

102. Kabat GC, Silvera SA, Miller AB, et al. A cohort study of reproductive and hormonal factors and renal cell cancer risk in women. Br J Cancer 2007; 96(5):845–9.

103. Altman D, Yin L, Johansson A, et al. Risk of renal cell carcinoma after hysterectomy. Arch Intern Med 2010;170(22):2011–6.

104. Chow WH, McLaughlin JK, Mandel JS, et al. Reproductive factors and the risk of renal cell cancer among women. Int J Cancer 1995;60(3):321–4.

105. Mattioli S, Truffelli D, Baldasseroni A, et al. Occupational risk factors for renal cell cancer: a case-control study in northern Italy. J Occup Environ Med 2002; 44(11):1028–36.

106. Pesch B, Haerting J, Ranft U, et al. Occupational risk factors for renal cell carcinoma: agent-specific results from a case-control study in Germany. MURC Study Group. Multicenter urothelial and renal cancer study. Int J Epidemiol 2000;29(6):1014–24.

107. Lynge E, Andersen A, Nilsson R, et al. Risk of cancer and exposure to gasoline vapors. Am J Epidemiol 1997;145(5):449–58.

108. Mandel JS, McLaughlin JK, Schlehofer B, et al. International renal-cell cancer study. IV. Occupation. Int J Cancer 1995;61(5):601–5.

109. Partanen T, Heikkila P, Hernberg S, et al. Renal cell cancer and occupational exposure to chemical agents. Scand J Work Environ Health 1991;17(4):231–9.
110. Boffetta P, Jourenkova N, Gustavsson P. Cancer risk from occupational and environmental exposure to polycyclic aromatic hydrocarbons. Cancer Causes Control 1997;8(3):444–72.
111. Kadamani S, Asal NR, Nelson RY. Occupational hydrocarbon exposure and risk of renal cell carcinoma. Am J Ind Med 1989;15(2):131–41.
112. Sharpe CR, Rochon JE, Adam JM, et al. Case-control study of hydrocarbon exposures in patients with renal cell carcinoma. CMAJ 1989;140(11):1309–18.
113. Cocco P, Hua F, Boffetta P, et al. Mortality of Italian lead smelter workers. Scand J Work Environ Health 1997;23(1):15–23.
114. Scott CS, Chiu WA. Trichloroethylene cancer epidemiology: a consideration of select issues. Environ Health Perspect 2006;114(9):1471–8.
115. Kelsh MA, Alexander DD, Mink PJ, et al. Occupational trichloroethylene exposure and kidney cancer: a meta-analysis. Epidemiology 2010;21(1):95–102.
116. Brauch H, Weirich G, Klein B, et al. VHL mutations in renal cell cancer: does occupational exposure to trichloroethylene make a difference? Toxicol Lett 2004;151(1):301–10.
117. Axwijk PH, Kluijt I, de Jong D, et al. Hereditary causes of kidney tumours. Eur J Clin Invest 2010;40(5):433–9.
118. Choyke PL, Glenn GM, Walther MM, et al. von Hippel-Lindau disease: genetic, clinical, and imaging features. Radiology 1995;194(3):629–42.
119. Maher ER. Inherited renal cell carcinoma. Br J Urol 1996;78(4):542–5.
120. Kim WY, Kaelin WG. Role of VHL gene mutation in human cancer. J Clin Oncol 2004;22(24):4991–5004.
121. Jacobsen J, Grankvist K, Rasmuson T, et al. Expression of vascular endothelial growth factor protein in human renal cell carcinoma. BJU Int 2004;93(3):297–302.
122. Van Poppel H, Nilsson S, Algaba F, et al. Precancerous lesions in the kidney. Scand J Urol Nephrol Suppl 2000;(205):136–65.
123. Czene K, Hemminki K. Kidney cancer in the Swedish Family Cancer Database: familial risks and second primary malignancies. Kidney Int 2002;61(5):1806–13.
124. Schlehofer B, Pommer W, Mellemgaard A, et al. International renal-cell-cancer study. VI. The role of medical and family history. Int J Cancer 1996;66(6):723–6.
125. Gago-Dominguez M, Yuan JM, Castelao JE, et al. Family history and risk of renal cell carcinoma. Cancer Epidemiol Biomarkers Prev 2001;10(9):1001–4.
126. Sweeney C, Farrow DC, Schwartz SM, et al. Glutathione S-transferase M1, T1, and P1 polymorphisms as risk factors for renal cell carcinoma: a case-control study. Cancer Epidemiol Biomarkers Prev 2000;9(4):449–54.
127. Semenza JC, Ziogas A, Largent J, et al. Gene-environment interactions in renal cell carcinoma. Am J Epidemiol 2001;153(9):851–9.
128. World Cancer Research Fund, American Institute for Cancer Research. Food, nutrition, physical activity, and the prevention of cancer: a global perspective. Washington, DC: American Institute for Cancer Research; 2007.

New Insights into the Biology of Renal Cell Carcinoma

Lianjie Li, PhD[a,b], William G. Kaelin Jr, MD[a,b],*

KEYWORDS

- Renal cell carcinoma • Clear-cell renal carcinoma
- Hypoxia-inducible factor • HIF-responsive gene products

Kidney cancer is one of the 10 most common forms of cancer in both men and women. Ninety percent or more of these cancers are believed to be of epithelial cell origin, and are referred to as renal cell carcinoma (RCC). RCCs can be further subdivided, based on their histologic appearance, into clear-cell renal carcinomas (~75%), papillary renal carcinomas (15%), chromophobe tumors (5%), and oncocytomas (5%).[1,2] Studies of hereditary kidney cancer families led to the identification of genes that, when mutated in the germline, confer an increased risk of these various histologic RCC subtypes and hence a glimpse at the molecular circuits that are deregulated in these different forms of RCC.[2] In practice, there is some overlap among the histologic subtypes (eg, a tumor with predominantly clear-cell features might contain areas more typical of papillary RCC). Similarly, there are some shared molecular features among these tumor types (see later discussion). This review focuses primarily on the most common form of RCC, clear-cell renal carcinoma, while making note of some recent advances in the other histologic subtypes.

CLEAR-CELL RCC GENETICS: ROLE OF THE VHL TUMOR SUPPRESSOR GENE

von Hippel-Lindau (VHL) disease is a hereditary cancer syndrome characterized by an increased risk of clear-cell RCC, retinal and central nervous system hemangioblastomas, and pheochromocytomas. Individuals with this disorder carry a defective copy of the *VHL* tumor suppressor gene, typically inherited from either parent but occasionally resulting from a de novo mutation. Tumor development in this setting is linked to inactivation of the remaining wild-type allele in a susceptible cell, either as a result of deletion, intragenic mutation, or hypermethylation.

[a] Howard Hughes Medical Institute (HHMI), 4000 Jones Bridge Road, Chevy Chase, MD 20815, USA
[b] Department of Medical Oncology, Dana-Farber Cancer Institute and Brigham and Women's Hospital, 450 Brookline Avenue, Boston, MA 02215, USA
* Corresponding author. Dana-Farber Cancer Institute, 450 Brookline Avenue, Mayer Building Room 457, Boston, MA 02215.
E-mail address: William_kaelin@dfci.harvard.edu

Hematol Oncol Clin N Am 25 (2011) 667–686
doi:10.1016/j.hoc.2011.04.004   **hemonc.theclinics.com**
0889-8588/11/$ – see front matter © 2011 Elsevier Inc. All rights reserved.

As might be predicted from this knowledge, *VHL* inactivation is also very common in sporadic clear-cell RCC. In most series about 50% of sporadic clear-cell RCC are unable to produce the normal (wild-type) VHL tumor suppressor protein (pVHL).[3] Typically this reflects a sporadic intragenic mutation of one copy of the *VHL* gene, which is located on chromosome 3p, in conjunction with loss of the remaining copy because of a large deletion affecting the other 3p arm. In other tumors this loss of wild-type pVHL is the consequence of transcriptional silencing of both the maternal and paternal copies of the *VHL* gene as a result of hypermethylation. A third group of clear-cell RCC have a gene expression signature typical of *VHL* inactivation without demonstrable *VHL* mutations or hypermethylation.[4] These tumors might theoretically have nonallelic mutations that indirectly affect *VHL* function, although to date no such mutations have been identified.[5]

In light of these considerations one would expect that the frequency of chromosome 3p loss would approximate the frequency of intragenic *VHL* mutations in clear-cell RCC; however, this is not the case. In particular, the frequency of chromosome 3p is consistently higher (often >90%) than the frequency of intragenic *VHL* mutations. There are several, nonmutually exclusive, possibilities to explain this conundrum. First, the failure to detect intragenic mutations in some tumors might be due to technical factors (ie, reflecting "false negatives"). If true, this would provide an alternative explanation for the existence of "*VHL*+/+" clear-cell RCC that display a *VHL*−/− gene expression signature. Indeed, there is some evidence that new sequencing technologies will reveal a higher *VHL* mutation rate in clear-cell RCC.[6,7] Second, chromosome 3p might harbor additional clear-cell RCC suppressor genes. In this regard, frequent inactivating mutations of the *PBRM1* gene, located on chromosome 3p21, were recently reported in clear-cell RCC.[8] This gene encodes a protein involved in the control of DNA packing into chromatin. Finally, it is possible that loss of one copy of *VHL* (haploinsufficiency) promotes clear-cell RCC in some settings, although there are presently no laboratory data to support the idea that *VHL* haploinsufficiency measurably alters the molecular pathways described later in this article.

Although *VHL* inactivation is an important event in the pathogenesis of many clear-cell RCC, it is not sufficient to cause this disease. This aspect has been most clearly documented by examining the kidneys of VHL patients, which often contain hundreds of preneoplastic lesions that have sustained loss of the remaining wild-type *VHL* allele, and yet few carcinomas.[9,10] Similarly, *VHL* inactivation in the murine kidney is not sufficient to cause RCC.[11] It appears that additional genetic events, occurring stochastically, are required to convert a *VHL*−/− preneoplastic lesion into clear-cell RCC.

Indeed, several nonrandom chromosomal changes, in addition to chromosome 3p loss, have been described in both sporadic and hereditary (VHL disease-associated) clear-cell RCC.[1,4,12] These alterations include frequent loss of chromosome 14q and gain of chromosome 5q. It is interesting that some clear-cell RCC contain unbalanced translocations of chromosomes 3 and 5, leading to loss of 3p and gain of 5q.[13] Recurrent amplifications and deletions in clear-cell RCC presumably harbor oncogenes and tumor suppressor genes, respectively, which play roles in the pathogenesis of clear-cell RCC.

Direct sequencing of kidney cancer genomes provides information that is complementary to technologies that measure changes in copy number (ie, amplifications and deletions). This approach has revealed that several chromatin-modifying enzymes, including the SETD2 histone methyltransferase, the JARID1C (also known as KDM5C) histone demethylase, and the UTX (also known as KMD6A) histone demethylase, are sometimes mutated in clear-cell RCC.[14]

Functions of the von Hippel-Lindau Tumor Suppressor Protein

The VHL tumor suppressor gene encodes 2 proteins by virtue of 2 alternative, in-frame, start codons. The shorter form lacks 53 N-terminal amino acid residues that are present in the long form. For simplicity, both forms here are referred to as "pVHL" because they behave similarly in most biochemical and biological assays performed to date, and because all of the *VHL* mutations identified in clear-cell carcinoma so far would be predicted to affect both pVHL isoforms. pVHL resides primarily in the cytoplasm but dynamically shuttles between the nucleus and the cytoplasm, and has also been detected in association with the endoplasmic reticulum and mitochondria.[15–17]

pVHL is the substrate recognition component of an E3 ubiquitin ligase complex that regulates hypoxia-inducible factor (HIF) (**Fig. 1**).[18] HIF is a heterodimeric DNA-binding transcription factor consisting of an unstable α subunit and a stable β subunit. When oxygen is present the α subunit becomes hydroxylated on one (or both) of two conserved prolyl residues by members of the EgIN (also called PHD) prolyl hydroxylase family.[18] Once prolyl hydroxylated, the α subunit is recognized by pVHL, polyubiquitinated, and destroyed by the proteasome. Under low oxygen conditions, or in cells lacking wild-type pVHL, the α subunit is stabilized, dimerizes with a β subunit, and transcriptionally activates 100 to 200 genes, many of which are involved in acute or chronic adaptation to hypoxia. Examples of such genes include *VEGF*, which promotes angiogenesis, *EPO*, which promotes erythropoiesis, and a suite of genes that promote glucose uptake and glycolysis.

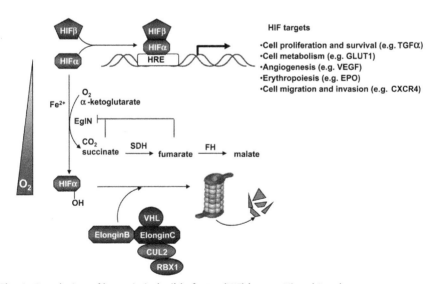

Fig. 1. Regulation of hypoxia-inducible factor (HIF) by von Hippel-Landau tumor suppressor protein (pVHL). Under normoxic conditions, HIFα is hydroxylated by EgIN prolyl hydroxylases. In addition to O_2, this reaction also requires α-ketoglutarate, which is converted to succinate, and reduced iron. Succinate dehydrogenase (SDH) converts succinate to fumarate, which is further converted to malate by fumarate hydratase (FH). Accumulation of succinate and fumarate can inhibit HIFα hydroxylation. Hydroxylated HIFα is recognized by pVHL, the substrate recognition subunit of an E3 ubiquitin ligase complex, polyubiquitinated, and degraded by the proteasome. Under hypoxic conditions, HIFα is stabilized, dimerizes with HIFβ, and activates target gene transcription. GLUT1, glucose transporter 1; HRE, hypoxia response element; TGFα, transforming growth factor α; VEGF, vascular endothelial growth factor.

There are 3 HIFα genes in the human genome (HIF1α, HIF2α, and HIF3α). HIF1α is ubiquitously expressed whereas the expression of HIF2α is more restricted. Both HIF1α and HIF2α can bind to specific DNA sequences (hypoxia-responsive elements) and activate transcription. HIF1α and HIF2α share many target genes, but it is also becoming increasingly clear that some genes are preferentially activated by one or the other. Multiple HIF3α splice variants have been described, many of which might actually serve to interfere with the function of HIF1α and HIF2α.[19–21]

Many lines of evidence point to a pivotal role of HIF, and especially HIF2α, in pVHL-defective clear-cell RCC. The risk of developing clear-cell RCC linked to germline *VHL* mutations mirrors the degree to which those mutations deregulate HIF.[22] In preclinical models HIF2α, but not HIF1α, can override the tumor suppressor activity of pVHL and elimination of HIF2α, but not HIF1α, is sufficient to suppress tumor formation by pVHL-defective clear-cell renal carcinoma cells.[23–28] Moreover, HIF2α appears to account for much or all of the pathology observed in mice that have been engineered to lack pVHL in certain tissues.[29–32] In further support of the importance of HIF2α, pVHL-defective clear-cell RCC produce both HIF1α and HIF2α or, informatively, HIF2α alone.[33,34] Close examination of preneoplastic renal lesions in patients with VHL disease suggests that the appearance of HIF2α, rather than HIF1α, heralds malignant transformation,[9] and a recent study linked the risk of developing clear-cell RCC to single-nucleotide polymorphisms affecting HIF2α.[35] Collectively these studies underscore that pVHL-defective clear-cell RCC are driven, at least partly, by a surfeit of HIF2α activity.

The EgIN prolyl hydroxylases require, in addition to oxygen, the metabolite 2-oxo-glutarate (also called α-ketoglutarate) to hydroxylate HIFα.[18] During the hydroxylation reaction, 2-oxoglutarate is converted to succinate. Succinate can be converted by succinate dehydrogenase (SDH) to fumarate, which in turn can be converted to malate by fumarate hydratase (FH). Inactivating SDH and FH mutations, which lead to an increase in succinate and fumarate, respectively, have been linked to an increased risk of RCC.[36] This link has been most clearly demonstrated by the increased risk of papillary RCC observed in kindreds bearing FH mutations. Succinate and fumarate can inhibit EgIN activity in vitro and in vivo, leading to HIF activation.[37–41] These findings suggest that HIF deregulation, whether due to inactivation of VHL, SDH, or FH, is a feature of RCC.

pVHL has several other functions that, although incompletely understood at a biochemical level, seem to be at least partly HIF-independent and which might be relevant to tumorigenesis (**Fig. 2**).[42] These functions include roles in the

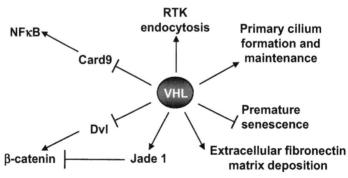

Fig. 2. HIF-independent functions of VHL. See text for details. NF-κB, nuclear factor κB; RTK, receptor tyrosine kinase.

assembly of an extracellular fibronectin matrix,[43–46] receptor internalization,[47–50] microtubule stability,[51–54] nerve growth factor signaling,[55] senescence,[56] and maintenance of the primary cilium,[10,57,58] which is a specialized structure on the surface of cells that serves as a sensory antenna (eg, responding to changes in adjacent fluid dynamics). This latter function is particularly intriguing because visceral cysts, including renal cysts, are a prominent feature of VHL disease and are also seen in several other unrelated diseases, such as Bardet-Biedl syndrome, that affect the primary cilium (so-called ciliopathies).[59,60] Whether these disparate pVHL functions relate to its function as part of an E3 ubiquitin ligase is not known. In this regard it is perhaps noteworthy that the other core components of the pVHL ubiquitin ligase complex, such as elongin B, elongin C, and Cul2, are not frequently mutated in clear-cell RCC.[5] This fact might reflect the importance of pVHL-independent functions of these proteins in cellular homeostasis or the importance of ubiquitin ligase–independent functions of pVHL in tumorigenesis (or both).

Recent studies suggest that pVHL regulates, at least indirectly, the nuclear factor κB (NF-κB) transcription factor. pVHL acts as an adaptor molecule that promotes the inhibitory phosphorylation of the NF-κB agonist Card9 by casein kinase II, thereby suppressing NF-κB activity.[61] In addition, HIF itself can activate NF-κB in some contexts whereas NF-κB can promote the transcription of HIF1α.[62–64] In keeping with the aforementioned, NF-κB activity is increased in clear-cell RCC and might contribute to the resistance of this tumor to many forms of therapy.[63,65–67] In addition, HIF and NF-κB share several target genes and hence might cooperate to promote the development of clear-cell RCC.

pVHL, in addition to regulating HIF and NF-κB, regulates the Wnt signaling pathway and hence the activity of the oncogenic transcription factor β-catenin. Several nonmutually exclusive mechanisms to account for suppression of Wnt signaling by pVHL have been proposed. pVHL promotes the ubiquitination of the Wnt signaling protein Disheveled (Dvl), which then interacts with SQSTM1/p62 and is subsequently degraded by the autophagy-lysosome pathway.[68] pVHL also stabilizes the candidate tumor suppressor protein Jade-1, which in turn is capable of targeting β-catenin for proteasomal degradation.[69] Finally, HIF1α itself modulates Wnt/β-catenin signaling in hypoxic embryonic stem (ES) cells by enhancing β-catenin activation and expression of the downstream effectors LEF-1 and TCF-1.[70] Thus pVHL inhibits, directly or indirectly, the oncogenic transcription factors HIF2α, NF-κB, and β-catenin. Conversely, Wnt signaling can affect *VHL* expression in some tissues.[71]

HIF AS A THERAPEUTIC TARGET IN RCC

The central role of HIFα, and particularly HIF2α, in pVHL-defective clear-cell RCC has spurred interest in the development of HIF antagonists for this disease. Unfortunately, however, there are very few examples of drug-like small organic molecules that are capable of inhibiting the function of DNA-binding transcription factors, with the notable exception of the steroid hormone receptors.

Inhibition of the mammalian target of rapamycin (mTOR) kinase decreases the transcription and translation of HIF1α, thereby lowering HIF1α protein levels.[72,73] This process might account for the observation that two rapamycin-like mTOR inhibitors ("rapalogs"), temsirolimus and everolimus, have activity in the treatment of clear-cell RCC (**Fig. 3**).[74–76] Unfortunately, these two drugs primarily inhibit mTOR when it is in the multiprotein complex called TORC1 rather than in the TORC2 complex. This aspect is important because HIF2α, which as noted is the HIFα paralog most closely linked to the pathogenesis of pVHL-defective clear-cell RCC, appears to be more

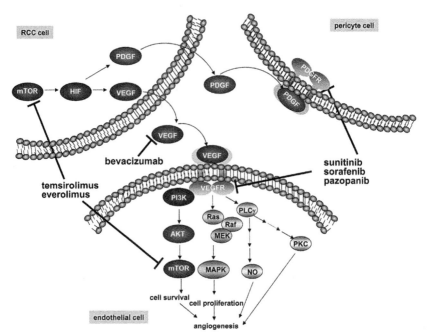

Fig. 3. Angiogenesis and targeted therapies in RCC. Inactivation of VHL in RCC cells lead to increased HIF activity. As a result, RCC cells secrete increased levels of vascular endothelial growth factor (VEGF) and platelet-derived growth factor (PDGF), which activate VEGF receptors and PDGF receptors to promote angiogenesis. Bevacizumab is a neutralizing antibody for VEGF. Sunitinib, sorafenib, and pazopanib act to block VEGF receptor and PDGF receptor activation. HIF protein levels are also influenced by mTOR kinase activity. Temsirolimus and everolimus block mTOR and thereby inhibit HIFα production. HIF, hypoxia-inducible factor; MAPK, mitogen-activated protein kinase; MEK, mitogen-activated protein kinase kinase; mTOR, mammalian target of rapamycin; NO, nitric oxide; PI3K, phosphatidylinositol 3-kinase; PKC, protein kinase C; PLCgγ, phospholipase-C gamma.

sensitive to TORC2 loss than to TORC1 loss.[77] Preclinical studies support the idea that adenosine triphosphate–competitive mTOR inhibitors, which inhibit both TORC1 and TORC2, will more effectively downregulate HIF2α and suppress tumor growth than do rapalogs.[78]

Several other drugs have been identified that, at least indirectly, are capable of downregulating HIF activity in cells. A cautionary note, however, is that HIFα, by virtue of having a high metabolic turnover rate (even in pVHL-defective cells), is very sensitive to decreases in its rate of transcription and translation. HIFα will therefore disappear more rapidly in response to drugs that are generally toxic than do many housekeeping proteins that are commonly used as specificity controls in evaluating putative HIF inhibitors. In short, it is possible that some drugs that have been reported to inhibit HIF actually have an inhibitory effect on transcription or translation in general, and would affect a variety of short-lived proteins.

HIF-RESPONSIVE GENE PRODUCTS
Vascular Endothelial Growth Factor

Kidney cancers are highly angiogenic tumors. In fact, renal angiograms were often used to diagnose this neoplasm prior to the availability of computed tomography.

The robust induction of angiogenesis by these tumors appears to be due, at least partly, to overproduction of vascular endothelial growth factor (VEGF), which is the product of a HIF-responsive gene. Accordingly, VEGF is normally induced by hypoxia but is constitutively produced in pVHL-defective tumors.[79,80] There has been a suggestion that VEGF might also act in an autocrine fashion to directly stimulate pVHL-defective tumors cells, although this idea remains controversial.[81]

Many VEGF inhibitors, including the neutralizing antibody bevacizumab and small molecules directed against the VEGF receptor VEGFR2 (also called KDR), such as sunitinib, sorafenib, and pazopanib, have been approved for the treatment of kidney cancer based on randomized clinical trial data (see **Fig. 3**).[82–85] In most studies about 70% of patients with kidney cancer will achieve some degree of tumor shrinkage when treated with a VEGF inhibitor, although the percentage of people achieving a partial response, as measured by RECIST criteria, varies considerably among the different agents. This finding might reflect differences in potency as well as the contribution of fortuitous "off-target" effects (see also later discussion). VEGF inhibitors have been approved for the treatment of metastatic kidney cancer based primarily on a significant improvement in terms of progression-free survival and a trend toward improved survival. The actual benefits of these agents in terms of overall survival are difficult to determine because control patients have typically been allowed to cross over to VEGF inhibitors at the time of disease progression.

There are conflicting reports as to whether *VHL* gene status influences the response to the existing VEGF inhibitors (ie, whether it can be used as a predictive biomarker).[86–89] These disparities might be due, at least partly, to technical factors such as the different methodologies used to identify *VHL* mutations in the different studies. In addition, the predictive value of *VHL* gene status might be diluted by the existence of *VHL*+/+ tumors that are phenotypically pVHL-defective, as described earlier. Suffice it to say that *VHL* gene status does not appear to be a robust predictive biomarker at present and should therefore not be used to guide therapeutic decision making, especially given the paucity of alternative agents.

Several second-generation KDR inhibitors that display improved potency and specificity are currently in development. It is hoped that these attributes will lead to enhanced clinical efficacy, reduced toxicity, and a greater ability to be combined with other agents. With respect to activity, however, there is already some evidence that there might be a limit to how completely VEGF signaling can be safely blocked in man. Microangiopathic changes, presumably reflecting damage to normal endothelial cells, have been reported in patients treated with a combination of two VEGF inhibitors.[90,91]

The vast majority of patients treated with a VEGF inhibitor will eventually become resistant to that agent and experience disease progression. Of interest, some of these patients will respond to a second, unrelated, VEGF inhibitor, suggesting that the patient's tumor remained VEGF dependent.[92] In other cases resistance to VEGF inhibition might, based on preclinical models, reflect activation of alternative angiogenic factors, such as fibroblast growth factor[93] and interleukin (IL)-8,[94] or to the ability of tumor cells to undergo a reversible epithelial-mesenchymal transition.[95]

Platelet-Derived Growth Factor

Platelet-derived growth factor (PDGF) B is another HIF target gene linked to angiogenesis. PDGF, which activates the PDGF receptor (PDGFR), stimulates the coverage of newly sprouting blood vessels by pericytes. In preclinical models, proliferating endothelial cells are less susceptible to VEGF withdrawal once they are provided with survival signals by such pericytes.[96–99] Accordingly dual inhibition of VEGF and PDGF should, in principle, be more effective than VEGF blockade alone. Several of the currently available KDR inhibitors do, in fact, have considerable activity against PDGFR. Whether this indeed contributes to their clinical activity is not known, however.

Transforming Growth Factor α and Epidermal Growth Factor Receptor

HIF induces the expression of the mitogenic transforming growth factor α (TGFα) and, at least indirectly, upregulates and activates its receptor, epidermal growth factor receptor (EGFR).[100–104] In addition, pVHL loss may potentiate EGFR signaling by decreasing its rate of internalization and recycling at the cell membrane.[50] EGFR is overexpressed and active in kidney cancers, and mouse models support an important role for EGFR in pVHL-defective tumor growth. Indeed, silencing EGFR suppresses tumor formation by *VHL*−/− RCC cells.[102] Nonetheless, the activity of EGFR inhibitors in the treatment of human kidney cancer has thus far been very disappointing.[105–107] A trivial explanation for this lack of a clinical response would be a failure to achieve a sufficient pharmacodynamic effect with the EGFR inhibitors tested so far. Another possibility relates to the potential importance of collateral signaling pathways. In particular, activation of c-Met confers partial resistance to EGFR inhibitors and, as discussed later, is frequently activated in pVHL-defective tumors.[108–110] Murine hepatocyte growth factor (HGF), the ligand for c-Met, does not activate human c-Met.[111,112] For this reason, the murine tumor xenograft studies performed to date with kidney cancer lines might have underestimated the potential influence of c-Met on EGFR dependence. A third, nonmutually exclusive, possibility is that the available kidney cancer lines became dependent on EGFR during adaptation to cell culture conditions.

Cyclin D

In renal epithelial cells, but not in the other epithelial cells tested thus far, HIF upregulates the expression of the cyclin D1 oncoprotein.[27,113–115] Cyclin D1 promotes cell cycle progression by activating Cdk4 and Cdk6, which phosphorylate and thereby inactivate the pRB tumor suppressor protein. Cdk6 is one of many genes located on a large chromosome 7 kidney cancer amplicon.[4] It is interesting that pVHL-defective clear-cell RCC appear to be hypersensitive to Cdk6 inhibition compared with isogenic, pVHL-proficient, control cells.[116] Several Cdk4/6 inhibitors are in clinical development.

Hepatocyte Growth Factor and c-Met

Several reports indicate that signaling by c-Met is enhanced by pVHL loss, although the exact mechanisms responsible are in dispute.[117–119] Some studies have reported that c-Met protein levels are increased by hypoxia and HIF,[120–122] whereas other studies have focused on the effect of pVHL loss on signaling events downstream of c-Met.[117–119] Of interest is that c-Met is mutationally activated in a subset of familial papillary renal cancers[36] and can, at least in certain settings, activate HIF.[123,124] This finding suggests that there is potential cross-talk between HIF and c-Met, and that there are molecular similarities between clear-cell and papillary renal cancer. Both c-Met and its ligand HGF are located on the large chromosome 7 amplicon described earlier,[4] and pVHL-defective cells appear to be hypersensitive to c-Met loss.[116] c-Met also plays a role in angiogenesis in addition to its potential cell autonomous role in clear-cell RCC. All of these considerations support the testing of c-Met inhibitors in clear-cell RCC.

Insulin-Like Growth Factor 2 and Insulin-Like Growth Factor 1 Receptor

HIF regulates the expression of insulin-like growth factor 2 (IGF2).[125] In addition, pVHL suppresses, in a HIF-independent manner, insulin-like growth factor 1 receptor (IGF1R) protein levels and downstream signaling.[126–128] The former has been linked to suppression of SP1 and sequestration of the HuR RNA-binding protein, and the latter to inhibition of protein kinase Cδ. IGF1R signaling can, in turn, upregulate HIF (particularly HIF1α).[125,129,130] Downregulation of IGFR sensitizes clear-cell RCC to conventional cytotoxics and to rapamycin-like drugs.[128] With respect to the latter, treatment of many cell types with rapalogs leads to a paradoxic increase in Akt activity due to loss of feedback inhibition of receptor tyrosine kinases such as IGFR,[131–133] providing a rationale for combining rapalogs with IGFR inhibitors.

Stromal Cell–Derived Factor and C-X-C Chemokine Receptor Type 4

Hypoxia and HIF increase the expression of the cytokine stromal cell–derived factor (SDF) and its receptor C-X-C chemokine receptor type 4 (CXCR4).[134,135] This cytokine-receptor pair has been implicated in tumor growth and invasion in other settings as well as in vasculogenesis, the process by which de novo blood vessels are formed through the recruitment of bone marrow–derived cells such as endothelial cell precursors and certain hematopoietic cells.[136] Preclinical studies in other tumor types suggest that blockade of VEGF and SDF would have additive effects.[137]

Interleukin-6

IL-6 functions as an autocrine growth factor in kidney cancer, and its expression is suppressed by pVHL.[114,138,139] Binding of IL-6 to its receptor, IL-6R, triggers receptor dimerization and phosphorylation by members of the Janus kinase families. Activation of IL-6R leads to STAT3 activation that promotes RCC cell proliferation.[140] Primary clear-cell RCCs produce high levels of IL-6 and frequently express IL-6R.[141,142] In addition, expression of IL-6R correlates with high serum IL-6 concentration and metastatic progression in this setting.[142] A clinical trial conducted in patients with progressive metastatic kidney cancer showed that CNOT328, a chimeric murine-human monoclonal antibody against IL-6, stabilized disease in more than 50% of the cases.[143]

RTK-Like Orphan Receptor 2

RTK-like orphan receptor 2 (ROR2) was identified in a biochemical screen for kinases that are induced and activated by pVHL loss in renal carcinoma cells.[144,145] ROR2 has an intracellular tyrosine kinase domain and an extracellular frizzled-like cysteine-rich domain that can act as a receptor for Wnt ligands. In preclinical models ROR2 promotes tumor cell invasiveness, at least partly through the upregulation of matrix metalloproteinase 2, soft agar growth, and orthotopic tumor formation.[144] These studies raise the possibility that targeting Wnt ligands or ROR2 itself will favorably alter the natural history of pVHL-defective clear-cell RCC.

Aurora Kinase A

pVHL inactivation leads to HIF-dependent induction of Nedd9 (also called renal carcinoma antigen NY-REN-1) and Aurora Kinase A,[146] which colocalize at the centrosome. Aurora A activation is Nedd9 dependent. Aurora A destabilizes ciliary microtubules through its ability to phosphorylate, and thereby activate, HDAC6, which deacetylates tubulin.[147] Suppression of Aurora Kinase A partially restores primary cilium formation, and impairs motility, in pVHL defective clear-cell RCC.[146]

Angiopoietin 4

The angiopoietins (Ang) and their receptor, TIE2, play an important role in angiogenesis.[148] Ang1 and Ang4 act as TIE2 agonists, and Ang2 is a TIE2 antagonist. Activation of TIE2 promotes the stabilization and maturation of vessels, whereas inhibition of TIE2 destabilizes blood vessels. In the latter context VEGF promotes sprouting of new blood vessels from the destabilized vessel wall, whereas loss of VEGF promotes endothelial cell death. These biological complexities have made it difficult to predict, a priori, the net effect of manipulating this system with respect to tumor angiogenesis. Nonetheless, pVHL has been reported to decrease the expression of Ang4 under normoxia, and blocking TIE2 blunts endothelial tube formation in response to pVHL-defective conditioned media in vitro.[149] The relationship between pVHL and Ang2 appears to be more complex, with pVHL seemingly required for the downregulation of Ang2 by hypoxia.[149,150] These findings support the exploration of TIE2 antagonists in conjunction with VEGF inhibitors for the treatment of clear-cell RCC.

Lactate Dehydrogenase A and Carbonic Anhydrase

HIF stimulates glycolysis and inhibits oxidative phosphorylation. The shift to glycolysis is accompanied by HIF-dependent increases in lactate dehydrogenase A, which converts pyruvate to lactate and carbonic anhydrases IX and XII, which help cells to accommodate the increased lactic acid load. These enzymes can be inhibited with drug-like small molecules, and preclinical studies suggest that such compounds would preferentially kill pVHL-defective tumor cells.[151,152]

Histone Methylases and Demethylases

HIF induces the expression of several histone demethylases including JMJD1A, JMJD2B, and JARID1B.[153-158] JMJD1A is, as expected, overexpressed in RCC, and its downregulation modestly suppresses tumor growth in vivo in preclinical models.[154] JARID1B (also called PLU-1) has been implicated as an oncoprotein in breast cancer, raising the possibility that it promotes RCC growth as well.[159] The identification of mutations affecting histone methylation in RCC also suggests that one or more enzymes that add or remove specific histone methyl marks will emerge as potential drug targets for this disease.[14]

SUMMARY

Inactivation of the *VHL* tumor suppressor gene is a frequent event in clear-cell renal carcinoma. The *VHL* gene product, pVHL, has many functions including serving as the substrate recognition subunit of a ubiquitin ligase complex that targets the HIF transcription factor for proteasomal degradation. HIF transcriptionally activates several genes implicated in clear-cell RCC pathogenesis, including VEGF. Multiple VEGF inhibitors have now been approved for this disease based on randomized clinical trial data. Two rapamycin-like mTOR inhibitors have also been approved for the treatment of metastatic kidney cancer. These drugs might operate by downregulating HIF in tumor cells, by downregulating VEGF signaling in endothelial cells, or perhaps both. Neither VEGF inhibitors nor mTOR inhibitors are curative for this disease, however. Further elucidation of the functions of pVHL and the genetic events that cooperate with *VHL* inactivation to cause clear-cell RCC will, it is hoped, yield additional molecular targets in this disease, as well as provide a conceptual foundation for effective combination therapies.

REFERENCES

1. Lopez-Beltran A, Carrasco JC, Cheng L, et al. 2009 update on the classification of renal epithelial tumors in adults. Int J Urol 2009;16(5):432–43.
2. Linehan WM, Zbar B. Focus on kidney cancer. Cancer Cell 2004;6(3):223–8.
3. Kim WY, Kaelin WG. Role of VHL gene mutation in human cancer. J Clin Oncol 2004;22:4991–5004.
4. Beroukhim R, Brunet JP, Di Napoli A, et al. Patterns of gene expression and copy-number alterations in von-Hippel Lindau disease-associated and sporadic clear cell carcinoma of the kidney. Cancer Res 2009;69(11):4674–81.
5. Clifford SC, Astuti D, Hooper L, et al. The pVHL-associated SCF ubiquitin ligase complex: molecular genetic analysis of elongin B and C, Rbx1 and HIF-1alpha in renal cell carcinoma. Oncogene 2001;20(36):5067–74.
6. Young AC, Craven RA, Cohen D, et al. Analysis of VHL gene alterations and their relationship to clinical parameters in sporadic conventional renal cell carcinoma. Clin Cancer Res 2009;15(24):7582–92.
7. Nickerson ML, Jaeger E, Shi Y, et al. Improved identification of von Hippel-Lindau gene alterations in clear cell renal tumors. Clin Cancer Res 2008; 14(15):4726–34.
8. Varela I, Tarpey P, Raine K, et al. Exome sequencing identifies frequent mutation of the SWI/SNF complex gene PBRM1 in renal carcinoma. Nature 2011; 469(7331):539–42.
9. Mandriota SJ, Turner KJ, Davies DR, et al. HIF activation identifies early lesions in VHL kidneys: evidence for site-specific tumor suppressor function in the nephron. Cancer Cell 2002;1(5):459–68.
10. Montani M, Heinimann K, von Teichman A, et al. VHL-gene deletion in single renal tubular epithelial cells and renal tubular cysts: further evidence for a cyst-dependent progression pathway of clear cell renal carcinoma in von Hippel-Lindau disease. Am J Surg Pathol 2010;34(6):806–15.
11. Rankin EB, Tomaszewski JE, Haase VH. Renal cyst development in mice with conditional inactivation of the von Hippel-Lindau tumor suppressor. Cancer Res 2006;66(5):2576–83.
12. Klatte T, Rao PN, de Martino M, et al. Cytogenetic profile predicts prognosis of patients with clear cell renal cell carcinoma. J Clin Oncol 2009;27(5):746–53.
13. Pei J, Feder MM, Al-Saleem T, et al. Combined classical cytogenetics and microarray-based genomic copy number analysis reveal frequent 3;5 rearrangements in clear cell renal cell carcinoma. Genes Chromosomes Cancer 2010;49(7):610–9.
14. Dalgliesh GL, Furge K, Greenman C, et al. Systematic sequencing of renal carcinoma reveals inactivation of histone modifying genes. Nature 2010; 463(7279):360–3.
15. Lee S, Neumann M, Stearman R, et al. Transcription-dependent nuclear-cytoplasmic trafficking is required for the function of the von Hippel-Lindau tumor suppressor protein. Mol Cell Biol 1999;19(2):1486–97.
16. Schoenfeld A, Davidowitz E, Burk R. Endoplasmic reticulum/cytosolic localization of von Hippel-Lindau gene products is mediated by a 64-amino acid region. Int J Cancer 2001;91:457–67.
17. Shiao YH, Resau JH, Nagashima K, et al. The von Hippel-Lindau tumor suppressor targets to mitochondria. Cancer Res 2000;60(11):2816–9.
18. Kaelin WG Jr, Ratcliffe PJ. Oxygen sensing by metazoans: the central role of the HIF hydroxylase pathway. Mol Cell 2008;30(4):393–402.

19. Makino Y, Cao R, Svensson K, et al. Inhibitory PAS domain protein is a negative regulator of hypoxia-inducible gene expression. Nature 2001;414(6863): 550–4.

20. Maynard MA, Evans AJ, Hosomi T, et al. Human HIF-3alpha4 is a dominant-negative regulator of HIF-1 and is down-regulated in renal cell carcinoma. FASEB J 2005;19(11):1396–406.

21. Maynard MA, Qi H, Chung J, et al. Multiple splice variants of the human HIF-3 alpha locus are targets of the von Hippel-Lindau E3 ubiquitin ligase complex. J Biol Chem 2003;278(13):11032–40.

22. Li L, Zhang L, Zhang X, et al. Hypoxia-inducible factor linked to differential kidney cancer risk seen with type 2A and type 2B VHL mutations. Mol Cell Biol 2007;27(15):5381–92.

23. Kondo K, Klco J, Nakamura E, et al. Inhibition of HIF is necessary for tumor suppression by the von Hippel-Lindau protein. Cancer Cell 2002;1(3):237–46.

24. Kondo K, Kim WY, Lechpammer M, et al. Inhibition of HIF2alpha is sufficient to suppress pVHL-defective tumor growth. PLoS Biol 2003;1(3):439–44.

25. Zimmer M, Doucette D, Siddiqui N, et al. Inhibition of hypoxia-inducible factor is sufficient for growth suppression of VHL-/- tumors. Mol Cancer Res 2004;2(2): 89–95.

26. Maranchie JK, Vasselli JR, Riss J, et al. The contribution of VHL substrate binding and HIF1-alpha to the phenotype of VHL loss in renal cell carcinoma. Cancer Cell 2002;1(3):247–55.

27. Raval RR, Lau KW, Tran MG, et al. Contrasting properties of hypoxia-inducible factor 1 (HIF-1) and HIF-2 in von Hippel-Lindau-associated renal cell carcinoma. Mol Cell Biol 2005;25(13):5675–86.

28. Biswas S, Troy H, Leek R, et al. Effects of HIF-1alpha and HIF2alpha on growth and metabolism of clear-cell renal cell carcinoma 786-0 xenografts. J Oncol 2010;2010:757908.

29. Kim WY, Safran M, Buckley MR, et al. Failure to prolyl hydroxylate hypoxia-inducible factor alpha phenocopies VHL inactivation in vivo. EMBO J 2006; 25(19):4650–62.

30. Moslehi J, Minamishima YA, Shi J, et al. Loss of hypoxia-inducible factor prolyl hydroxylase activity in cardiomyocytes phenocopies ischemic cardiomyopathy. Circulation 2010;122(10):1004–16.

31. Rankin EB, Rha J, Unger TL, et al. Hypoxia-inducible factor-2 regulates vascular tumorigenesis in mice. Oncogene 2008;27:5354–8.

32. Rankin EB, Rha J, Selak MA, et al. HIF-2 regulates hepatic lipid metabolism. Mol Cell Biol 2009;29:4527–38.

33. Maxwell P, Weisner M, Chang GW, et al. The von Hippel-Lindau gene product is necessary for oxygen-dependent proteolysis of hypoxia-inducible factor a subunits. Nature 1999;399:271–5.

34. Gordan JD, Lal P, Dondeti VR, et al. HIF-alpha effects on c-Myc distinguish two subtypes of sporadic VHL-deficient clear cell renal carcinoma. Cancer Cell 2008;14:435–46.

35. Purdue MP, Johansson M, Zelenika D, et al. Genome-wide association study of renal cell carcinoma identifies two susceptibility loci on 2p21 and 11q13.3. Nat Genet 2011;43(1):60–5.

36. Linehan WM, Srinivasan R, Schmidt LS. The genetic basis of kidney cancer: a metabolic disease. Nat Rev Urol 2010;7(5):277–85.

37. Sudarshan S, Sourbier C, Kong HS, et al. Fumarate hydratase deficiency in renal cancer induces glycolytic addiction and hypoxia-inducible transcription

factor 1alpha stabilization by glucose-dependent generation of reactive oxygen species. Mol Cell Biol 2009;29(15):4080–90.

38. Isaacs JS, Jung YJ, Mole DR, et al. HIF overexpression correlates with biallelic loss of fumarate hydratase in renal cancer: novel role of fumarate in regulation of HIF stability. Cancer Cell 2005;8(2):143–53.

39. Pollard PJ, Spencer-Dene B, Shukla D, et al. Targeted inactivation of fh1 causes proliferative renal cyst development and activation of the hypoxia pathway. Cancer Cell 2007;11(4):311–9.

40. Pollard PJ, Briere JJ, Alam NA, et al. Accumulation of Krebs cycle intermediates and over-expression of HIF1alpha in tumours which result from germline FH and SDH mutations. Hum Mol Genet 2005;14(15):2231–9.

41. Dahia PL, Ross KN, Wright ME, et al. A HIF1alpha regulatory loop links hypoxia and mitochondrial signals in pheochromocytomas. PLoS Genet 2005;1(1): 72–80.

42. Kaelin WG. von Hippel-Lindau disease. Annu Rev Pathol 2007;2:145–73.

43. Stickle NH, Chung J, Klco JM, et al. pVHL modification by NEDD8 is required for fibronectin matrix assembly and suppression of tumor development. Mol Cell Biol 2004;24(8):3251–61.

44. He Z, Liu S, Guo M, et al. Expression of fibronectin and HIF-1alpha in renal cell carcinomas: relationship to von Hippel-Lindau gene inactivation. Cancer Genet Cytogenet 2004;152(2):89–94.

45. Ohh M, Yauch RL, Lonergan KM, et al. The von Hippel-Lindau tumor suppressor protein is required for proper assembly of an extracellular fibronectin matrix. Mol Cell 1998;1:959–68.

46. Tang N, Mack F, Haase VH, et al. pVHL function is essential for endothelial extracellular matrix deposition. Mol Cell Biol 2006;26(7):2519–30.

47. Hsouna A, Nallamothu G, Kose N, et al. Drosophila von Hippel-Lindau tumor suppressor gene function in epithelial tubule morphogenesis. Mol Cell Biol 2010;30(15):3779–94.

48. Champion KJ, Guinea M, Dammai V, et al. Endothelial function of von Hippel-Lindau tumor suppressor gene: control of fibroblast growth factor receptor signaling. Cancer Res 2008;68(12):4649–57.

49. Hsu T, Adereth Y, Kose N, et al. Endocytic function of von Hippel-Lindau tumor suppressor protein regulates surface localization of fibroblast growth factor receptor 1 and cell motility. J Biol Chem 2006;281(17):12069–80.

50. Wang Y, Roche O, Yan MS, et al. Regulation of endocytosis via the oxygen-sensing pathway. Nat Med 2009;15(3):319–24.

51. Hergovich A, Lisztwan J, Barry R, et al. Regulation of microtubule stability by the von Hippel-Lindau tumour suppressor protein pVHL. Nat Cell Biol 2003;5(1):64–70.

52. Lolkema MP, Mans DA, Snijckers CM, et al. The von Hippel-Lindau tumour suppressor interacts with microtubules through kinesin-2. FEBS Lett 2007; 581(24):4571–6.

53. Schermer B, Ghenoiu C, Bartram M, et al. The von Hippel-Lindau tumor suppressor protein controls ciliogenesis by orienting microtubule growth. J Cell Biol 2006;175(4):547–54.

54. Thoma CR, Matov A, Gutbrodt KL, et al. Quantitative image analysis identifies pVHL as a key regulator of microtubule dynamic instability. J Cell Biol 2010; 190(6):991–1003.

55. Lee S, Nakamura E, Yang H, et al. Neuronal apoptosis linked to EgIN3 prolyl hydroxylase and familial pheochromocytoma genes: developmental culling and cancer. Cancer Cell 2005;8(2):155–67.

56. Young AP, Schlisio S, Minamishima YA, et al. VHL loss actuates a HIF-independent senescence programme mediated by Rb and p400. Nat Cell Biol 2008;10(3):361–9.

57. Lutz MS, Burk RD. Primary cilium formation requires von Hippel-Lindau gene function in renal-derived cells. Cancer Res 2006;66(14):6903–7.

58. Thoma CR, Frew IJ, Hoerner CR, et al. pVHL and GSK3beta are components of a primary cilium-maintenance signalling network. Nat Cell Biol 2007;9(5): 588–95.

59. Singla V, Reiter JF. The primary cilium as the cell's antenna: signaling at a sensory organelle. Science 2006;313(5787):629–33.

60. Zhang Q, Taulman PD, Yoder BK. Cystic kidney diseases: all roads lead to the cilium. Physiology (Bethesda) 2004;19:225–30.

61. Yang H, Minamishima YA, Yan Q, et al. pVHL acts as an adaptor to promote the inhibitory phosphorylation of the NF-kappaB agonist Card9 by CK2. Mol Cell 2007;28(1):15–27.

62. An J, Rettig MB. Mechanism of von Hippel-Lindau protein-mediated suppression of nuclear factor kappa B activity. Mol Cell Biol 2005;25(17):7546–56.

63. An J, Fisher M, Rettig MB. VHL expression in renal cell carcinoma sensitizes to bortezomib (PS-341) through an NF-kappaB-dependent mechanism. Oncogene 2005;24(9):1563–70.

64. Pantuck AJ, An J, Liu H, et al. NF-kappaB-dependent plasticity of the epithelial to mesenchymal transition induced by Von Hippel-Lindau inactivation in renal cell carcinomas. Cancer Res 2010;70(2):752–61.

65. Oya M, Takayanagi A, Horiguchi A, et al. Increased nuclear factor-kappa B activation is related to the tumor development of renal cell carcinoma. Carcinogenesis 2003;24(3):377–84.

66. Oya M, Ohtsubo M, Takayanagi A, et al. Constitutive activation of nuclear factor-kappaB prevents TRAIL-induced apoptosis in renal cancer cells. Oncogene 2001;20(29):3888–96.

67. Qi H, Ohh M. The von Hippel-Lindau tumor suppressor protein sensitizes renal cell carcinoma cells to tumor necrosis factor-induced cytotoxicity by suppressing the nuclear factor-kappaB-dependent antiapoptotic pathway. Cancer Res 2003;63(21):7076–80.

68. Gao C, Cao W, Bao L, et al. Autophagy negatively regulates Wnt signalling by promoting Dishevelled degradation. Nat Cell Biol 2010;12(8):781–90.

69. Chitalia VC, Foy RL, Bachschmid MM, et al. Jade-1 inhibits Wnt signalling by ubiquitylating beta-catenin and mediates Wnt pathway inhibition by pVHL. Nat Cell Biol 2008;10(10):1208–16.

70. Mazumdar J, O'Brien WT, Johnson RS, et al. O_2 regulates stem cells through Wnt/beta-catenin signalling. Nat Cell Biol 2010;12(10):1007–13.

71. Giles RH, Lolkema MP, Snijckers CM, et al. Interplay between VHL/HIF1-alpha and Wnt/beta-catenin pathways during colorectal tumorigenesis. Oncogene 2006.

72. Brugarolas J, Kaelin WG Jr. Dysregulation of HIF and VEGF is a unifying feature of the familial hamartoma syndromes. Cancer Cell 2004;6(1):7–10.

73. Amornphimoltham P, Patel V, Leelahavanichkul K, et al. A retroinhibition approach reveals a tumor cell-autonomous response to rapamycin in head and neck cancer. Cancer Res 2008;68(4):1144–53.

74. Hudes G, Carducci M, Tomczak J, et al. A phase 3, randomized, 3-arm study of temsirolimus (TEMSR) or interferon-alpha (IFN) or the combination of TEMSR + IFN in the treatment of first-line, poor-risk patients with advanced renal cell

carcinoma (adv RCC). JCO, 2006 ASCO Annual Meetings Proceedings Part I. Atlanta (GA), June 2–6, 2006;24:LBA4.

75. Motzer RJ, Escudier B, Oudard S, et al. Efficacy of everolimus in advanced renal cell carcinoma: a double-blind, randomised, placebo-controlled phase III trial. Lancet 2008;372(9637):449–56.

76. Motzer RJ, Escudier B, Oudard S, et al. RAD001 vs placebo in patients with metastatic renal cell carcinoma (RCC) after progression on VEGFr-TKI therapy: results from a randomized, double-blind, multicenter phase-III study. J Clin Oncol 2008;26 [abstract: LBA5026].

77. Toschi A, Lee E, Gadir N, et al. Differential dependence of HIF1alpha and HIF2alpha on mTORC1 and mTORC2. J Biol Chem 2008;283:34495–9.

78. Cho DC, Cohen MB, Panka DJ, et al. The efficacy of the novel dual PI3-kinase/mTOR inhibitor NVP-BEZ235 compared with rapamycin in renal cell carcinoma. Clin Cancer Res 2010;16(14):3628–38.

79. Iliopoulos O, Jiang C, Levy AP, et al. Negative regulation of hypoxia-inducible genes by the von Hippel-Lindau protein. Proc Natl Acad Sci U S A 1996;93:10595–9.

80. Gnarra JR, Zhou S, Merrill MJ, et al. Post-transcriptional regulation of vascular endothelial growth factor mRNA by the VHL tumor suppressor gene product. Proc Natl Acad Sci 1996;93:10589–94.

81. Fox SB, Turley H, Cheale M, et al. Phosphorylated KDR is expressed in the neoplastic and stromal elements of human renal tumours and shuttles from cell membrane to nucleus. J Pathol 2004;202(3):313–20.

82. Sternberg CN, Davis ID, Mardiak J, et al. Pazopanib in locally advanced or metastatic renal cell carcinoma: results of a randomized phase III trial. J Clin Oncol 2010;28(6):1061–8.

83. Motzer RJ, Hutson TE, Tomczak P, et al. Sunitinib versus interferon alfa in metastatic renal-cell carcinoma. N Engl J Med 2007;356(2):115–24.

84. Escudier B, Eisen T, Stadler WM, et al. Sorafenib in advanced clear-cell renal-cell carcinoma. N Engl J Med 2007;356(2):125–34.

85. Escudier B, Pluzanska A, Koralewski P, et al. Bevacizumab plus interferon alfa-2a for treatment of metastatic renal cell carcinoma: a randomised, double-blind phase III trial. Lancet 2007;370(9605):2103–11.

86. Gossage L, Eisen T. Alterations in VHL as potential biomarkers in renal-cell carcinoma. Nat Rev Clin Oncol 2010;7(5):277–88.

87. Cowey CL, Rathmell WK. VHL gene mutations in renal cell carcinoma: role as a biomarker of disease outcome and drug efficacy. Curr Oncol Rep 2009;11(2):94–101.

88. Choueiri TK, Vaziri SA, Jaeger E, et al. von Hippel-Lindau gene status and response to vascular endothelial growth factor targeted therapy for metastatic clear cell renal cell carcinoma. J Urol 2008;180(3):860–5 [discussion: 865–6].

89. Pena C, Lathia C, Shan M, et al. Biomarkers predicting outcome in patients with advanced renal cell carcinoma: results from sorafenib phase III treatment approaches in renal cancer global evaluation trial. Clin Cancer Res 2010;16(19):4853–63.

90. Feldman DR, Baum MS, Ginsberg MS, et al. Phase I trial of bevacizumab plus escalated doses of sunitinib in patients with metastatic renal cell carcinoma. J Clin Oncol 2009;27(9):1432–9.

91. Rini BI, Garcia JA, Cooney MM, et al. Toxicity of sunitinib plus bevacizumab in renal cell carcinoma. J Clin Oncol 2010;28(17):e284–5 [author reply: e286–7].

92. Rini BI, Michaelson MD, Rosenberg JE, et al. Antitumor activity and biomarker analysis of sunitinib in patients with bevacizumab-refractory metastatic renal cell carcinoma. J Clin Oncol 2008;26(22):3743–8.
93. Casanovas O, Hicklin DJ, Bergers G, et al. Drug resistance by evasion of anti-angiogenic targeting of VEGF signaling in late-stage pancreatic islet tumors. Cancer Cell 2005;8(4):299–309.
94. Huang D, Ding Y, Zhou M, et al. Interleukin-8 mediates resistance to antiangiogenic agent sunitinib in renal cell carcinoma. Cancer Res 2010;70(3):1063–71.
95. Hammers HJ, Verheul HM, Salumbides B, et al. Reversible epithelial to mesenchymal transition and acquired resistance to sunitinib in patients with renal cell carcinoma: evidence from a xenograft study. Mol Cancer Ther 2010;9(6): 1525–35.
96. Benjamin LE, Golijanin D, Itin A, et al. Selective ablation of immature blood vessels in established human tumors follows vascular endothelial growth factor withdrawal. J Clin Invest 1999;103(2):159–65.
97. Benjamin LE, Keshet E. Conditional switching of vascular endothelial growth factor (VEGF) expression in tumors: induction of endothelial cell shedding and regression of hemangioblastoma-like vessels by VEGF withdrawal. Proc Natl Acad Sci U S A 1997;94:8761–6.
98. Benjamin LE, Hemo I, Keshet E. A plasticity window for blood vessel remodelling is defined by pericyte coverage of the preformed endothelial network and is regulated by PDGF-B and VEGF. Development 1998;125(9):1591–8.
99. Bergers G, Song S, Meyer-Morse N, et al. Benefits of targeting both pericytes and endothelial cells in the tumor vasculature with kinase inhibitors. J Clin Invest 2003;111(9):1287–95.
100. Knebelmann B, Ananth S, Cohen H, et al. Transforming growth factor alpha is a target for the von Hippel-Lindau tumor suppressor. Cancer Res 1998;58: 226–31.
101. de Paulsen N, Brychzy A, Fournier M-C, et al. Role of transforming growth factor-alpha in VHL-/- clear cell renal carcinoma cell proliferation: a possible mechanism coupling von Hippel-Lindau tumor suppressor inactivation and tumorigenesis. Proc Natl Acad Sci U S A 2001;13:1387–92.
102. Smith K, Gunaratnam L, Morley M, et al. Silencing of epidermal growth factor receptor suppresses hypoxia-inducible factor-2-driven VHL-/- renal cancer. Cancer Res 2005;65(12):5221–30.
103. Franovic A, Gunaratnam L, Smith K, et al. Translational up-regulation of the EGFR by tumor hypoxia provides a nonmutational explanation for its overexpression in human cancer. Proc Natl Acad Sci U S A 2007;104(32):13092–7.
104. Franovic A, Holterman CE, Payette J, et al. Human cancers converge at the HIF-2alpha oncogenic axis. Proc Natl Acad Sci U S A 2009;106(50): 21306–11.
105. Rowinsky EK, Schwartz GH, Gollob JA, et al. Safety, pharmacokinetics, and activity of ABX-EGF, a fully human anti-epidermal growth factor receptor monoclonal antibody in patients with metastatic renal cell cancer. J Clin Oncol 2004; 22(15):3003–15.
106. Bukowski RM, Kabbinavar FF, Figlin RA, et al. Randomized phase II study of erlotinib combined with bevacizumab compared with bevacizumab alone in metastatic renal cell cancer. J Clin Oncol 2007;25(29):4536–41.
107. Dawson NA, Guo C, Zak R, et al. A phase II trial of gefitinib (Iressa, ZD1839) in stage IV and recurrent renal cell carcinoma. Clin Cancer Res 2004;10(23): 7812–9.

108. Bean J, Brennan C, Shih JY, et al. MET amplification occurs with or without T790M mutations in EGFR mutant lung tumors with acquired resistance to gefitinib or erlotinib. Proc Natl Acad Sci U S A 2007;104(52):20932–7.
109. Engelman JA, Zejnullahu K, Mitsudomi T, et al. MET amplification leads to gefitinib resistance in lung cancer by activating ERBB3 signaling. Science 2007; 316(5827):1039–43.
110. Stommel JM, Kimmelman AC, Ying H, et al. Coactivation of receptor tyrosine kinases affects the response of tumor cells to targeted therapies. Science 2007;318(5848):287–90.
111. Zhang YW, Staal B, Essenburg C, et al. MET kinase inhibitor SGX523 synergizes with epidermal growth factor receptor inhibitor erlotinib in a hepatocyte growth factor-dependent fashion to suppress carcinoma growth. Cancer Res 2010; 70(17):6880–90.
112. Rong S, Bodescot M, Blair D, et al. Tumorigenicity of the met proto-oncogene and the gene for hepatocyte growth factor. Mol Cell Biol 1992;12(11):5152–8.
113. Bindra RS, Vasselli JR, Stearman R, et al. VHL-mediated hypoxia regulation of cyclin D1 in renal carcinoma cells. Cancer Res 2002;62(11):3014–9.
114. Zatyka M, da Silva NF, Clifford SC, et al. Identification of cyclin D1 and other novel targets for the von Hippel-Lindau tumor suppressor gene by expression array analysis and investigation of cyclin D1 genotype as a modifier in von Hippel-Lindau disease. Cancer Res 2002;62(13):3803–11.
115. Baba M, Hirai S, Yamada-Okabe H, et al. Loss of von Hippel-Lindau protein causes cell density dependent deregulation of CyclinD1 expression through hypoxia-inducible factor. Oncogene 2003;22(18):2728–38.
116. Bommi-Reddy A, Almeciga I, Sawyer J, et al. Kinase requirements in human cells: III. Altered kinase requirements in VHL-/- cancer cells detected in a pilot synthetic lethal screen. Proc Natl Acad Sci U S A 2008;105(43): 16484–9.
117. Koochekpour S, Jeffers M, Wang P, et al. The von Hippel-Lindau tumor suppressor gene inhibits hepatocyte growth factor/scatter factor-induced invasion and branching morphogenesis in renal carcinoma cells. Mol Cell Biol 1999; 19:5902–12.
118. Nakaigawa N, Yao M, Baba M, et al. Inactivation of von Hippel-Lindau gene induces constitutive phosphorylation of MET protein in clear cell renal carcinoma. Cancer Res 2006;66(7):3699–705.
119. Peruzzi B, Athauda G, Bottaro DP. The von Hippel-Lindau tumor suppressor gene product represses oncogenic beta-catenin signaling in renal carcinoma cells. Proc Natl Acad Sci U S A 2006;103(39):14531–6.
120. Pennacchietti S, Michieli P, Galluzzo M, et al. Hypoxia promotes invasive growth by transcriptional activation of the met protooncogene. Cancer Cell 2003;3(4): 347–61.
121. Hara S, Nakashiro KI, Klosek SK, et al. Hypoxia enhances c-Met/HGF receptor expression and signaling by activating HIF-1alpha in human salivary gland cancer cells. Oral Oncol 2006;42(6):593–8.
122. Hayashi M, Sakata M, Takeda T, et al. Up-regulation of c-met protooncogene product expression through hypoxia-inducible factor-1alpha is involved in trophoblast invasion under low-oxygen tension. Endocrinology 2005;146(11): 4682–9.
123. Tacchini L, Dansi P, Matteucci E, et al. Hepatocyte growth factor signalling stimulates hypoxia inducible factor-1 (HIF-1) activity in HepG2 hepatoma cells. Carcinogenesis 2001;22(9):1363–71.

124. Tacchini L, De Ponti C, Matteucci E, et al. Hepatocyte growth factor-activated NF-kappaB regulates HIF-1 activity and ODC expression, implicated in survival, differently in different carcinoma cell lines. Carcinogenesis 2004;25(11): 2089–100.

125. Feldser D, Agani F, Iyer NV, et al. Reciprocal positive regulation of hypoxia-inducible factor 1alpha and insulin-like growth factor 2. Cancer Res 1999; 59(16):3915–8.

126. Yuen JS, Cockman ME, Sullivan M, et al. The VHL tumor suppressor inhibits expression of the IGF1R and its loss induces IGF1R upregulation in human clear cell renal carcinoma. Oncogene 2007;26(45):6499–508.

127. Datta K, Nambudripad R, Pal S, et al. Inhibition of insulin-like growth factor-I-mediated cell signaling by the von Hippel-Lindau gene product in renal cancer. J Biol Chem 2000;275(27):20700–6.

128. Yuen JS, Akkaya E, Wang Y, et al. Validation of the type 1 insulin-like growth factor receptor as a therapeutic target in renal cancer. Mol Cancer Ther 2009; 8(6):1448–59.

129. Fukuda R, Hirota K, Fan F, et al. Insulin-like growth factor 1 induces hypoxia-inducible factor 1-mediated vascular endothelial growth factor expression, which is dependent on MAP kinase and phosphatidylinositol 3-kinase signaling in colon cancer cells. J Biol Chem 2002;277(41):38205–11.

130. Treins C, Giorgetti-Peraldi S, Murdaca J, et al. Insulin stimulates hypoxia-inducible factor 1 through a phosphatidylinositol 3-kinase/target of rapamycin-dependent signaling pathway. J Biol Chem 2002;277(31):27975–81.

131. O'Reilly KE, Rojo F, She QB, et al. mTOR inhibition induces upstream receptor tyrosine kinase signaling and activates Akt. Cancer Res 2006; 66(3):1500–8.

132. Wan X, Harkavy B, Shen N, et al. Rapamycin induces feedback activation of Akt signaling through an IGF-1R-dependent mechanism. Oncogene 2007;26(13): 1932–40.

133. Manning BD, Logsdon MN, Lipovsky AI, et al. Feedback inhibition of Akt signaling limits the growth of tumors lacking Tsc2. Genes Dev 2005;19(15): 1773–8.

134. Staller P, Sulitkova J, Lisztwan J, et al. Chemokine receptor CXCR4 downregu-lated by von Hippel-Lindau tumour suppressor pVHL. Nature 2003;425(6955): 307–11.

135. Zagzag D, Krishnamachary B, Yee H, et al. Stromal cell-derived factor-1alpha and CXCR4 expression in hemangioblastoma and clear cell-renal cell carci-noma: von Hippel-Lindau loss-of-function induces expression of a ligand and its receptor. Cancer Res 2005;65(14):6178–88.

136. Petit I, Jin D, Rafii S. The SDF-1-CXCR4 signaling pathway: a molecular hub modulating neo-angiogenesis. Trends Immunol 2007;28(7):299–307.

137. Kioi M, Vogel H, Schultz G, et al. Inhibition of vasculogenesis, but not angiogen-esis, prevents the recurrence of glioblastoma after irradiation in mice. J Clin Invest 2010;120(3):694–705.

138. Miki S, Iwano M, Miki Y, et al. Interleukin-6 (IL-6) functions as an in vitro autocrine growth factor in renal cell carcinomas. FEBS Lett 1989;250(2):607–10.

139. Gogusev J, Barbey S, Nezelof C. Modulation of c-myc, c-myb, c-fos, c-sis and c-fms proto-oncogene expression and of CSF-1 transcripts and protein by phor-bol diester in human malignant histiocytosis DEL cell line with 5q 35 break point. Anticancer Res 1993;13(4):1043–7.

140. Horiguchi A, Oya M, Marumo K, et al. STAT3, but not ERKs, mediates the IL-6-induced proliferation of renal cancer cells, ACHN and 769P. Kidney Int 2002; 61(3):926–38.
141. Takenawa J, Kaneko Y, Fukumoto M, et al. Enhanced expression of interleukin-6 in primary human renal cell carcinomas. J Natl Cancer Inst 1991;83(22): 1668–72.
142. Costes V, Liautard J, Picot MC, et al. Expression of the interleukin 6 receptor in primary renal cell carcinoma. J Clin Pathol 1997;50(10):835–40.
143. Rossi JF, Negrier S, James ND, et al. A phase I/II study of siltuximab (CNTO 328), an anti-interleukin-6 monoclonal antibody, in metastatic renal cell cancer. Br J Cancer 2010;103(8):1154–62.
144. Wright TM, Brannon AR, Gordan JD, et al. Ror2, a developmentally regulated kinase, promotes tumor growth potential in renal cell carcinoma. Oncogene 2009;28(27):2513–23.
145. Wright TM, Rathmell WK. Identification of Ror2 as a hypoxia-inducible factor target in von Hippel-Lindau-associated renal cell carcinoma. J Biol Chem 2010;285(17):12916–24.
146. Xu J, Li H, Wang B, et al. VHL inactivation induces HEF1 and Aurora kinase A. J Am Soc Nephrol 2010;21(12):2041–6.
147. Pugacheva EN, Jablonski SA, Hartman TR, et al. HEF1-dependent Aurora A activation induces disassembly of the primary cilium. Cell 2007;129(7):1351–63.
148. Huang H, Bhat A, Woodnutt G, et al. Targeting the ANGPT-TIE2 pathway in malignancy. Nat Rev Cancer 2010;10(8):575–85.
149. Yamakawa M, Liu LX, Belanger AJ, et al. Expression of angiopoietins in renal epithelial and clear cell carcinoma cells: regulation by hypoxia and participation in angiogenesis. Am J Physiol Renal Physiol 2004;287(4):F649–57.
150. Currie MJ, Gunningham SP, Turner K, et al. Expression of the angiopoietins and their receptor Tie2 in human renal clear cell carcinomas; regulation by the von Hippel-Lindau gene and hypoxia. J Pathol 2002;198(4):502–10.
151. Xie H, Valera VA, Merino MJ, et al. LDH-A inhibition, a therapeutic strategy for treatment of hereditary leiomyomatosis and renal cell cancer. Mol Cancer Ther 2009;8(3):626–35.
152. Cianchi F, Vinci MC, Supuran CT, et al. Selective inhibition of carbonic anhydrase IX decreases cell proliferation and induces ceramide-mediated apoptosis in human cancer cells. J Pharmacol Exp Ther 2010;334(3):710–9.
153. Pollard P, Loenarz C, Mole D, et al. Regulation of Jumonji-domain-containing histone demethylases by hypoxia-inducible factor (HIF)-1alpha. Biochem J 2008;416(3):387–94.
154. Krieg AJ, Rankin EB, Chan D, et al. Regulation of the histone demethylase JMJD1A by hypoxia-inducible factor 1 alpha enhances hypoxic gene expression and tumor growth. Mol Cell Biol 2010;30(1):344–53.
155. Yang J, Jubb AM, Pike L, et al. The histone demethylase JMJD2B is regulated by estrogen receptor alpha and hypoxia, and is a key mediator of estrogen induced growth. Cancer Res 2010;70(16):6456–66.
156. Beyer S, Kristensen MM, Jensen KS, et al. The histone demethylases JMJD1A and JMJD2B are transcriptional targets of hypoxia-inducible factor HIF. J Biol Chem 2008;283(52):36542–52.
157. Wellmann S, Bettkober M, Zelmer A, et al. Hypoxia upregulates the histone demethylase JMJD1A via HIF-1. Biochem Biophys Res Commun 2008;372(4): 892–7.

158. Xia X, Lemieux ME, Li W, et al. Integrative analysis of HIF binding and transactivation reveals its role in maintaining histone methylation homeostasis. Proc Natl Acad Sci U S A 2009;106(11):4260–5.

159. Yamane K, Tateishi K, Klose RJ, et al. PLU-1 is an H3K4 demethylase involved in transcriptional repression and breast cancer cell proliferation. Mol Cell 2007; 25(6):801–12.

Imaging in Renal Cell Carcinoma

Katherine M. Krajewski, MD[a,b,]*, Angela A. Giardino, MD[a,b],
Katherine Zukotynski, MD[a,b], Annick D. Van den Abbeele, MD[a,b],
Ivan Pedrosa, MD[c]

KEYWORDS

• Imaging • Renal cell carcinoma • Management • Diagnosis

Renal cell carcinoma (RCC) accounts for about 3% of all adult cancers and 85% to 90% of all renal malignancies.[1] Approximately 46,000 new cases of RCC were diagnosed in 2008.[2] An estimated 50% to 60% of RCCs are found incidentally when diagnostic imaging is performed for an unrelated indication.[1] As a result, renal tumor size and stage at presentation has steadily decreased in the United States in recent years,[3] and the number of cases presenting with the classic triad of hematuria, flank pain, and an abdominal mass is declining.

The differential diagnosis of a renal mass includes both benign and malignant entities. Although RCC is the most common renal neoplasm and several pathologic subtypes of RCC show typical imaging features, tissue sampling or surgical resection is usually required to make a definitive diagnosis. However, imaging may permit the diagnosis of some benign lesions (eg, angiomyolipoma) and can help in the management of masses suspicious for RCC.

MODALITY-SPECIFIC CHARACTERIZATION OF RENAL MASSES

Detection of vascularity in a renal mass is the most reliable finding to characterize a renal lesion as a neoplasm.[4,5] Based on this premise, cross-sectional imaging studies are tailored primarily to detection of blood flow (Doppler ultrasound [US]) or enhancement after contrast administration (contrast-enhanced computed tomography [CT] and magnetic resonance imaging [MRI]) in a renal mass as an indicator of tumor vascularity. The characterization of cystic renal masses is also based on detection of complex solid components within the cyst. The presence of enhancing

[a] Department of Imaging, Dana-Farber Cancer Institute, 450 Brookline Avenue, Boston, MA 02215, USA
[b] Department of Radiology, Brigham and Women's Hospital and Harvard Medical School, Boston, MA 02215, USA
[c] Department of Radiology, Beth Israel Deaconess Medical Center and Harvard Medical School, Boston, MA 02215
* Corresponding author. Department of Imaging, Dana-Farber Cancer Institute, 450 Brookline Avenue, Boston, MA 02215.
E-mail address: kmkrajewski@partners.org

Hematol Oncol Clin N Am 25 (2011) 687–715
doi:10.1016/j.hoc.2011.04.005
0889-8588/11/$ – see front matter © 2011 Elsevier Inc. All rights reserved.

thick septa and/or nodules indicates a neoplasm, whereas cysts that contain more than a few thin septa may require imaging follow-up.[4] A classification for characterization of cystic masses based on radiologic features (ie, the Bosniak classification), was originally developed to guide management of such lesions according to CT features, but may be applicable to lesions characterized by US and MRI as well.[6]

US

US is frequently used as the initial imaging modality to assess renal disorders because of the lack of radiation, low cost, and availability, and is particularly helpful for characterizing cystic renal masses. Benign simple cysts may be diagnosed confidently by US when lesions are anechoic and thin walled with posterior acoustic enhancement. Cystic lesions with more complex features may require imaging follow-up or surgical intervention. Doppler US evaluation yields additional important information regarding the vascularity of a lesion. A lesion of variable echogenicity and demonstrable blood flow is consistent with a solid neoplasm (**Fig. 1**). Except for a highly echogenic lesion in which a diagnosis of angiomyolipoma is suspected (usually confirmed with CT or MRI), these findings usually indicate the need for surgical resection. Similarly, a vascularized mural nodule in an otherwise cystic lesion is highly suspicious for malignancy. Doppler US is also helpful for interrogation of patency of the renal vein and characterization of tumor thrombus, when present, by detecting blood flow within the thrombus.[7]

CT

Contrast-enhanced, multiphasic, multidetector CT (MDCT) is the most commonly used imaging modality in the detection, characterization, and staging of RCC (**Fig. 2**).[1] MDCT assessment of renal mass improves with dynamic imaging during the corticomedullary, nephrographic, and excretory phases. The corticomedullary phase helps to differentiate the RCC subtypes based on tumor vascularity and provides valuable information about the vascular renal anatomy for planning a partial/radical nephrectomy. The nephrographic phase is optimal for detecting enhancement in a renal mass and improves the visualization of small renal masses. The excretory phase allows for delineation of the collecting system and its relationship with the renal mass. New MDCT protocols using dual-phase administration strategies of contrast may provide equivalent information with fewer acquisitions and, hence, decreased radiation to the patient.[8] MDCT is also useful in the demonstration of macroscopic fat within a mass, which allows for the diagnosis of angiomyolipoma,

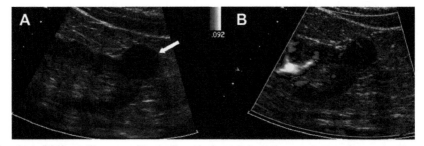

Fig. 1. A 57-year-old man with moderate thrombocytosis, presenting for evaluation of splenic size by US. (A) Sagittal US of the left kidney reveals an incidental hypoechoic, exophytic renal mass (*arrow*). Low-level internal echoes and lack of posterior acoustic enhancement are suggestive of a solid mass. (B) Power Doppler confirms the presence of blood flow within the mass, which is therefore characterized as a solid neoplasm. Partial nephrectomy was performed, and histopathologic analysis revealed grade 2 papillary RCC.

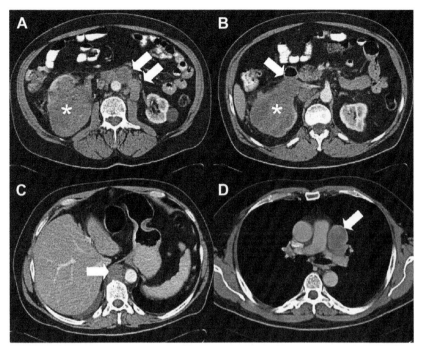

Fig. 2. A 61-year-old man with papillary RCC staged with contrast-enhanced CT. (*A*) Axial image shows a large right renal mass (*asterisk*) replacing most of the right kidney, with enlarged retroperitoneal nodes representing nodal metastases (*arrows*). (*B*) Tumor extends into the right renal vein (*arrow*). Retrocrural (*arrow* in *C*) and mediastinal (*arrow* in *D*) adenopathy are also seen, representing distant nodal metastases.

a benign lesion included in the differential diagnosis of a renal mass.[9] MDCT is also widely used for surveillance following nephrectomy and percutaneous thermal ablation, to evaluate metastatic disease, and to monitor treatment response.

MRI

MRI is a modality suited to renal mass characterization because of its superior soft tissue contrast. Noncontrast T1-weighted and T2-weighted MRI, including chemical shift imaging, permit detection of both bulk fat (as in benign angiomyolipomas) and intravoxel fat (as in clear cell RCC [**Fig. 3**]) or angiomyolipomas with minimal fat.[10,11] Furthermore, the exquisite sensitivity of MRI for small amounts of gadolinium-based contrast agents is particularly suited for the detection of enhancement within a renal lesion (see **Fig. 3**), which can be facilitated with the generation of subtracted images. When paired with high-resolution three-dimensional MRI, the sensitivity to detect solid, nodular enhancing components within a renal cyst is unparalleled; when present, these have excellent positive predictive value for malignancy, correlating with RCC in 95% of such lesions.[12] MRI is also useful in the locoregional staging through the assessment of regional lymph nodes and is superior to CT for the detection of tumor thrombus in the renal vein and inferior vena cava.[13]

Positron Emission Tomography

Positron emission tomography (PET) with ^{18}F-labeled fluoro-2-deoxy-2-glucose (FDG) provides an alternative to contrast-enhanced approaches by showing metabolically

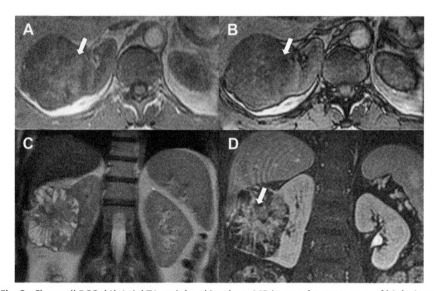

Fig. 3. Clear cell RCC. (*A*) Axial T1-weighted in-phase MR image shows an area of high signal in the right renal mass (*arrow*) that significantly drops in intensity on the axial T1-weighted opposed-phase image (*arrow* in *B*), representing intravoxel fat. Coronal single-shot fast-spin echo T2-weighted image (*C*) shows a heterogeneously hyperintense right renal mass with avid enhancement of the central portion (*arrow* in *D*) on the coronal gadolinium-enhanced three-dimensional (3D) fat-saturated gradient recalled echo (GRE) T1-weighted image. Histopathologic analysis after nephrectomy confirmed clear cell RCC.

active disease, and is helpful for the diagnosis and follow-up of patients with many types of cancer. Although RCC can have intense FDG uptake, uptake is often mild and similar in intensity to adjacent renal parenchyma. Furthermore, excreted radiotracer in the renal collecting system may obscure renal masses. Therefore, a negative study does not exclude malignancy.[14–16] Published studies report a broad range of accuracy rates for primary tumors and staging, likely because of variability in the degree of tumor uptake, likely secondary to differences in primary tumor differentiation,[17] patient populations, and low accuracy in comparison to CT.[18] To date, the role of FDG-PET in the initial detection and diagnosis of RCC is therefore limited. However, FDG-PET seems to show some promise for the detection of distant metastases (**Fig. 4**) and local recurrence, and may be occasionally complementary to other cross-sectional imaging techniques.[18,19] A study by Majhail and colleagues[20] suggested that, despite high specificity, FDG-PET is not a sensitive imaging modality for the evaluation of metastatic RCC and may not adequately characterize small metastatic lesions.

FDG-PET may be useful as a biomarker of metabolic tumor response to therapy, such as with sunitinib therapy in both soft tissue and skeletal lesions. Metabolic response by FDG-PET after 1 cycle of sunitinib therapy was predictive of later response as evaluated by Response Evaluation Criteria in Solid Tumors (RECIST) on CT.[14–16,21–23] Other investigators found that PET response at 16 weeks predicts outcome, which is not the case at 4 weeks.[24] Recent reports have indicated that intense FDG uptake may indicate a worse outcome compared with less intensely FDG-avid RCC lesions,[25] and that FDG-PET may be useful in the postoperative surveillance of advanced RCC.[26]

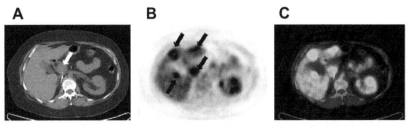

Fig. 4. A 62-year-old woman with history of papillary RCC after radical right nephrectomy. (*A*) Noncontrast CT, (*B*) FDG-PET, and (*C*) fused images show FDG-avid recurrent metastatic disease in the liver and periportal lymph nodes (*arrows*). Lesions are seen best on PET images, with liver lesions difficult to discern on the noncontrast CT.

IMAGING FINDINGS IN DISTINCT HISTOPATHOLOGIC SUBTYPES OF RCC

The World Health Organization classification of RCC includes clear cell, papillary, chromophobe, collecting duct, medullary, and unclassified categories. Imaging and pathologic features vary among the RCC subtypes, and pathologic diagnosis is important because of differences in biologic behavior, response to current therapies, and prognosis.

Clear cell is the most common RCC subtype, accounting for about 70% to 75% of cases, characterized by glycogen-rich and lipid-rich clear cells histologically.[1] Most sporadic clear cell RCCs show inactivating somatic mutations of the von Hippel-Lindau gene.[27] On CT imaging, clear cell RCC is typically hypervascular and heterogeneous because of central necrosis (**Fig. 5**), hemorrhage, and/or foci of calcification.[28] On MRI, typical features of clear cell RCC may include the loss of signal on opposed-phase images caused by intracellular lipid, a rim of tumor surrounding central necrosis and/or hemorrhage, and avid enhancement, particularly in the corticomedullary phase, in contrast with other RCC subtypes.[29,30] A pseudocapsule of low signal intensity on T1-weighted images and T2-weighted images may be present, and disruption of this pseudocapsule is more common in high-grade clear cell neoplasms.[31] Predominantly cystic masses with fluid contents similar in appearance to that of simple cysts on T2-weighted imaging, but with variable amounts of enhancing thick septae and nodularity, correlate with low-grade clear cell histology.[32] Vascular involvement, with extension into the renal vein and inferior vena cava (IVC), may occur and, together with the presence of retroperitoneal collaterals and tumor

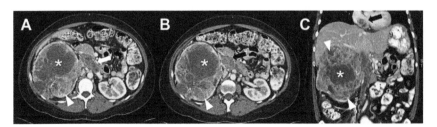

Fig. 5. A 39-year-old woman with back pain and leg swelling. Axial (*A, B*) and coronal (*C*) contrast-enhanced CT images show a large right renal mass with features typical of clear cell RCC, including central necrosis (*asterisk*) and peripheral heterogeneously hyperenhancing tissue (*arrowheads*). Note extensive tumor thrombus extending into the left renal vein (*arrow* in A), inferior vena cava (*arrow* in B), and the right atrium (*arrow* in C). Nephrectomy was performed and histopathology showed clear cell RCC, grade IV.

necrosis, are predictive of high-grade histology in clear cell RCC.[32] Hematogenous metastases primarily involve the lungs, liver, and bones. Lymph node metastases are reported in about one-sixth of cases.[1] In general, clear cell RCC has a poorer prognosis than other histologic subtypes.

Papillary RCC is the second most common histologic subtype, accounting for 10% to 15% of cases, with 2 subtypes described based on histologic appearance and behavior. However, distinction of the 2 papillary subtypes at imaging is usually not possible. On CT imaging, these tumors are often homogeneous and hypoenhancing compared with adjacent renal parenchyma.[11] On MRI, papillary RCC often manifests as a small peripheral mass that is hypointense on T2-weighted images because of intratumoral hemosiderin.[33,34] Papillary RCC frequently undergoes internal hemorrhage leading to another characteristic appearance on MRI: cystic mass with hyperintense fluid content on T1-weighted images and enhancing papillary projections arising from the wall of the cyst.[35] Dynamic contrast-enhanced MRI shows low-level, progressive enhancement (**Fig. 6**), which allows for accurate differentiation from the characteristically hypervascular clear cell carcinomas.[29,30] Metastasis from papillary RCC shows similar features and tends to be hypovascular. Compared with clear cell RCC, tumor extension into the renal vein and IVC is less common; visceral metastasis is less frequent, with lung most common; and nodal involvement is more prevalent.[2]

Chromophobe RCC accounts for 5% of RCC.[1] Birt-Hogg-Dube syndrome is associated with chromophobe RCC and oncocytomas.[1] On CT imaging, these tumors tend to be large and homogeneous.[36] Chromophobe RCCs typically lack hemorrhage and necrosis pathologically[37] and this reflects in their imaging appearance; these tumors, unlike clear cell RCC, can grow to a large size without undergoing central necrosis. Perinephric extension and renal vein involvement occurs infrequently. On MRI, chromophobe RCCs may be heterogeneous in appearance, similar to clear cell tumors, but enhancement tends to be more moderate, between that of clear cell and papillary subtypes.[30] Recently, a characteristic segmental enhancement inversion in contrast-enhanced MDCT and MRI has been described both for oncocytomas and chromophobe RCC, but is not present in other RCC subtypes or angiomyolipoma.[38,39] This

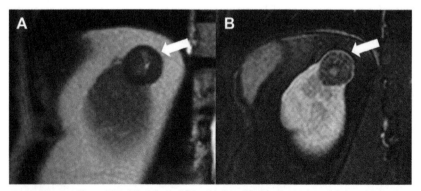

Fig. 6. MRI in papillary RCC. (*A*) Coronal T2-weighted half-Fourier single-shot fast-spin echo image shows an exophytic right upper pole renal mass (*arrow*) that is predominantly hypointense relative to adjacent renal cortex with mild central hyperintensity representing a small focus of central necrosis. (*B*) Coronal gadolinium-enhanced T1-weighted 3D fat-saturated spoiled gradient echo image shows predominant hypoenhancement of the mass relative to the renal cortex, with a small focus of centrally increased signal. Magnetic resonance features are typical of papillary RCC, confirmed pathologically.

enhancement pattern is characterized by increased enhancement in a segment within the mass during the corticomedullary phase that becomes less enhanced during the later phases, whereas a less-enhanced segment during the corticomedullary phase becomes hyperenhanced during the excretory phase. Patients with chromophobe RCC have a greater propensity for liver metastases compared with other subtypes.[40]

Other uncommon types of RCC include collecting duct (Bellini) tumors, medullary RCC, multilocular cystic RCC, and unclassified types.[29,36] Collecting duct tumors are central and infiltrative, and are associated with a poor prognosis. Medullary RCC are indistinguishable from collecting duct tumors but occur characteristically in young patients with sickle cell trait.[36] Multilocular cystic RCC are predominately cystic masses with multiple septae and carry excellent prognosis. By definition, these neoplasms do not contain solid elements within the cyst, although mildly thickened, irregular septations are commonly seen.[35] It is challenging to differentiate these from benign complex cysts and/or multilocular cystic nephroma by imaging. Enhancing mural or septal nodules are a feature of the more common cystic subtype of clear cell RCC. Typical imaging features of unclassified types have not yet been described.

Overall, there are limited data about the ability to predict the histologic diagnosis based on imaging findings. In a retrospective study, Sheir and colleagues[41] found different levels of enhancement on contrast-enhanced CT examinations, with the highest accuracy for the diagnosis of clear cell subtype when using a cutoff value in attenuation of 83.5 Hounsfield units (HU) on images acquired during the corticomedullary phase and 64.5 HU for images acquired during the excretory phase, respectively. In another retrospective analysis of 198 renal masses evaluated by CT, including some benign lesions, Zhang and colleagues[28] found that clear cell RCC was characterized by a mixed enhancement pattern with areas of hyperenhancement and low attenuation, whereas other types of RCC were characterized by homogeneous or peripheral enhancement. A classification based on the appearance of malignant tumors on MRI, or MRI phenotype, was proposed by Pedrosa and colleagues.[32] The reported sensitivity and specificity for the diagnosis of clear cell subtype using this classification were of 93% and 75%, respectively. Similarly, the sensitivity and specificity for the diagnosis of papillary subtype were 80% and 94%, respectively. Sun and colleagues[30] found excellent diagnostic accuracy to differentiate clear cell from papillary histology on dynamic contrast-enhanced MRI, with a reported sensitivity and specificity of 93% and 96% respectively, when using a cutoff of 84% change in signal intensity during the corticomedullary phase compared with precontrast images.

Hereditary RCC and Other Associations

Hereditary RCC syndromes refer to multisystem syndromes with an increased predisposition to multiple tumors, including RCCs.[1] Ten hereditary RCC syndromes have been described, all with autosomal dominant inheritance of increased cancer susceptibility. The most commonly known syndromes include von Hippel-Lindau disease, hereditary papillary RCC, and tuberous sclerosis. A syndrome may be suspected when there is a family or individual history of renal tumors, bilateral or multiple tumors, or early onset.[42] MRI surveillance and follow-up may be favored in these patients, to avoid the cumulative radiation associated with multiple CT examinations in a young patient, although specific follow-up schedules have not been established. Detailed delineation of the anatomy and tumor extent is crucial in these patients to facilitate nephron-sparing surgical resections because they frequently require repeated surgical procedures during their life span.

STAGING, MANAGEMENT, AND SURVEILLANCE

Because surgery plays a central role in the management of RCC and many cancers in general, it is logical that staging systems have incorporated detailed categorization of locoregional disease extent to facilitate resection. In the 1960s, the Robson classification was developed to stage renal cell cancers, a widely used system with a focus on the degree of primary tumor spread into adjacent tissues, in which stage I tumors were confined to the renal capsule; stage II tumors extended to the perirenal fat or ipsilateral adrenal gland; stage III tumors had vascular (A) or nodal (B) extension, or both (C); and stage IV indicated distant disease.[43] The Robson classification has been replaced by tumor, node, metastasis (TNM) staging, commonly used in cancer staging today worldwide. The obvious advantage of the TNM system maintained by the International Union Against Cancer is the widespread, standardized application of this system allowing disease study and continual refinement and evolution of the staging system in response to new developments.[44] From a practical point of view, the TNM classification provides important prognostic information about the likelihood of disease progression.

In the seventh edition[45] (2010) of the TNM classification (**Table 1**), the T staging indicating the size of the primary tumor was defined as follows: T1 to 2 disease is organ confined (T1a$\leq$4 cm, T1b 4–7 cm, T2a 7–10 cm, T2b>10 cm). Stage T3a indicates extension to the perinephric tissue, renal sinus, or renal vein, whereas T3b tumors extend to the infradiaphragmatic IVC and T3c tumors extend to the supradiaphragmatic IVC or into the vessel wall at any level. T4 disease indicates extension beyond Gerota fascia or directly into the ipsilateral adrenal gland. N1 indicates disease in regional lymph node(s) (eg, adjacent to the renal vasculature, para-aortic for left-sided masses or paracaval for right-sided masses). M1 disease represents distant disease and includes nonregional lymph nodes. Recent updates in the seventh edition include the division of T2a and T2b disease, incorporating renal vein and perinephric involvement into T3a, and advancing adrenal involvement to T4 disease. A recent validation study of the seventh edition indicates opportunities for further improvements in TNM staging, with overlap in prognosis associated with some stages and heterogeneous outcomes in others.[46]

CT and MRI offer noninvasive preoperative staging and surgical planning in patients with renal masses suspicious for RCC. The role of preoperative imaging is to identify tumor features that render a patient amenable to a particular treatment approach and to assess for distant disease (**Fig. 7**). Small renal masses may be managed with nephron-sparing partial nephrectomy, thermal ablation, or, in some cases, active surveillance. Therefore, important components of the radiologic report include the size and position of the renal mass within the kidney, specifically whether it is largely exophytic or if it extends into the renal sinus, for appropriate surgical planning.[47] Evidence and extent of renal vein/IVC involvement must be described. The presence and location of suspicious adenopathy should also be detailed.

Some small renal tumors (particularly those <4 cm) are also amenable to alternative, minimally invasive, thermal ablative therapies, specifically cryoablation and radiofrequency ablation (RFA). Cryoablation involves tissue freezing to temperatures to −20 to −50°C with visible ice ball formation,[48] whereas RFA involves tissue heating to temperatures greater than 50°C with coagulation necrosis.[49] These ablation strategies can be applied via open, laparoscopic, or percutaneous approaches, although small exophytic masses that spare the renal hilum, located away from the main renal vasculature and ureter, are best suited to the percutaneous technique. Percutaneous ablations are performed using US, CT, or magnetic resonance (MR) guidance (**Fig. 8**).

Table 1
TNM of RCC

	Definitions of TNM
Primary tumor	
TX	Primary tumor cannot be assessed
T0	No evidence of primary tumor
T1	Tumor ≤7 cm in greatest dimension; limited to the kidney
T1a	Tumor ≤4 cm in greatest dimension; limited to the kidney
T1b	Tumor >4 cm but ≤7 cm in greatest dimension; limited to the kidney
T2	Tumor >7 cm in greatest dimension; limited to the kidney
T2a	Tumor >7 cm but ≤10 cm in greatest dimension; limited to the kidney
T2b	Tumor >10 cm; limited to the kidney
T3	Tumor extends into major veins or perinephric tissues but not into the ipsilateral adrenal gland and not beyond Gerota fascia
T3a	Tumor grossly extends into the renal vein or its segmental (muscle-containing) branches, or tumor invades perirenal and/or renal sinus fat but not beyond Gerota fascia
T3b	Tumor grossly extends into the vena cava below the diaphragm
T3c	Tumor grossly extends into the vena cava above the diaphragm or invades the wall of the vena cava
T4	Tumor invades beyond Gerota fascia (including contiguous extension into the ipsilateral adrenal gland)
Regional lymph nodes	
NX	Regional lymph nodes cannot be assessed
N0	No regional lymph node metastasis
N1	Metastasis in regional lymph node(s)
Distant metastasis	
M0	No distant metastasis
M1	Distant metastasis

From The American Joint Committee on Cancer (AJCC). Cancer staging handbook. 7th edition. Chicago (IL): Springer Science and Business Media LLC www.springerlink.com; 2010. p. 553; with permission.

Some advantages of percutaneous ablations include the least invasive approach, tamponade effect of Gerota fascia, and, for cryoablation specifically, direct visualization of the entire ice ball via CT or MRI, consistent pattern of tissue ablation, and associated decreased risk of injury to the urinary tract or other adjacent tissues.[50] In a meta-analysis of percutaneous and surgical approaches to ablation, major complications were decreased in percutaneously treated patients, with equally effective treatment in the groups.[51] However, more than 1 treatment is sometimes needed for effective treatment in percutaneously treated patients with residual viable tumor after an initial ablation. Imaging features of successful ablation and long-term efficacy remain undefined, although tumor shrinkage with time and absence of internal enhancement have been associated with effective ablation.[52–54] However, long-term imaging follow-up is necessary to monitor potential recurrent disease.

As percutaneous thermal RCC ablation becomes increasingly common, the role of percutaneous biopsy of small renal masses continues to evolve. When percutaneous ablation techniques are applied, small renal masses are typically biopsied before

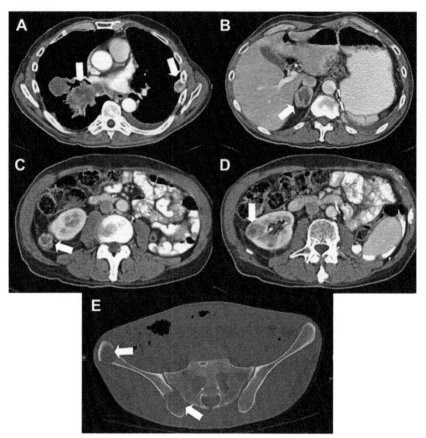

Fig. 7. CT of typical sites of RCC metastasis (*arrows*) includes (*A*) lung and pleura, (*B*) adrenal gland, (*C*) retroperitoneum, (*D*) kidney, and (*E*) bone.

ablation to ascertain the pathologic diagnosis,[53,55] because benign masses and other masses such as lymphoma do not merit ablation. In patients with a history of another malignancy or synchronous nonrenal primary malignancy, percutaneous biopsy may affirm or exclude the diagnosis of RCC. Because the imaging features of benign and malignant masses overlap, biopsy can be informative but should be used when its results have the potential to change the patient's management. However, percutaneous biopsies can be inconclusive in up to 3% to 20% of cases,[56] and sampling error is a consideration, particularly in predominantly cystic and necrotic lesions. For these reasons, the role of biopsy in renal masses is still controversial.[47]

Patients who undergo surgical resection or ablation of their primary RCC are monitored for the development of recurrent or metastatic disease by serial imaging. At the authors' institutions, patients receiving percutaneous ablation are frequently monitored with MRI, whereas those undergoing surgery are followed by either CT or MRI. The most frequent surveillance occurs in the first 3 years following nephrectomy, in which 85% of metastases have been reported to occur.[40] Patients may be imaged every 6 months for 3 years following nephrectomy and then yearly, although this may vary among different institutions. When CT is used, the chest is typically imaged during the arterial phase after contrast administration to facilitate detection of mediastinal

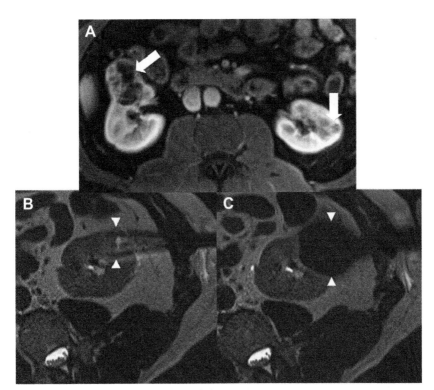

Fig. 8. A 52-year-old man with bilateral RCC. Axial gadolinium-enhanced 3D fat-saturated GRE T1-weighted image (*A*) shows bilateral enhancing renal masses (compared with precontrast images, not shown), larger on the right (*white arrows*). The patient underwent a partial nephrectomy for the right mass, which was confirmed as clear cell RCC at histopathology, and elected MRI-guided percutaneous cryoablation for the small left renal tumor. Axial single-shot fast-spin echo T2-weighted images (*B, C*) during the procedure performed in a wide-bore 3 Tesla MRI, with the patient in the right posterior oblique position, show cryoablation applicator placement (*arrowheads* in *B*) around the hyperintense tumor and the hypointense ice ball (*arrowheads* in *C*) encompassing the tumor during treatment. (*Courtesy of* Kemal Tuncali, MD.)

lymphadenopathy, whereas the abdomen and pelvis are imaged during the portal venous phase. Detection of liver metastasis is improved if the images of the liver are acquired in the arterial and portal venous phases. With the development and metastatic disease and initiation of systemic therapy, timing of CT follow-up is dictated by the particular drug regimen.[40]

METASTATIC DISEASE AND ASSESSING RESPONSE TO THERAPY

Between 20% and 30% of patients with RCC show metastatic disease at the time of diagnosis (**Fig. 9**),[1] and up to 25% to 50% diagnosed with locoregional disease eventually develop metastases.[57,58] Thus, systemic therapy is indicated in a significant proportion of patients. However, metastatic RCC (mRCC) is notoriously insensitive to cytotoxic chemotherapies. Before 2005, interleukin-2 and interferon-α were standard therapies for metastatic RCC, with few patients benefiting from treatment.[59]

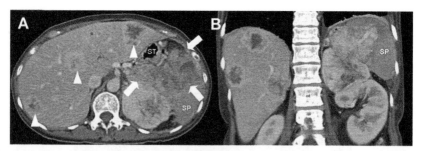

Fig. 9. A 55-year-old woman with metastatic RCC at presentation. Axial image (*A*) and coronal reconstruction (*B*) of a contrast-enhanced CT examination show a large, heterogeneous, infiltrating enhancing mass of the left kidney (*arrows*) with several liver metastases (*arrowheads*). Note the close proximity and possible invasion of the stomach (ST) and spleen (SP). Gastric wall biopsy confirmed the diagnosis. The patient was not considered a good candidate for antiangiogenic therapies given bowel involvement.

Since that time, targeted therapies have revolutionized the care of such patients, offering a significant clinical benefit.[60–63]

As surgical indications in metastatic RCC continue to evolve, imaging studies become more crucial in the detection of metastatic disease. The survival benefit of cytoreductive nephrectomy in the setting of metastatic disease was established in the era of interferon therapy in patients well enough to undergo surgery before systemic treatment,[64,65] and it is still commonly used in patients with stage IV disease in whom most of the tumor burden is at the site of the primary tumor.[66] Therefore, detailed description of the primary mass and renal vasculature remains relevant in this setting. Surgery is also a consideration in selected patients with oligometastatic disease who have already undergone nephrectomy (**Fig. 10**), because, in selected cases, complete removal of metastases has been associated with improved survival.[67]

At present, therapies targeted to vascular endothelial growth factor (VEGF) have become a standard treatment of patients with metastatic RCC. Because these therapies induce tumor necrosis[68] with sometimes little tumor shrinkage, the RECIST 1.0 criteria and its recent modification (RECIST version 1.1), based on changes in CT tumor size, may not serve as best indicators of response to therapy in this setting.[69,70] Many patients who benefit from targeted therapies do not achieve the 30% decrease in the sum long axis diameter (SLD) of target lesions to be considered as having a partial response by RECIST (**Fig. 11**[71]), and the few patients who achieve this response category do so in the course of several cycles of therapy. This situation results in prolonged uncertainty for patients with stable disease, who have been shown to have as much chance of improved progression-free survival (PFS) as not.[72] Several groups have examined a variety of size and density parameters on CT to best delineate responders and nonresponders earlier in the treatment course. The definition and validation of early posttherapy imaging changes (EPTIC) is desirable to identify patients likely to achieve a prolonged benefit after initiation of therapy, to minimize toxicities to patients not achieving a benefit, and to permit these patients to be considered for an alternate therapy.

Various size changes in metastatic target lesions have been investigated in patients on VEGF-targeted therapies to determine indicators of treatment benefit. Such size variation thresholds were systematically assessed in a large cohort of patients with mRCC treated with sunitinib.[72] In this study, the investigators evaluated a range of

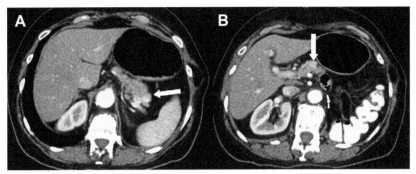

Fig. 10. A 57-year-old woman with recurrent clear cell RCC. Axial contrast-enhanced CT images of the upper abdomen acquired during the arterial phase (*A, B*) show subtle new hypervascular nodules (*arrows*) in the pancreas. The patient underwent distal pancreatectomy and splenectomy, which confirmed the presence of pancreatic metastases. The patient had no evidence of metastatic disease elsewhere.

size change thresholds from −45% to +10% change in the SLD of target lesions and found that the −10% (ie, decrease in SLD of 10% compared with baseline) threshold best differentiated responders and nonresponders on this therapy; responders experienced longer median PFS (11.1 months) than nonresponders (5.6 months). Furthermore, 73% of responders achieved the −10% threshold after the first cycle of treatment, and 93% reached it in 2 cycles, permitting early posttherapy imaging assessment in this particular setting.

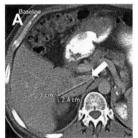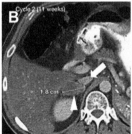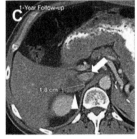

Fig. 11. Stable disease and inherent challenges in tumor measurement by RECIST guidelines. In this figure entitled "Example of partial response according to RECIST guidelines in a patient treated with sunitinib," the original measurement of 3 cm retrocaval adenopathy at baseline (*A*) includes the inferior vena cava (IVC; *arrows* in A–C). A repeated measurement of the mass performed by the investigators and excluding the IVC (*black line*) results in a 2.4-cm-long axis at baseline. After initiation of therapy, the lesion measures 1.8 cm at cycle 2 (*B*) and 1.8 cm at 1-year follow-up (*C*). Although this decrease in size was interpreted as partial response, it represents a 25% decrease in the long axis measurement or stable disease according to RECIST criteria if the measurement excluding the IVC were used. However, there is obvious interval decrease in attenuation within the metastatic adenopathy after treatment, suggestive of treatment-induced necrosis (*white arrowheads* in B and C). The Choi criteria would indicate partial response in this case, which illustrates the challenges in assessing response by RECIST. (*From* Motzer RJ, Rini BI, Bukowski RM, et al. Sunitinib in patients with metastatic renal cell carcinoma. JAMA 2006;295(21):2516–24. © 2006 American Medical Association. All rights reserved; with permission.)

The 10% decrease in SLD is 1 component of the Choi criteria (ie, 10% decrease in size or 15% decrease in target lesion density compared with baseline), originally developed for patients with gastrointestinal stromal tumors undergoing therapy with imatinib.[73,74] Recently, van der Veldt and colleagues[75] applied the Choi criteria to 55 patients with mRCC treated with sunitinib, with the Choi criteria better predicting PFS and overall survival (OS) than the RECIST criteria at the time of the first imaging follow-up. The Choi criteria may be applicable to other antiangiogenic therapies (**Fig. 12**). The investigators concluded that these combined size and density criteria define patients with treatment benefit but that the criteria would not change management, because the Choi criteria did not allow the identification of patients with early disease progression.[75]

Other groups have sought to incorporate size and density changes in target lesions in response to VEGF-targeted therapies to best characterize patients with treatment benefit early in the course of therapy. The size and attenuation CT (SACT) criteria and the subsequent, refined morphology, attenuation, size, and structure (MASS) criteria were developed to describe size and density changes in patients with mRCC responding to first-line sorafenib or sunitinib therapy.[76,77] These criteria combine a host of radiologic assessments to define patients with PFS greater than 250 days, an arbitrarily selected time point. These criteria incorporate 20% decrease in tumor size into a favorable response criterion associated with PFS greater than 250 days; several other criteria indicate indeterminate or unfavorable responses. The complexity of the criteria and measurements are limitations to routine clinical use. The combination of reduction in tumor size and arterial phase density has been correlated to time to progression in a retrospective study of a small cohort of 20 evaluable patients. The usefulness of these diagnostic criteria needs further investigation.[78]

Our group has evaluated EPTIC with different approaches including RECIST, Choi, tumor shrinkage, and changes in CT tumor density in a retrospective analysis of 70 patients with mRCC treated with VEGF-targeted therapies.[79] At the first CT follow-up

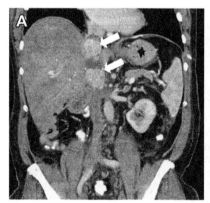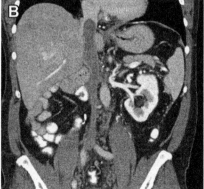

Fig. 12. A 55-year-old man with prior right nephrectomy for clear cell RCC and recurrent RCC limited to the IVC. Coronal reconstruction (*A*) of contrast-enhanced CT obtained at baseline shows enhancing tumor thrombus in the IVC (*arrows*). Coronal reconstruction (*B*) of contrast-enhanced CT obtained 6 weeks after initiation of pazopanib therapy shows markedly decreased density of the tumor thrombus, which indicates an antiangiogenic effect, without a definitive evidence of change in size. This case illustrates the limitations of RECIST criteria for assessing response to therapy, whereas changes in density in this case would be characterized as partial response when using the Choi criteria.

after initiation of therapy, only a 10% decrease in SLD of target lesions was statistically significant in predicting time to treatment failure and OS, whereas responses by RECIST, Choi, and other thresholds were not predictive. The findings merit further, prospective investigation.

Pretreatment tumor enhancement, an estimate of tumor vascularity, was recently evaluated as an imaging predictor of outcome in the targeted therapy setting. In a retrospective study of 46 patients treated with sunitinib or sorafenib, pretreatment enhancement in individual metastatic lesions was associated with RECIST response and time to progression in the individual lesions.[80] Specifically, lesions with greater than 125 HU on pretherapy early arterial phase images had nearly a complete response, and lesions with the least enhancement (<30 HU) rapidly progressed, with variable responses in the individual metastases in more than half of the patients. Although patients are generally evaluated for response to therapy on a more global, whole-body scale, these data provide insight into the patients and lesions best suited to the VEGF-targeted therapies and may permit development of lesion-specific treatment strategies.

Mammalian target of rapamycin (mTOR) inhibitors such as everolimus and temsirolimus are agents that are approved by the US Food and Drug Administration and commonly used in second-line therapy for patients with metastatic RCC, offering prolonged PFS and OS, respectively.[81,82] Temsirolimus can be administered as a first-line therapy in poor-risk patients. These therapies inhibit the mTOR serine-threonine kinase, involved in cell metabolism, growth, proliferation, and angiogenesis. Most patients treated with everolimus achieve stable disease status by RECIST, with only 1.8% achieving partial response,[81] providing another opportunity to assess early imaging markers of response to therapy in this setting. For mTOR-directed therapy, decreased tumor glucose uptake, as shown by FDG-PET imaging, is a clear pharmacodynamic marker,[83,84] but may not be predictive. The preclinical suggestion that baseline FDG-PET uptake is predictive of benefit from mTOR-directed therapy is being evaluated in a prospective trial (clinicaltrials.gov NCT00529802). In addition, patients may develop radiographic evidence of mTOR inhibitor–related pneumonitis manifesting as ground glass and/or patchy consolidation in the lungs during the course of therapy (**Fig. 13**).[85]

FUTURE DIRECTIONS

In recent years, technical improvements have allowed for a paradigm shift in oncologic imaging from the traditional morphologic evaluation of tumors (ie, measurements of tumor size and extent) toward a physiologic or functional assessment of tumors, including evaluation of tumor perfusion, oxygenation, and diffusion characteristics.[86–90] Several of these functional imaging techniques are being applied to provide noninvasive characterization of RCC biology, aggressiveness, and responsiveness to therapy, including dynamic contrast-enhanced (DCE) imaging, arterial spin labeling (ASL), and novel PET tracers. DCE protocols have been used in combination with US, CT, and MRI to evaluate tumor vascularity and response to antiangiogenic therapy in a variety of primary tumor types, including RCC.[16] Each of these approaches, with their inherent advantages and limitations, are discussed.

DCE Techniques

DCE-US is a diagnostic imaging tool primarily used in Europe and Asia that is now being applied to early response evaluation in patients with mRCC treated with antiangiogenic agents.[91] A small bolus of microbubbles is injected intravenously and

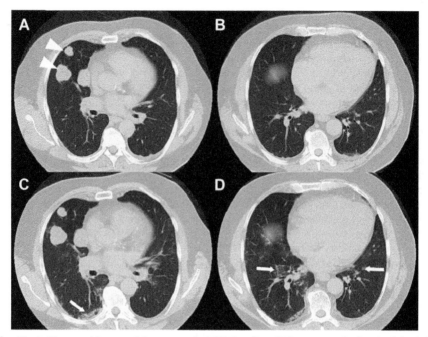

Fig. 13. A 67-year-old man with metastatic RCC. Baseline CT images at the level of the hila (*A*) and base of the lungs (*B*) show 2 large pulmonary metastases (*arrowheads* in *A*) and otherwise clear lungs. (*C, D*) Follow-up CT images obtained 2 months after initiation of everolimus therapy show stable metastatic disease but development of new ground glass densities in both lower lobes (*arrows*). The patient was afebrile and complained of shortness of breath. The drug was eventually held for proteinuria and symptomatic pneumonitis, toxicities attributed to therapy.

remains in the intravascular compartment, with continuous imaging of the target lesion with US during a 3-minute raw data collection period. This process yields a quantitative time-intensity curve, from which a host of vascular parameters in an individual lesion can be calculated. Advantages include the low relative cost compared with other functional techniques, lack of radiation exposure, usefulness of the contrast agent in patients with renal dysfunction (ie, microbubbles are eliminated through the lung), and in those with allergy to other types of contrast. However, brain and lung metastases are not amenable to evaluation because US waves do not adequately penetrate bone and gas. Furthermore, microbubble-based US contrast agents have not yet been approved by the US Food and Drug Administration for this application, limiting its use within the United States.

Recently, perfusion changes in RCC metastases on DCE-US were correlated to response to antiangiogenic treatment (**Fig. 14**). In 30 patients with mRCC randomized to sorafenib or placebo, good responders were identified at 3 weeks after initiation of therapy as having greater than 10% decrease in contrast uptake and stability or decrease in tumor volume compared with baseline, whereas poor responders showed persistent tumor vascularity at the same time point.[92] In this cohort, there was a statistically significant difference in PFS and OS in the good versus poor responders. In a phase I trial of sorafenib in combination with interferon-α-2a in the treatment of 13 patients with unresectable or metastatic RCC or melanoma, good responders with

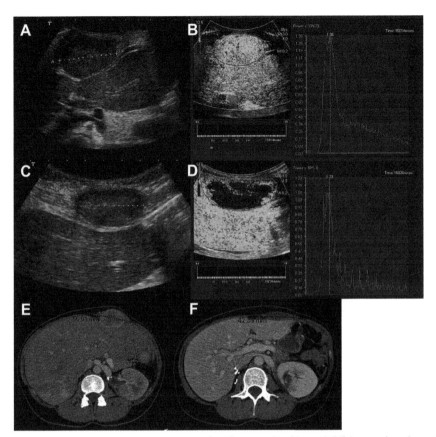

Fig. 14. Patient with metastatic RCC treated with a tyrosine kinase inhibitor and evaluated by DCE-US. Baseline gray-scale US (*A*) and DCE-US image with time-intensity curve (*B*) shows a vascular metastasis along the hepatic capsule of the left lobe. Note the rapid rise of the time-intensity curve, indicating intense vascularity in the mass. Follow-up gray-scale (*C*) and DCE-US images with time-intensity curve (*D*) obtained 7 days after initiation of therapy show no substantial difference in peak enhancement, although the mean enhancement in the entire lesion is dramatically decreased (indicated by decreased area under the curve), likely secondary to therapy-induced central necrosis. Note the central devascularized area of necrosis, which is only evident after administration of contrast (*D*) and imperceptible on the gray-scale images (*C*). Contrast-enhanced axial CT images obtained at baseline (*E*) and 3 months after treatment (*F*) show significant decrease in the size and density of the metastasis, representing response to therapy. (*Courtesy of* Nathalie Lassau, MD, PhD.)

prolonged PFS/OS were differentiated from poor responders by DCE-US, with good response indicated by greater than or equal to 20% decrease in contrast uptake with stability/decrease in tumor volume, or greater than or equal to 30% decrease in volume without change in uptake.[93] In another trial of 38 patients with mRCC, DCE-US parameters at day 15 of sunitinib treatment correlated with RECIST response after 2 cycles of therapy, PFS and OS.[94] In these examples, DCE-US was predictive of response earlier in the course of therapy than traditional assessment by RECIST after at least 1 cycle of therapy.

Dynamic contrast-enhanced CT (DCE-CT) has been recently applied to patients with mRCC treated with antiangiogenic therapies. DCE-CT is performed in a localized region of interest before, during, and after administration of a bolus of iodinated contrast material. Several perfusion variables including tumor blood flow (TBF), tumor blood volume (TBV), and mean transit time (MTT) can be extrapolated from the raw data using different available software packages.[95] Because iodinated contrast agents diffuse variably between the intravascular and extravascular space depending on the vascular permeability in the tumor bed, these quantitative assessments of tumor vascularity are derived from a series of assumptions regarding compartmental tracer kinetics.[96] In one study performed in patients with mRCC treated with sunitinib or sorafenib, DCE-CT showed a significant decrease in TBF and TBV after the first cycle of therapy. Baseline perfusion parameters were higher in those with partial response by RECIST; however, there was no significant correlation between baseline perfusion or changes in perfusion after therapy and PFS or OS.[97]

Dynamic contrast-enhanced MRI (DCE-MRI) has also been examined in patients with mRCC. In this technique, diffusion of contrast media from the intravascular space into the extracellular space permits quantitative assessment of the tumor microvasculature. Similar to DCE-CT, quantitative measurements of tumor perfusion in DCE-MRI techniques using extravascular contrast agents are based on assumptions regarding compartmental tracer kinetics. A series of T1-weighted MR images are acquired before, during, and for several minutes following the administration of a bolus of gadolinium-based contrast media. Several values are then determined based on these data points, including intratumoral vascular fraction, TBF, vascular permeability-surface area product and accessible extravascular-extracellular space.[95,98] These calculations are dependent both on the MRI acquisition protocol and the compartment model used to analyze the data, which are not standardized, limiting broad application and reproducibility. Furthermore, the relative contribution of vessel leakiness (ie, permeability) and TBF to the overall signal intensity changes observed on DCE-MRI studies is frequently unknown, making the calculation of tumor perfusion challenging and possibly erroneous. Recent reports in animal studies have illustrated a potential advantage of using gadolinium-based intravascular contrast agents, which do not diffuse into the extravascular space because of their large size, for evaluation of tumor vascularity with DCE-MRI.[99,100]

In DCE-MRI, the transfer constant (K^{trans}) between the intravascular and extravascular space is a commonly cited measure of interest. A change of more than 40% in K^{trans} from baseline to follow-up has been proposed as consistent with a drug effect in pharmacodynamic studies.[16,101] Two reports evaluating K^{trans} in sorafenib-treated patients with mRCC have offered divergent conclusions. In 15 patients treated with sorafenib in a phase II study, K^{trans} decreased significantly during treatment (60.3%) and both K^{trans} at baseline and the decrease in K^{trans} after therapy were significantly associated with PFS.[102] However, these patients had higher response rates and time to progression than the overall phase II population. In another report, changes in K^{trans} and the area under the contrast concentration versus time curve 90 seconds after contrast injection ($IAUC_{90}$) in patients with mRCC correlated with the administered dose of sorafenib, indicating its usefulness as a pharmacodynamic biomarker, although these 2 variables did not correlate with PFS and, therefore, were not considered predictive biomarkers. However, the investigators indicated a potential association between high baseline K^{trans} and a prolonged time to progression or death, which requires further investigation.[103]

Each of the dynamic techniques is limited by the necessity of intravenous contrast administration with high spatial and temporal resolution imaging of single metastases performed per single contrast bolus administration. Because marked heterogeneity can exist within and between individual metastases in any single patient, observations and measurements referable to a single metastasis may not apply to the patient as a whole. In addition, imaging protocols and parameters must be standardized in equipment from various vendors and across institutions, and reproducibility must be assessed.

Other MRI Techniques

ASL is an MRI technique that provides blood flow quantification within tissue without the use of intravenous contrast material. Water protons in flowing arterial blood are labeled using alterations in the magnetic field. When these protons flow into a target lesion, the signal intensity in the mass is altered and the difference in signal intensity within the target lesion between 2 similar images acquired with and without the labeling represents blood flow (**Fig. 15**). Advantages of ASL imaging include the ability to obtain repeated measurements without exogenous contrast material or radiation, and, compared with contrast-enhanced techniques using extravascular contrast agents, there is no ambiguity regarding the contribution of permeability to signal intensity; blood flow is directly proportional to signal intensity on ASL. The limited availability of the ASL techniques and preferable application to high-flow tumors are limitations for its widespread use.

ASL was recently evaluated in 10 patients with mRCC treated with PTK787 (vatalanib), where ASL blood flow changes at 1 month correlated with time to progression and size changes at 4 months.[104] ASL has also been evaluated in animal tumor models of RCC, where minimal blood flow at baseline in sorafenib-resistant Caki-1 xenografts

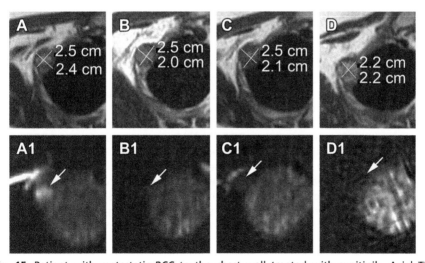

Fig. 15. Patient with metastatic RCC to the chest wall treated with sunitinib. Axial T2-weighted half-Fourier single-shot fast-spin echo (*top*) and arterial spin-labeled perfusion (*bottom*) images obtained at baseline (*A, A1*), 2 weeks (*B, B1*), after cycle 2 (*C, C1*), and after cycle 4 (*D, D1*). At baseline, intense tumor vascularity is indicated by hyperintense signal in the ASL image (*arrow* in *A1*). On subsequent follow-up MRI, the target lesion is stable in size (bidirectional measurements in *A–D*). However, absence of signal in ASL images suggests decreased tumor vascularity (*arrows* in *B1–D1*) likely caused by maintained antiangiogenic effect. Note the background signal intensity in the lung reflecting pulmonary arterial perfusion, which serves as internal control for assessing tumor perfusion on ASL images.

correlated with poor response to sorafenib therapy.[105] In addition, high signal on ASL highlighted the viable portions of tumor at histopathology and necrotic areas showed low signal intensity on ASL. Furthermore, a decrease in ASL signal intensity within viable areas of tumor after initiation of therapy correlated with decreased microvascular density (CD34 stains).[105] These data support the use of ASL as a method for monitoring tumor angiogenesis in RCC.

Diffusion-weighted imaging (DWI) is an MRI technique garnering interest largely in the assessment and characterization of primary tumors. It is an imaging technique in which diffusion of water molecules is restricted in highly cellular areas (tumor) in contrast with less cellular (nontumor) tissues or the extracellular space. Water diffusion and the apparent diffusion coefficient (ADC) can be determined using the DWI data, which allow for quantitative characterization of tumors. Recently, high-grade clear cell RCCs have been found to show higher levels of restricted diffusion/lower ADC, in contrast with lower grade clear cell tumors, which show less restricted water diffusion.[106] However, to the best of our knowledge, changes in water diffusion/ADC that may indicate response to therapy in RCC have not yet been defined (**Fig. 16**).

Other MRI techniques have been used in the assessment of mRCC but are not widely used. For example, in a study using magnetic resonance spectroscopy (MRS) in mRCC, a significantly lower ratio of signal was found at a 5.4-ppm frequency shift compared with that at 1.3 ppm in metastatic RCC compared with that in healthy tissue.[107] The latter may be correlated with the lipid content in the voxel. The usefulness of this finding as a marker for renal malignancy and therapy monitoring has not yet been evaluated.

Future PET Applications

Besides FDG, the most common PET radiotracer used in clinical practice today, several other PET radiotracers have been developed, including ^{11}C-labeled acetate (^{11}C-acetate), ^{18}F-labeled fluorothymidine (^{18}F-FLT), ^{18}F-labeled fluoromisonidazole (^{18}F-MISO), and ^{15}O-labeled water.

[11]C-acetate uptake is related to the cell membrane phospholipid metabolism, which is increased in malignant cells with increased cellular growth. ^{18}F-FLT uptake may reflect cellular proliferation and ^{18}F-MISO can be used to image tumor hypoxia. ^{15}O-labeled water permits quantification of tumor perfusion and may be used to monitor response to antiangiogenic medications. There are several studies that have reported ^{11}C-acetate uptake in RCC.[108–110] Overall, the value of these PET radiotracers for the evaluation and management of patients with RCC is still a topic of research. Ultimately, it is hoped that these radiotracers will have a higher sensitivity and specificity for primary RCC compared with FDG, helping to characterize the tumor by imaging key molecules and molecular processes, assess response to therapy including molecular-targeted therapy, and affect patient management. Although there are promising preliminary results, more data are needed to bring these radiotracers into clinical practice.

Targeted therapeutic agents such as bevacizumab can be radiolabeled to evaluate tumor uptake, perform kinetic modeling of uptake, and predict tumor response.[111–114] Research is also underway to develop monoclonal antibodies labeled with PET radiotracers (immuno-PET) to target RCC antigens for imaging (radioimmunoscintigraphy) and therapy (radioimmunotherapy). An example of a monoclonal antibody being investigated for use in patients with RCC is the radioiodinated antibody G250 and its chimeric form cG250. This monoclonal antibody binds to the antigen carbonic anhydrase IX (CAIX), a transmembrane glycoprotein expressed in clear cell RCC. CAIX is synthesized following the loss of the tumor suppressor gene VHL, and is typically

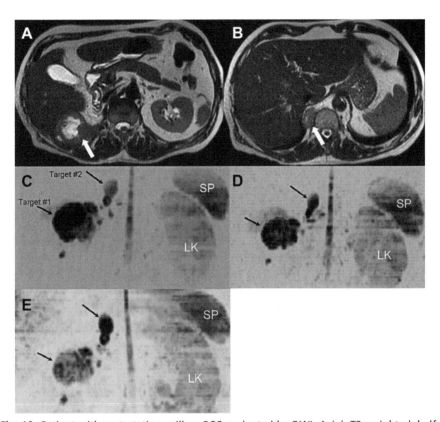

Fig. 16. Patient with metastatic papillary RCC evaluated by DWI. Axial, T2-weighted, half-Fourier, single-shot, fast-spin echo images (*A, B*) in the upper abdomen show metastatic lesions in the right nephrectomy bed (*arrow* in *A*, target lesion #1) and retrocrural region (*arrow* in *B*, target lesion #2). Baseline DWI (*C*) shows restricted diffusion in both target lesions. Note progressive decrease in the size of target lesion #1 accompanied by a progressive increase in water diffusion (ie, brighter signal) on DWI obtained at 2 weeks and after cycle 2 of therapy with sunitinib. In contrast, target lesion #2 shows only transient decrease in size at 2 weeks followed by an increase in size after cycle 2; these findings are associated with a progressive decrease in water diffusion (ie, darker signal) in this lesion. The pathophysiology behind the DWI findings and the potential use of this technique for monitoring response to targeted therapies merits further study. SP, spleen; LK, left kidney (*D, E*).

found in clear cell RCC tumors. The monoclonal antibody G250 (girentuximab) labeled with a positron-emitting radionuclide is being tested in clinical trials as a diagnostic agent to assess whether it can distinguish clear cell from non–clear cell renal carcinomas in patients with renal masses (**Fig. 17**). Data from a phase I study showed encouraging results with 94% sensitivity and 100% specificity for clear cell RCC and suggest that I-124-cG250 may help stratify patients with renal masses.[115] A pivotal phase III study (REDECT) enrolled 266 patients between May 2008 and September 2009. Results from G250 were compared with standard PET-CT scans as well as pathologic reports from all of the tumors. In a preliminary presentation, the study reported a preliminary sensitivity of 86% and specificity of 87% with an excellence side effects profile, most of them being postoperative complications.[116]

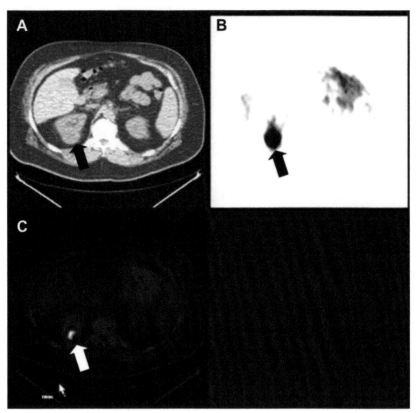

Fig. 17. Patient with a 4-cm right renal mass imaged with cG250 immuno-PET. Axial CT (*A*) shows a 4-cm mass of the right upper renal pole (*arrow*). There is increased uptake of iodine 124 (^{124}I)-cG250 in the mass in PET and fused PET-CT images (*arrows* in *B* and *C*, respectively), indicating clear cell histology. (*Courtesy of* Chaitanya Divgi, MD.)

SUMMARY

Imaging is a powerful tool in the detection, diagnosis, characterization, and management of RCC. Because smaller lesions are incidentally detected, minimally invasive ablation techniques and even surveillance can be considered in the appropriate clinical settings, in addition to the established surgical standard of care. Multiple imaging modalities provide complimentary information in RCC diagnosis, staging, and management. Targeted therapies in the metastatic disease setting have spurred great interest in the imaging assessment of response to therapy, and imaging techniques are in development to answer newly posed clinical questions. The role of imaging in RCC management will continue to expand to meet growing clinical and therapeutic needs.

REFERENCES

1. Choudhary S, Sudarshan S, Choyke PL, et al. Renal cell carcinoma: recent advances in genetics and imaging. Semin Ultrasound CT MR 2009;30(4):315–25.

2. Vikram R, Ng CS, Tamboli P, et al. Papillary renal cell carcinoma: radiologic-pathologic correlation and spectrum of disease. Radiographics 2009;29: 741–54.
3. Chow WH, Devesa SS, Warren JL, et al. Rising incidence of renal cell cancer in the United States. JAMA 1999;281:1628–31.
4. Bosniak MA. The current radiological approach to renal cysts. Radiology 1986; 158:1–10.
5. Bosniak MA. The small (less than or equal to 3.0 cm) renal parenchymal tumor: detection, diagnosis, and controversies. Radiology 1991;179:307–17.
6. Israel GM, Hindman N, Bosniak MA. Evaluation of cystic renal masses: comparison of CT and MR imaging by using the Bosniak classification system. Radiology 2004;231:365–71.
7. Habboub HK, Abu-Yousef HM, Williams RD, et al. Accuracy of color Doppler sonography in assessing venous thrombus extension in renal cell carcinoma. AJR Am J Roentgenol 1997;168(1):267–71.
8. Chow LC, Kwan SW, Olcott EW, et al. Split-bolus MDCT urography with synchronous nephrographic and excretory phase enhancement. AJR 2007;189(2): 314–22.
9. Bosniak MA, Megibow AJ, Hulnick DH, et al. CT diagnosis of renal angiomyolipoma: the importance of detecting small amounts of fat. AJR 1988;151(3): 497–501.
10. Israel GM, Hindman N, Hecht E, et al. The use of opposed-phase chemical shift MRI in the diagnosis of renal angiomyolipomas. AJR 2005;184:1868–72.
11. Zhang J, Lefkowicz RA, Bach A. Imaging of kidney cancer. Radiol Clin North Am 2007;45(1):119–47.
12. Adey GS, Pedrosa I, Rofsky NR, et al. Lower limits of detection using magnetic resonance imaging for solid components in cystic renal neoplasms. Urology 2008;71:47–51.
13. Semelka RC, Shoenut JP, Magro CM, et al. Renal cancer staging: comparison of contrast-enhanced CT and gadolinium-enhanced fat-suppressed spin-echo and gradient-echo MR imaging. J Magn Reson Imaging 1993;3(4):597–602.
14. Lawrentschuk N, Davis ID, Bolton DM, et al. Functional imaging of renal cell carcinoma. Nat Rev Urol 2010;7:258–66.
15. Lawrentschuk N, Bolton DM, Davis ID, et al. Renal cell cancer and positron emission tomography- an evolving diagnostic and therapeutic relationship. Current Medical Imaging Reviews 2007;3:17–26.
16. van der Veldt AA, Meijerink MR, van den Eertwegh AJ, et al. Targeted therapies in renal cell cancer: recent developments in imaging. Target Oncol 2010;5: 95–112.
17. Avril N, Dambha F, Murray I, et al. The clinical advances of fluorine-2-D-deoxy-glucose – positron emission tomography/computed tomography in urological cancers. Int J Urol 2010;17(6):501–11.
18. Aide N, Cappele O, Bottet P, et al. Efficiency of [18F]FDG PET in characterising renal cancer and detecting distant metastases: a comparison with CT. Eur J Nucl Med Mol Imaging 2003;30(9):1236–45.
19. Kang DE, White JR, Zuger JH, et al. Clinical use of fluorodeoxyglucose F 18 positron emission tomography for detection of renal cell carcinoma. J Urol 2004;171(5):1806–9.
20. Majhail NS, Urbain J, Albani JM, et al. F-18 fluorodeoxyglucose positron emission tomography in the evaluation of distant metastases from renal cell carcinoma. J Clin Oncol 2003;21(21):3995–4000.

21. Revheim ME, Winge-Main AK, Hagen G, et al. Combined positron emission tomography/computed tomography in sunitinib therapy assessment of patients with metastatic renal cell carcinoma. Clin Oncol (R Coll Radiol) 2011;23(5): 339–43.

22. Minamimoto R, Nakaigawa N, Tateishi U, et al. Evaluation of response to multi-kinase inhibitor in metastatic renal cell carcinoma by FDG PET/contrast-enhanced CT. Clin Nucl Med 2010;35:918–23.

23. Vercellino L, Bousquet G, Baillet G, et al. 18F-FDG PET/CT imaging for an early assessment of response to sunitinib in metastatic renal carcinoma: preliminary study. Cancer Biother Radiopharm 2009;24(1):137–44.

24. Powles T, Chowdhury S, Avril N, et al. Sequential FDG-PET/CT as a surrogate marker of response to sunitinib in metastatic clear cell renal cancer. J Clin Oncol 2011;29(Suppl 7) [abstract: 301].

25. Namura K, Minamimoto R, Yao M, et al. Impact of maximum standardized uptake value (SUVmax) evaluated by 18-Fluoro-2-deoxy-D-glucose positron emission tomography/computed tomography (18F-FDG-PET/CT) on survival for patients with advanced renal cell carcinoma: a preliminary report. BMC Cancer 2010;10:667–73.

26. Park JW, Jo MK, Lee HM. Significance of 18F-fluorodeoxyglucose positron-emission tomography/computed tomography for the postoperative surveillance of advanced renal cell carcinoma. BJU Int 2009;103(5):615–9.

27. Kaelin WG. Kidney cancer: now available in a new flavor. Cancer Cell 2008; 14(6):423–4.

28. Zhang J, Lefkowitz RA, Ishill NM, et al. Solid renal cortical tumors: differentiation with CT. Radiology 2007;244(2):494–504.

29. Sun MR, Pedrosa I. Magnetic resonance imaging of renal masses. Semin Ultrasound CT MR 2009;30:326–51.

30. Sun MR, Ngo L, Genega EM, et al. Renal cell carcinoma: dynamic contrast-enhanced MR imaging for differentiation of tumor subtypes - correlation with pathologic findings. Radiology 2009;250(3):793–802.

31. Yamashita Y, Watanabe O, Miyazaki T, et al. Cystic renal cell carcinoma. Acta Radiol 1994;35(1):19–24.

32. Pedrosa I, Chou MT, Ngo L, et al. MR classification of renal masses with pathologic correlation. Eur Radiol 2008;18:365–75.

33. Roy C, Sauer B, Lindner V, et al. Imaging of papillary renal neoplasms: potential application for characterization of small renal masses. Eur Radiol 2007;17:193–200.

34. Yoshimitsu K, Kakihara D, Irie H, et al. Papillary renal carcinoma: diagnostic approach by chemical shift gradient-echo and echo-planar MR imaging. J Magn Reson Imaging 2006;23:339–44.

35. Pedrosa I, Sun MR, Spencer M, et al. MR Imaging of renal masses: correlation with findings at surgery and pathologic analysis. Radiographics 2008;28: 985–1003.

36. Prasad SR, Humphrey PA, Catena JR, et al. Common and uncommon histologic subtypes of renal cell carcinoma: imaging spectrum with pathologic correlation. Radiographics 2006;26:1795–810.

37. Quaia E, Bussani R, Cova M, et al. Radiologic–pathologic correlations of intra-tumoral tissue components in the most common solid and cystic renal tumors. Pictorial review. Eur Radiol 2005;15(8):1734–44.

38. Kim JI, Cho JY, Moon KC. Segmental enhancement inversion at biphasic multi-detector CT: characteristic finding in small renal oncocytoma. Radiology 2009; 252(2):441–8.

39. Rosenkrantz AB, Hindman N, Fitzgerald EF, et al. MRI features of renal oncocytoma and chromophobe renal cell carcinoma. AJR 2010;195(6):W421–7.
40. Griffin N, Grant LA, Bharwani N, et al. Computed tomography in metastatic renal cell carcinoma. Semin Ultrasound CT MR 2009;30(4):359–66.
41. Sheir KZ, El-Azab M, Mosbah A, et al. Differentiation of renal cell carcinoma subtypes by multislice computerized tomography. J Urol 2005;174(2):451–5.
42. Verine J, Pluvinage A, Bousquet G, et al. Hereditary renal cancer syndromes: an update of a systematic review. Eur Urol 2010;58:701–10.
43. Robson CJ. Radical nephrectomy for renal cell carcinoma. J Urol 1963;89: 37–42.
44. Mueller-Lisse UG, Mueller-Lisse UL, Meindl T, et al. Staging of renal cell carcinoma. Eur Urol 2007;17:2268–77.
45. Kidney. In: Edge SB, Byrd DR, Compton CC, editors. AJCC cancer staging handbook. 7th edition. New York: Springer; 2010. p. 553.
46. Novara G, Ficarra V, Antonelli A, et al. Validation of the 2009 TNM version in a large multi-institutional cohort of patients treated for renal cell carcinoma: are further improvements needed? Eur Urol 2010;58:588–95.
47. Heuer R, Gill IS, Guazzoni G, et al. A critical analysis of the actual role of minimally invasive surgery and active surveillance for kidney cancer. Eur Urol 2010; 57:223–32.
48. Tatli S, Acar M, Tuncali K, et al. Percutaneous cryoablation techniques and clinical applications. Diagn Interv Radiol 2010;16:90–5.
49. Hines-Peralta A, Goldberg SN. Review of radiofrequency ablation for renal cell carcinoma. Clin Cancer Res 2004;10:6328s–34s.
50. Hinshaw JL, Shadid AM, Nakada SY, et al. Comparison of percutaneous and laparoscopic cryoablation for the treatment of solid renal masses. AJR 2008; 191:1159–68.
51. Hui GC, Tuncali K, Tatli S, et al. Comparison of percutaneous and surgical approaches to renal tumor ablation: metaanalysis of effectiveness and complication rates. J Vasc Interv Radiol 2008;19(9):1311–20.
52. Kawamoto S, Soloman SB, Bluemke DA, et al. Computed tomography and magnetic resonance imaging appearance of renal neoplasms after radiofrequency ablation and cryoablation. Semin Ultrasound CT MR 2009;30:67–77.
53. Uppot RN, Silverman SG, Zagoria RJ, et al. Imaging-guided percutaneous ablation of renal cell carcinoma: a primer of how we do it. AJR 2009;192:1558–70.
54. Smith S, Gillams A. Imaging appearances following thermal ablation. Clin Radiol 2008;63:1–11.
55. Tuncali K, vanSonnenberg E, Shankar S, et al. Evaluation of patients referred for percutaneous ablation of renal tumors: importance of a preprocedural diagnosis. AJR 2004;183:575–82.
56. Remzi M, Marberger M. Renal tumor biopsies for evaluation of small renal tumors: why, in whom, and how? Eur Urol 2009;55:359–67.
57. Rabinovich RA, Zelefsky MJ, Gaynor JJ, et al. Patterns of failure following surgical resection of renal cell carcinoma: implications for adjuvant local and systemic therapy. J Clin Onc 1994;12(1):206–12.
58. Janzen NK, Kim HL, Figlin RA, et al. Surveillance after radical or partial nephrectomy for localized renal cell carcinoma and management of recurrent disease. Urol Clin North Am 2003;30:843–52.
59. Negrier S, Escudier B, Lasset C, et al. Recombinant human interleukin-2, recombinant human interferon alfa-2a, or both in metastatic renal-cell carcinoma. Groupe Français d'Immunothérapie. N Engl J Med 1998;338:1272–8.

60. Yang JC, Haworth L, Sherry RM, et al. A randomized trial of bevacizumab, an anti-vascular endothelial growth factor antibody, for metastatic renal cell carcinoma. N Engl J Med 2003;349:427–34.
61. Motzer RJ, Hutson TE, Tomczak P, et al. Sunitinib versus interferon alfa in metastatic renal-cell carcinoma. N Engl J Med 2007;356:115–24.
62. Escudier B, Eisen T, Stadler WM, et al. Sorafenib in advanced renal cell carcinoma. N Engl J Med 2007;356:125–34.
63. Motzer RJ, Michaelson MD, Rosenberg J, et al. Sunitinib efficacy against advanced renal cell carcinoma. J Urol 2007;178:1883–7.
64. Mickisch GHJ, Garin A, van Poppel H, et al. Radical nephrectomy plus interferon-alfa-based immunotherapy compared with interferon alfa alone in metastatic renal-cell carcinoma: a randomized trial. Lancet 2001;358:966–70.
65. Flanigan RC, Salmon SE, Blumenstein BA, et al. Nephrectomy followed by interferon alfa-2b compared with interferon alfa-2b alone for metastatic renal-cell cancer. N Engl J Med 2001;345:1655–9.
66. Choueiri TK, Xie W, Kollmannsberger C, et al. The impact of cytoreductive nephrectomy on survival of patients with metastatic renal cell carcinoma receiving vascular endothelial growth factor targeted therapy. J Urol 2011; 185:60–6.
67. Breau RH, Blute ML. Surgery for renal cell carcinoma metastases. Curr Opin Urol 2010;20(5):375–81.
68. Baccala A, Hedfepeth R, Kaouk J, et al. Pathological evidence of necrosis in recurrent renal mass following treatment with sunitinib. Int J Urol 2007;14: 1095–7.
69. Therasse P, Arbuck SG, Eisenhauer EA, et al. New guidelines to evaluate the response to treatment in solid tumors. European Organization for Research and Treatment of Cancer, National Cancer Institute of the United States, National Cancer Institute of Canada. J Natl Cancer Inst 2000;92(3):205–16.
70. Eisenhauer EA, Therasse P, Bogaerts J, et al. New response evaluation criteria in solid tumours: revised RECIST guideline (version 1.1). Eur J Cancer 2009;45: 228–47.
71. Motzer RJ, Rini BI, Bukowski RM, et al. Sunitinib in patients with metastatic renal cell carcinoma. JAMA 2006;295(21):2516–24.
72. Thiam R, Fournier LS, Trinquart L, et al. Optimizing the size variation threshold for the CT evaluation of response in metastatic renal cell carcinoma treated with sunitinib. Ann Oncol 2010;21(5):936–41.
73. Benjamin RS, Choi H, Macapinlac HA, et al. We should desist using RECIST, at least in GIST. J Clin Oncol 2007;25:1760–4.
74. Choi H, Charnsangavej C, Faria SC, et al. Correlation of computed tomography and positron emission tomography in patients with metastatic gastrointestinal stromal tumor treated at a single institution with imatinib mesylate: proposal of new computed tomography response criteria. J Clin Oncol 2007;25:1753–9.
75. van der Veldt AA, Meijerink MR, van den Eertwegh AJ, et al. Choi response criteria for early prediction of clinical outcome in patients with metastatic renal cell carcinoma treated with sunitinib. Br J Cancer 2010;102:803–9.
76. Smith AD, Leiber ML, Shah SN. Assessing tumor response and detecting recurrence in metastatic renal cell carcinoma on targeted therapy: importance of size and attenuation on contrast-enhanced CT. AJR 2010;194:157–65.
77. Smith AD, Shah SN, Rini BI, et al. Attenuation, size and structure (MASS) criteria: assessing response and predicting clinical outcome in metastatic renal cell carcinoma on antiangiogenic targeted therapy. AJR 2010;194:1470–8.

78. Nathan PD, Vinayan A, Stott D, et al. CT response assessment combining reduction in both size and arterial phase density correlates with time to progression in metastatic renal cancer patients treated with targeted therapies. Cancer Biol Ther 2010;9(1):15–9.

79. Krajewski KM, Guo M, Van den Abbeele AD, et al. Comparison of four early posttherapy imaging changes (EPTIC; RECIST 1.0, tumor shrinkage, computed tomography tumor density, Choi criteria) in assessing outcome to vascular endothelial growth factor-targeted therapy in patients with advanced renal cell carcinoma. Eur Urol 2011;59(5):856–62.

80. Han KS, Jung DC, Choi JF, et al. Pretreatment assessment of tumor enhancement on contrast-enhanced computed tomography as a potential predictor of treatment outcome in metastatic renal cell carcinoma patients receiving antiangiogenic therapy. Cancer 2010;116(10):2332–42.

81. Motzer RJ, Escudier B, Oudard S, et al. Phase 3 of everolimus for metastatic renal cell carcinoma. Cancer 2010;116:4256–65.

82. Hudes G, Carducci M, Tomczak P, et al. Temsirolimus, interferon alfa, or both for advanced renal-cell carcinoma. N Engl J Med 2007;356:2271–81.

83. Cejka D, Kuntner C, Preusser M, et al. FDG uptake is a surrogate marker for defining the optimal biological dose of the mTOR inhibitor everolimus in vivo. Br J Cancer 2009;100:1739–45.

84. Ma WW, Jacene H, Song D, et al. [18F] Fluorodeoxyglucose positron emission tomography correlates with Akt pathway activity but is not predictive of clinical outcome during mTOR inhibitor therapy. J Clin Oncol 2009;27:2697–704.

85. White DA, Camus P, Endo M, et al. Noninfectious pneumonitis after everolimus therapy for advanced renal cell carcinoma. Am J Respir Crit Care Med 2010; 182:396–403.

86. Palmowski M, Schifferdecker I, Zwick S, et al. Tumor perfusion assessed by dynamic contrast-enhanced MRI correlates to the grading of renal cell carcinoma: initial results. Eur J Radiol 2010;74(3):e176–80.

87. De Bazelaire C, Rofsky NM, Duhamel G, et al. Arterial spin labeling blood flow magnetic resonance imaging for the characterization of metastatic renal cell carcinoma. Acad Radiol 2005;12(3):347–57.

88. Gilad AA, Israely T, Dafni H, et al. Functional and molecular mapping of uncoupling between vascular permeability and loss of vascular maturation in ovarian carcinoma xenografts: the role of stroma cells in tumor angiogenesis. Int J Cancer 2005;117(2):202–11.

89. Hahn OM, Yang C, Medved M, et al. Dynamic contrast-enhanced magnetic resonance imaging pharmacodynamic biomarker study of sorafenib in metastatic renal carcinoma. J Clin Oncol 2008;26(28):4572–8.

90. Taouli B, Thakur RK, Mannelli L, et al. Renal lesions: characterization with diffusion-weighted imaging versus contrast-enhanced MR imaging. Radiology 2009;251(2):398–407.

91. Lassau N, Chebil M, Chami L, et al. Dynamic contrast-enhanced ultrasonography: a new toll for the early evaluation of antiangiogenic treatment. Target Oncol 2010;5:53–8.

92. Lamuraglia M, Escudier B, Chami L, et al. To predict progression-free survival and overall survival in metastatic renal cancer treated with sorafenib: pilot study using dynamic contrast-enhanced Doppler ultrasound. Eur J Cancer 2006;42:2472–9.

93. Escudier B, Lassau N, Angevin E, et al. Phase I trial of sorafenib in combination with IFN alfa-2a in patients with unresectable and/or metastatic renal cell carcinoma or malignant melanoma. Clin Cancer Res 2007;13:1801–9.

94. Lassau N, Koscielny S, Albiges L, et al. Metastatic renal cell carcinoma treated with sunitinib: early evaluation of treatment response using dynamic contrast-enhanced ultrasonography. Clin Cancer Res 2010;16(4):1216–25.

95. Rosen MA, Schnall MD. Dynamic contrast-enhanced magnetic resonance imaging for assessing tumor vascularity and vascular effects of targeted therapies in renal cell carcinoma. Clin Cancer Res 2007;13(2 pt 2):770s–6s.

96. Sheiman RG, Sitek A. CT perfusion imaging: know its assumptions and limitations. Radiology 2008;246(2):649 [author reply: 649–50].

97. Fournier LS, Oudard S, Thiam R, et al. Metastatic renal carcinoma: evaluation of antiangiogenic therapy with dynamic contrast-enhanced CT. Radiology 2010; 256:511–8.

98. Tofts PS, Brix G, Buckley DL, et al. Estimating kinetic parameters from dynamic contrast-enhanced T-weighted MRI of a diffusable tracer: standardized quantities and symbols. J Magn Reson Imaging 1999;10:223–32.

99. Brasch RC, Daldrup H, Shames D, et al. Macromolecular contrast media-enhanced MRI estimates of microvascular permeability correlate with histopathologic tumor grade. Acad Radiol 1998;5(Suppl 1):S2–5.

100. Roberts TP, Turetschek K, Preda A, et al. Tumor microvascular changes to antiangiogenic treatment assessed by MR contrast media of different molecular weights. Acad Radiol 2002;9(Suppl 2):S511–3.

101. Jackson A, O'Connor JP, Parker GJ, et al. Imaging tumor vascular heterogeneity and angiogenesis using dynamic contrast-enhanced magnetic resonance imaging. Clin Cancer Res 2009;13:3449–59.

102. Flaherty KT, Rosen MA, Heitjan DF, et al. Pilot study of DCE-MRI to predict progression-free survival with sorafenib therapy in renal cell carcinoma. Cancer Biol Ther 2008;7:496–501.

103. Hahn OM, Yang C, Medved M, et al. Dynamic contrast-enhanced magnetic resonance imaging pharmacodynamic biomarker study of sorafentib in metastatic renal carcinoma. J Clin Oncol 2008;26:4572–8.

104. de Bazelaire C, Alsop DC, George D, et al. MRI measured tumor blood flow change following antiangiogenic therapy with PTK787/ZK 222584 correlates with clinical outcome in patients with metastatic renal cell carcinoma. Clin Cancer Res 2008;14:5548–54.

105. Schor-Bardach R, Alsop DC, Pedrosa I, et al. Does arterial spin labeling MRI measured tumor perfusion correlate with response of renal cell cancer to antiangiogenic therapy in a mouse model? Radiology 2009;51(3):731–42.

106. Rosenkrantz AB, Niver BE, Fitzgerald EF, et al. Utility of the apparent diffusion coefficient for distinguishing clear cell renal cell carcinoma of low and high nuclear grade. AJR 2010;195:W344–51.

107. Katz-Brull R, Rofsky NM, Morrin MM, et al. Decreases in free cholesterol and fatty acid unsaturation in renal cell carcinoma demonstrated by breath-hold magnetic resonance spectroscopy. Am J Physiol Renal Physiol 2005;288:F637–41.

108. Shreve P, Chiano PC, Humes HD, et al. Carbon-11-acetate PET imaging in renal disease. J Nucl Med 1995;36:1595–601.

109. Maleddu A, Pantaleo MA, Castellucci P, et al. 11C-Acetate PET for early prediction of sunitinib response in metastatic renal cell carcinoma. Tumori 2009;95:382–4.

110. Oyama N, Okazawa H, Kusukawa N, et al. 11C-acetate PET imaging for renal cell carcinoma. Eur J Nucl Med Mol Imaging 2009;36:422–7.

111. Rosso L, Brock CS, Gallo JM, et al. A new model for prediction of drug distribution in tumor and normal tissues: pharmacokinetics of temozolomide in glioma patients. Cancer Res 2009;69:120–7.

112. van der Veldt AA, Luurtsema G, Lubberink M, et al. Individualized treatment planning in oncology: role of PET and radiolabelled anticancer drugs in predicting tumor resistance. Curr Pharm Des 2008;14:2914–31.

113. Nagengast WB, De Vries EG, Hospers GA, et al. In vivo VEGF imaging with radiolabeled bevacizumab in a human ovarian tumor xenograft. J Nucl Med 2007; 48:1313–9.

114. Nagengast WB, De Korte MA, Oude M, et al. 89Zr-Bevacizumab PET of early antiangiogenic tumor response to treatment with HSP90 inhibitor NVP-AUY922. J Nucl Med 2010;51:761–7.

115. Divgi C, Pandit-Taskar N, Jungbluth A, et al. Preoperative characterization of clear-cell renal carcinoma using iodine-124-labelled antibody chimeric G250 (124I-cG250) and PET in patients with renal masses: a phase I trial. Lancet Oncol 2007;8:304–10.

116. Divgi C. Molecular imaging for phenotypic characterization of urologic cancers: implication for management and targeted therapy (G250 PET). ASCO 2010 Genitourinary Cancers Symposium. San Francisco (CA), March 5–7, 2010.

Small Renal Masses: Risk Prediction and Contemporary Management

Yuka Yamaguchi, MD[a], Matthew N. Simmons, MD, PhD[b],
Steven C. Campbell, MD, PhD[b],*

KEYWORDS

- Renal cell carcinoma • Small renal mass • Biopsy
- Nephrectomy • Thermal ablation • Active surveillance

Renal cell carcinoma (RCC) accounts for approximately 4% of cancers and 2% of cancer mortality in the United States.[1] In the past, most patients presented with advanced-stage disease and symptoms of gross hematuria, flank pain, and palpable mass. Over the past two decades, renal masses have been increasingly diagnosed as an incidental finding due to the increased use of cross-sectional imaging. At present, more than 60% of renal cancers are discovered in patients undergoing evaluation for unrelated conditions, a fact which has prompted some investigators to term this the "radiologist's tumor."[2,3] Small renal mass (SRM) specifically refers to a contrast-enhancing renal lesion measuring less than or equal to 4 cm which corresponds to the American Joint Committee on Cancer clinical staging designation of T1a. The incidence of SRMs increased twofold between 1993 and 2003, and the percentage of patients who initially presented with tumors less than or equal to 3 cm increased from 33% to 43% over this period.[4] This trend is expected to continue. As a result the SRM has become a frequently encountered clinical dilemma.

Increased rates of renal surgery for T1a tumors have paralleled a rise in detection.[5] It is expected that the shifts in both early detection and increased use of curative-intent surgery will result in improved oncologic and overall survival of patients with RCC. However, cancer-specific mortality has not decreased, with at least one study suggesting that mortality rates have increased for local-stage disease.[5–7] This rising

Financial Disclosures: The authors have nothing to disclose.
[a] Department of Urology, Cleveland Clinic, Glickman Urological and Kidney Institute, 9500 Euclid Avenue, Room Q10-1, Cleveland, OH 44195, USA
[b] Center for Urologic Oncology, Cleveland Clinic, Glickman Urological and Kidney Institute, 9500 Euclid Avenue, Room Q10-1, Cleveland, OH 44195, USA
* Corresponding author.
E-mail address: campbes3@ccf.org

Hematol Oncol Clin N Am 25 (2011) 717–736
doi:10.1016/j.hoc.2011.04.007
0889-8588/11/$ – see front matter © 2011 Elsevier Inc. All rights reserved.

hemonc.theclinics.com

mortality has called the current paradigm of aggressive surgical therapy for SRMs into question. The observation that early detection and early intervention are not resulting in improved survival rates suggests that nononcologic risk factors weigh heavily on the overall survival of patients treated for SRMs.[8–11] There has been a trend toward declining health and increasing age of patients presenting with SRMs. Most patients with incidental SRMs are between 60 and 70 years of age; 20% to 30% of patients with SRMs have preexisting chronic kidney disease (CKR); glomerular filtration rate (GFR) less than 60 mL/min per 1.73 m^2. Many patients have significant comorbidities, including hypertension and cardiovascular disease.[12] These patients are at higher risk for postoperative morbidity and mortality, and are at high risk of development of postoperative CKD.

Radical nephrectomy (RN) had long been held as the mainstay of treatment for RCC, regardless of tumor size. In the 1980s, partial nephrectomy (PN) emerged as an alternative to RN that provided equivalent oncologic control with the added benefit of functional preservation. Over the past two decades, a wealth of data has accrued that attests to the oncologic safety and superior functional outcomes of PN. There has been a steady shift toward use of PN, especially for SRMs. American Urologic Association guidelines published in 2009 specify PN as the reference standard for management of clinical T1 masses given the importance of functional preservation.[13] PN is associated with lower risk of development of CKD compared with RN, but can still result in clinically significant functional decline in high-risk patients. Huang and colleagues[14] reported that 65% of patients had new-onset CKD within 3 years after RN versus 20% in the PN population. In certain patients with SRMs, oncologic risk may be outweighed by competing causes of mortality.

Contemporary data from pathologic studies has revealed that 20% of SRMs are benign, whereas only 20% harbor potentially aggressive features.[15,16] In this regard, the therapeutic index of RN or PN may be low for the majority of SRMs. By focusing radical therapy on patients with potentially aggressive disease, the net impact of surgery can be optimized. As a result, there has been renewed interest in development of novel radiologic and pathologic techniques that may allow for reliable diagnosis and risk assessment of kidney tumors. In this article, the authors discuss the pathobiology and natural history of SRMs, clinical risk assessment, the role of biopsy, outcomes of current standard treatments, and current recommendations for management based on recent guidelines published by the American Urological Association.

PATHOLOGIC FEATURES OF SRMs

The kidney can give rise to a variety of neoplasms, all of which can be found in SRMs. Benign tumors include fat-poor angiomyolipoma, oncocytoma, metanephric adenoma, cystic nephroma, and a variety other nonmalignant histologies. Malignant tumors consist predominantly of RCC, but non-RCC tumors such as transitional cell carcinomas, sarcomas, and metastatic tumors are also occasionally encountered. RCC consists of a heterogenous group of tumors with varied aggressiveness and tumor architecture. Clear cell (conventional) RCC comprises 70% of tumors, whereas papillary (chromophil) and chromophobe subtypes comprise 15% and 5%, respectively.[17] Of the common RCC subtypes, clear cell and papillary type II tumors have the highest risk for metastatic progression. Other RCC subtypes such as collecting duct carcinoma and medullary carcinoma can be particularly aggressive, although fortunately rare.

Histologic analysis of kidney tumors serves as the definitive basis for prognosis and clinical management. **Table 1** outlines several contemporary pathologic studies that have looked specifically at pathologic features of SRMs. These studies represent the

Table 1
Contemporary SRM pathology data

Author	N	Percent Benign	Percent Indolent	Percent Aggressive	Percent Metastatic	Aggressiveness Criteria
Frank[24] (2003)	947	23%	64%	13%	NA	FG $\geq$3
Remzi[72] (2006)	287	20%	58%	22%	5%	Stage $\geq$T3a or metastatic
Schlomer[73] (2006)	206	23%	52%	25%	NA	FG $\geq$3
Pahernik[74] (2007)	663	17%	70%	13%	3%	FG $\geq$3, stage $\geq$T3a or metastatic
Lane[22] (2007)	862	20%	56%	24%	NA	FG $\geq$3 or stage $\geq$T3a
Mean Values		20%	60%	20%	4%	

Abbreviations: FG, Fuhrman Grade; NA, Not Available.

current clinical picture of SRM presentation, as the majority of tumors (60%–70%) in these studies were both incidentally detected and asymptomatic. Data from these studies confirm that 20% of SRMs are benign, that 20% are potentially aggressive RCC, and that 60% are potentially indolent RCC. These studies defined potential aggressiveness based on presence of high-risk pathologic features including Fuhrman nuclear grade greater than or equal to 3; presence of type II papillary, sarcomatoid or collecting duct histology; presence of invasion into the renal sinus capsule or vasculature (ie, Stage ≥T3a); or presence of metastasis at the time of diagnosis. Retrospective studies have shown clear associations between these high-risk pathologic features and advanced tumor stage and metastasis.

Although histologic phenotype and Fuhrman nuclear grade is relied on to predict tumor behavior, it must be recognized that these prognostic features are limited. The assumption is that the clinical behavior of two clear cell Fuhrman grade 3 tumors will be similar based on shared pathologic features and information obtained from retrospective clinical outcomes studies. However, a recent study by Dalgliesh and colleagues[18] illustrates the potential inaccuracy of phenotypic features to predict tumor behavior. The investigators conducted a large-scale genetic sequencing analysis in 101 clear cell RCC tumors, and found substantial variability in gene expression and mutation patterns. Although these tumors appear the same histologically, their clinical courses can be highly variable. This and other studies suggest that discerning genetic and molecular analysis along with clinical correlation will be required to more accurately predict tumor behavior.[19,20]

NATURAL HISTORY OF SRMs

The second series of important studies relating to the pathobiology of SRMs has focused on active surveillance (AS) of solid stage T1 lesions. **Table 2** summarizes data from several larger contemporary AS studies. These data refer specifically to solid-enhancing SRMs that do not demonstrate evidence of aggressiveness at the time of study initiation. Most studies have followed patients for only 2 to 3 years, although emerging studies include follow-up as long as 5 years. In general, it was observed that SRMs grow slowly with an average diameter increase of 3 mm/year. In these studies, the incidence of de novo metastatic progression during the observation period was low at 0% to 5%.

Contemporary AS studies have provided important data; however, they have significant limitations. Patient selection bias is present as those selected for these studies are older, less healthy, and have tumors that are considered low risk upon initiation of observation. In this regard, AS study data may pertain only to this low-risk subset of SRMs. There are no objective parameters that define clinically significant tumor growth or change in appearance. "Surveillance failure," defined as conversion from observation to intervention, is not necessarily indicative of disease progression because treatment initiation is based on subjective indications such as patient emotional burden, surgeon anxiety, and economic factors. Another limitation is that pathologic information is not available for a significant percentage of patients in these studies. Most patients do not undergo initial biopsy when recruited into AS and the only patients with post-surveillance pathology data are those that underwent treatment. This precludes prospective correlation of pathologic features with clinical behavior. Although current AS studies are not ideal, they do provide a loose framework for the general clinical behavior profile for select SRMs. It should be emphasized that these data may not be generalized to all SRMs.

Table 2
SRM active surveillance & natural history

Author (Year)	N	Mean cm Tumor Size	Mean cm/y Growth Rate	Mean Months Follow-up	Metastatic Progression (%)
Bosniak et al,[28] (1995)	40	1.73	0.36	39.0	0
Kato et al,[32] (2004)	18	2.0	0.42	26.9	0
Lamb et al,[75] (2004)	36	7.2	0.39	27.7	1 (2.8%)
Volpe et al,[16] (2005)	32	2.48	0.10	38.9	0
Wehle et al,[76] (2004)	29	1.83	0.12	32.0	0
Abouassaly et al,[77] (2008)	110	2.5[a]	0.26	24.0[a]	0
Kouba et al,[78] (2007)	46	2.92	0.70	35.8	0
Kunkle et al,[31] (2007)	106	2.0[a]	0.19[a]	29.0[a]	1 (1.1%)
Youssif et al,[79] (2007)	41	2.2	0.21	47.6	2 (5.7%)
Crispen et al,[30] (2008)	173	2.45	0.285	31.0	2 (1.3%)
Rosales et al,[80] (2010)	223	2.8[a]	0.34[a]	35.0[a]	4 (1.9%)
Mean values		2.7	0.31	33.0	1.2%

[a] Median values rather than mean values.

SRM RISK ASSESSMENT

Radiologic imaging is the primary means by which kidney tumors are clinically evaluated. Cross-sectional imaging with CT scan or MRI allows for anatomic analysis of the kidney, tumor, vasculature, and adjacent structures. A three-phase study with non-contrast, arterial, and delayed excretory phases is ideal. Any lesion with enhancement of greater than or equal to 15 Hounsfield units (HU) on CT scan imaging is considered suspicious for RCC, whereas renal lesions demonstrating less than 10 HU of enhancement are predominantly benign. MRI with administration of gadolinium contrast is an acceptable alternative for evaluation of kidney tumors in patients with iodine contrast allergy and, at some institutions, MRI is the preferred routine imaging modality. Gadolinium should not be administered to patients with stage 4 CKD (ie, GFR $\leq$30 mL/min/1.73m^2) due to the risk for nephrogenic systemic fibrosis, a severe and potentially irreversible condition.[21] Once it is established that the mass is a solid, contrast-enhancing, kidney tumor, it is assumed RCC until proven otherwise by pathologic analysis.

Demographic Risk Features

Patient demographic factors can provide insight into the clinical behavior of SRMs. Patients with multifocal small kidney tumors may have heritable syndromes such as von Hippel-Lindau (VHL), the familial form of clear cell RCC. Management strategy in patients with VHL and most familial syndromes of RCC is critical given the high incidence of de novo tumor growth and risk for CKD that can be associated with multiple surgical interventions, thus observation of tumors less than 3 cm is accepted practice. For sporadic RCC, age and gender appear to correlate with likelihood of malignancy. Younger women with contrast-enhancing solid SRMs have a benign tumor rate of 40% to 50%, which is much higher than for males.[22] DeRoche and colleagues[23] reported the rate of benign tumors in females at 27% compared with 15% for males. The rate of malignancy in this study for tumors less than or equal to 3.5 cm was both age and gender-dependent. SRM malignancy rates in patients less than 68 years of age were 87% for males and 69% for females. Younger patients of African descent with sickle cell trait are a special consideration because they have a predilection for medullary RCC. In this demographic, aggressive management of a SRM is advisable. Although demographic and clinical correlates may associate with certain tumors types, they are by no means diagnostic. For any SRM the likelihood of RCC is high, and these tumors are best managed surgically.

Tumor Size

Tumor size has been shown to correlate with malignancy and high nuclear grade.[24,25] Two large studies have reported that for every 1 cm increase in tumor diameter there is a 16% to 17% increase in the odds of malignancy.[24,25] In these studies, 38% to 46% of tumors measuring less than or equal to 1 cm were benign compared with 6% to 7% of tumors greater than or equal to 7 cm. The risk of high nuclear grade (ie, Fuhrman nuclear grade $\geq$3) disease also increases in relation to tumor size. Among clear cell RCC, each 1 cm increase in tumor size increased the odds of high grade disease by 32%.[25] Variability in these data reinforce that all tumors should be assumed to be malignant regardless of size until proven otherwise on pathologic analysis.

When considering enrollment of a patient into an AS protocol it is generally agreed that smaller tumors are "safer" to observe than larger ones. One group has described surveillance outcomes in patients with T1a versus T1b-T2 masses.[26,27] Failure of surveillance was defined as progression to metastatic disease or conversion from surveillance to delayed treatment. Of 41 patients with pT1a tumors, only one failed surveillance (2%), and none progressed to metastasis. In contrast, of 42 patients with T1b-T2 tumors, 14% failed surveillance and 6% progressed to metastasis disease. No study has yet been conducted to assess the risk differential within the 0 to 4 cm size range, but it is likely that similar trends would be observed. Most urologic oncologists would entertain the idea of surveillance for masses measuring 1 to 2 cm in appropriate scenarios and would elect to proceed to treatment once these masses reached the 3 to 4 cm range.

Tumor Growth Rate

Tumors that demonstrate rapid growth on serial imaging studies are assumed clinically aggressive. Bosniak and colleagues[28] examined 40 cT1a incidental kidney tumors over a period of approximately 3 years and found the median tumor diameter growth rate to be 0.36 cm per year. No patients with a growth rate less than or equal to 0.35 cm/y exhibited metastatic progression within the 3 year study period. Similar studies have shown equivalent data with mean tumor growth rates ranging from 0.2 to 0.4 cm per year and no progression to metastatic disease in slow growing tumors.[29–31] Although slow growth rate was associated with decreased metastatic rates, it did not correlate with malignancy rates. Kunkle and colleagues[31] followed 106 enhancing masses for a minimum of 12 months and found that the proportion of malignant tumors was equivalent in tumors with and without growth, 89% versus 83% ($P = .56$), respectively. Kato and colleagues[32] found similar malignancy rates in slow and fast growing tumors, but did find a difference in the proportion of high Fuhrman nuclear grade greater than or equal to 3 cm in the latter group. Among masses that were malignant, high-grade tumors had a faster growth rate (0.93 cm/y) compared with low-grade tumors (0.28–0.37 cm/y). As more data emerge, a greater understanding of the relationship between tumor growth rate and metastatic potential will develop.

Tumor Enhancement and Morphology

Anatomic features that may signify aggressive tumor behavior include tumor morphology and contrast-enhancement characteristics. An invasive or infiltrative appearance is strongly associated with high-grade or sarcomatoid differentiation and poor prognosis.[33] A homogeneous appearance suggests preservation of tissue organization, uniform histology, and ordered vascularity. Heterogenous enhancement suggests poor differentiation, loss of organization, central necrosis, and aberrant vascularization. Zhang and colleagues[34] examined 193 tumors and found that 79% to 88% of tumors with heterogeneous appearance had clear cell RCC pathology. In contrast papillary and chromophobe tumors tended to have more homogenous appearance. These features can enhance tumor evaluation, but are too nonspecific to be used in isolation to guide clinical management.

Much attention has been paid to diagnostic potential of the degree of contrast enhancement. The basis for this is the observation that tumors of specific histology have different vascular organization. Contrast enhancement tends to be lowest in papillary RCC compared with other solid tumors. Alshumrani and colleagues[35] examined 46 cT1 tumors and found contrast enhancement in clear cell RCC, oncocytoma, and papillary RCC tumors to be 65 HU, 80 HU, and 16 HU, respectively. Similarly, Sun and colleagues[36] examined dynamic contrast-enhanced MRIs in 122 patients. Clear cell RCC had the greatest signal-intensity change (205.6% in corticomedullary phase and 247.1% in nephrographic phase), which was significantly higher than in papillary RCC (32.1% and 96.6%, respectively; $P<.001$).[36] They reported 93% sensitivity and 96% specificity to distinguish between papillary and clear cell RCC using these parameters. The importance of accurately detecting these features is diminished because nearly half of papillary RCC tumors behave as aggressively as clear cell RCC. Type II papillary tumors exhibit 5 year cancer specific mortality rates double that of type I papillary RCC.[37] Although tumor enhancement and complexity may suggest a specific tumor type or behavior, radiologic appearance is nonspecific and should be interpreted with caution.

RENAL MASS BIOPSY

Biopsy-based pathologic analysis could potentially augment traditional tumor evaluation and further optimize SRM management. Tumor biopsy is central to diagnosis and management of cancers of the breast, prostate, thyroid, and skin, to name only a few. However, its routine use for evaluation of kidney tumors has been limited. Concerns over false negative results, potential complications, and the belief that biopsy may not change eventual management have relegated biopsy to limited scenarios. This mindset regarding renal mass biopsy (RMB) persists and a recent survey of urologists in the United Kingdom highlighted the belief that biopsy was not useful in the evaluation of renal masses. In this survey, 43% of consultant urologists never used biopsy during evaluation of an indeterminate renal mass and 23% only used biopsy for a select patient group.[38] New data from modern RMB have shown significant improvements in diagnostic accuracy of RMB, and are challenging long-held beliefs regarding its utility.

RMB is currently indicated when tissue diagnosis at biopsy could potentially change management of the mass.[39] Well established indications for RMB include a kidney tumor in the presence of a known extrarenal primary malignancy, suspicion of lymphoma or abscess, or in select cases where tumors display an infiltrative growth pattern. RMB in these cases can rule out metastasis, lymphoma, infection, or other disease entities whose treatment is fundamentally different than that for RCC. The role for RMB of SRMs has been increasingly debated. RMB in its current state can reliably distinguish benign versus malignant pathology and, in most cases, is able to diagnose histology and Fuhrman nuclear grade. RMB can also be useful to guide decision-making regarding initiation of AS in high-risk patients in whom identification of potentially aggressive features would justify the risks of surgery.

RMB Techniques

There is no consensus protocol for the manner in which RMB is conducted. Two distinct methods for tissue collection include core biopsy needle sampling and fine-needle aspiration (FNA). Core biopsies are typically acquired using an 18-gauge needle, and technique for tissue collection has been shown to influence diagnostic accuracy of SRMs. In T1a tumors, Wunderlich and colleagues[40] reported that the accuracy of a central core was 83.3%, whereas that of a peripheral core was 75%. An increase in accuracy to 97% was observed if both central and peripheral core biopsies were obtained. The current recommendation is to obtain two to three core samples from both the central and peripheral regions of the tumor.[40] FNA allows for tissue collection using multiple needle passes through the tumor under negative pressure. This allows for enrichment of cellular aspirates from the tumor, which are evaluated using cytologic techniques. With appropriate tissue handling, specimens from either type of biopsy can be prepared for molecular analysis. In general, core needle biopsy has increased diagnostic accuracy compared with FNA and is recommended as the preferred method for tissue acquisition. Some investigators advocate combined core and FNA biopsy because this is associated with greater sensitivity and accuracy than either technique in isolation.[41,42]

Diagnostic Accuracy of RMB

Current high-resolution, real-time CT scan-guided imaging has resulted in dramatic improvement in sampling accuracy of tumors and their subcomponents. Improved techniques for tissue processing have led to improved accuracy of histologic and Fuhrman nuclear grade evaluation. **Table 3** summarizes data from several contemporary RMB studies. The historical noninformative rate of RMB was on the order of 20% to 40% and its accuracy to obtain the correct pathologic diagnosis ranged from 70% to 80%.[43–45] In contemporary series, the noninformative rate has decreased to as low as 2% to 8%. Accuracy to distinguish between benign and malignant pathology is 97% for informative biopsies and accuracy to define the correct histologic subtype has increased to approximately 93%. Most importantly, the false negative rate has decreased to 1%.[46–52] Noninformative biopsies can be attributed to inadequate tissue acquisition or the presence of ambiguous oncocytic histology, which still represents a major challenge in this field. In cases where the first biopsy renders nondiagnostic results, a second biopsy has been advocated and has a reported success rate of 75% to 100%.[53]

There are few studies regarding the value of biopsy specifically in SRMs, with most studies examining RMB success rates for tumors over a wide size range. In general, it has been reported that small tumors are associated with decreased biopsy sensitivity and increased failure rates. One study demonstrated that there was an increase in biopsy failures in lesions smaller than 3 cm (37% vs 9%, $P = .006$).[54] Rybicki and colleagues[55] reported an increased false negative rate in masses less than 3 cm and greater than 6 cm (60% and 44%, respectively) versus masses between 4 and 6 cm (negative predictive value of 89%). On average, SRMs have less necrosis and heterogeneity because they have not outgrown their blood supply, but they can be more difficult to target due to their smaller size.

Complications of RMB

Complications of RMB consist of hemorrhage, pseudoaneurysm formation, infection, adjacent organ injury, pneumothorax, and tract seeding. Contemporary series demonstrate that complications of RMB are rare, with minor and major complication rates of 5% and 1%, respectively. Hemorrhagic complications can be managed with conservative measures such as bed rest and transfusion in the vast majority of cases. Patients should stop anticoagulation drugs such as aspirin or IIa/IIIb inhibitors 7 to 10 days before biopsy to allow for normalization of coagulation parameters. This can be problematic as a large percentage of patients who are candidates for AS have a history of stroke or cardiovascular disease. In these patients, the risk of cessation of anticoagulation medications must be balanced by the potential benefit of the proposed biopsy. Fear of tumor seeding of the biopsy tract has been a concern, but appears to be extremely rare with only six cases reported in the literature and no cases reported since 1994. Current practice is to conduct RMB via a coaxial dilator to minimize the risk of bleeding and needle-tract seeding.

The Future of RMB

It is likely that a shift will occur in which RMB forms a primary basis for SRM evaluation. As RMB technique improves, concerns over reliability of tissue acquisition will diminish. Molecular profiling of tumor tissue will likely identify new biomarkers with superior accuracy, sensitivity, and specificity to predict clinical tumor behavior, even for the challenging "oncocytic tumor." Several studies have provided a glimpse of things to come using techniques such as proteomic evaluation, comparative

Table 3
Contemporary CT-guided core renal mass biopsy data summary

Author	N	Informative Rate[a]	Benign/Malignant Accuracy[b]	Histologic Accuracy[b]	Nuclear Grade Accuracy[b]	Complication Rate[c]
Beland[81] (2007)	58	90%	98%	NA	NA	0%
Schmibauer[48] (2008)	78	97%	95%	91%	76%	6%
Lebret[82] (2007)	119	79%	92%	86%	46%	0%
Maturen[83] (2007)	152	96%	97%	NA	NA	2%
Reichelt[84] (2007)	30	84%	100%	NA	NA	3%
Somani[85] (2007)	70	87%	100%	100%	NA	1%
Schmidbauer[48] (2008)	78	97%	96%	98%	76%	1%
Shannon[49] (2008)	235	78%	100%	98%	98%	1%
Volpe[42] (2008)	100	84%	100%	93%	68%	3%
Masoom[86] (2009)	31	100%	97%	97%	NA	NA
Wang[52] (2009)	110	91%	100%	NA	NA	7%
Blumenfeld[47] (2010)	81	98%	97%	88%	43%	NA
Veltri[51] (2011)	45	92%	91%	93%	NA	6%
Mean Values		90%	97%	94%	68%	2.7%

Abbreviation: NA, Not Available.
[a] Percent of biopsies providing diagnostic information.
[b] Percent correlation of biopsy with definitive surgical pathology results for informative biopsies.
[c] Includes both minor and major events.

genomic hybridization, and gene-expression analysis. Additional discoveries relating to micro-RNAs, epigenetic processes, and posttranslation modification are also revealing insights into the pathobiology of RCC, and are allowing for identification of new markers for disease aggressiveness. A future when RMB-based analysis plays a primary role in clinical management is foreseen.

SRM: TREATMENT OPTIONS AND OUTCOMES

For healthy patients who are acceptable surgical candidates, the current standard of care for SRMs is nephron-sparing surgery. These patients stand to benefit from tumor removal and typically exhibit minimal functional decrease as the result of ischemic injury or functional parenchymal volume loss. Unfortunately, a significant percentage of patients are poor surgical candidates and the oncologic benefit of surgery must be weighed against potential harm associated with the intervention, including loss of renal function. A recent study showed that, in patients with bilateral tumors, the amount of functional parenchymal volume decrease after surgery was specifically associated with decreased overall survival. Patients with final GFR of less than 60 ml/min/1.73 m^2 had significantly decreased overall survival that was not cancer-related.[56] Management of patients with kidney tumors is multifactorial. Patient factors to consider include age, performance status, comorbidities, and preexisting CKD. Tumor-related factors to consider include tumor size, stage, appearance, and growth rate. Some of these patients will experience acute kidney injury as a result of PN, and a significant percentage may develop CKD and its harmful sequelae. Balanced counseling of patients regarding the relative risks and benefits of treatment is paramount, and risk assessment of SRMs can contribute significantly to optimal management. Current treatment options for SRMs are discussed in brief with emphasis on their role in the management of SRMs.

RN

RN remains the standard of care for locally advanced or infiltrative high-risk tumors, but it should only play a marginal role in the management of SRMs. With open technique, the tumor and its investing perinephric fat are removed via a flank, subcostal, or thoracoabdominal incision. The introduction of laparoscopic technique has significantly decreased morbidity associated with RN while maintaining equivalent oncologic efficacy. Because of its popular appeal, decreased morbidity, and low complication rate, laparoscopic RN is performed routinely in community practice. This is problematic because it constitutes overtreatment in most cases of SRMs, and is associated with increased risk for development of CKD and CKD-related disease.[57] Ideally, RN would be reserved only for cT1a tumors situated in a central position that could not be removed without irreparable disruption of the renal vessels or collecting system. In reality, these comprise a very small minority of SRMs.

PN

Evidence regarding CKD has pushed PN to the forefront as the reference standard for clinical T1 renal masses.[13] PN allows for complete extirpation of the tumor with maximal preservation of the remaining normal kidney parenchyma. PN has the same oncologic efficacy as RN, with 5-year recurrence-free and metastatic progression-free survival rates as high as 98% and 97%, respectively.[58] PN can be conducted using open, laparoscopic, or robotic techniques. Technical expertise is requisite for all PN techniques to ensure oncologic safety and to minimize the potential for complications. Advantages of the open approach include wider exposure and the ability to apply ice to extend the safety limit of the ischemic period. The advantages of laparoscopic and robotic PN include decreased morbidity and faster recuperation time. **Fig. 1** illustrates essential elements in the technique for PN. This involves mobilization of the kidney, identification and careful excision of the tumor and a small margin of normal parenchyma, reconstruction of the renal vessels and collecting system, and hemostatic closure of the renal capsule. Ischemia is induced by clamping the renal artery and vein during excision and reconstruction to minimize blood loss and to allow for visualization of the tissues within a bloodless field. The accepted safe limit for warm ischemia duration is 20 to 25 minutes, but patients with preexisting CKD may exhibit functional decline with shorter warm ischemia times.[59,60] The majority of patients with ischemia-induced kidney injury exhibit normalization of function in the weeks to months after surgery. Older patients with preexisting CKD and additional risk factors such as diabetes, hypertension, and obesity appear to be more susceptible to ischemic injury, and suffer permanent decline in function specifically as a result of ischemic insult.[59] The major determinant of permanent functional decline appears to be renal parenchymal volume decrease, which is associated with increased tumor size and depth within the kidney.[61,62]

One potential downside of PN is an increased risk of local or urologic complications when compared with other treatment modalities, because PN requires a reconstruction that must heal. Postoperative bleeding is the most serious complication, occurring in about 1% to 2% of cases with a centrally located tumor. This is typically managed with superselective embolization, which is highly efficacious and typically associated with minimal loss of renal function. Urine leak is found in 3% to 5% of cases and will almost always heal with prolonged drainage, occasionally complemented by ureteral stent placement to facilitate antegrade drainage. Reoperation for this complication is uncommon.

Although a gradual increase in the implementation of PN has been noted, Miller and colleagues[63] reported that only 20% of renal masses 2 to 4 cm treated surgically were managed with PN from 2000 to 2001. PN is now being used more frequently, but RN still predominates. Reasons for this disconnect have been the popularization of laparoscopic RN, the increased technical complexity of PN with its higher rate of local complications, and possible concerns regarding cancer control that persist in the community. Concerns raised regarding the under-use of PN led an American Urologic Association

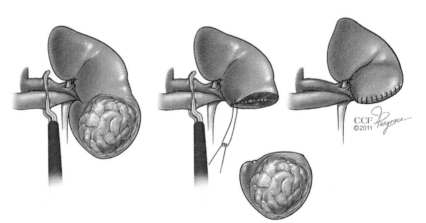

Fig. 1. PN technique and outcome. (*Courtesy of* Cleveland Clinic Foundation, Cleveland, OH; with permission.)

to commission a panel to provide guidelines for the management of clinical stage T1 renal masses. One of the main statements of this panel emphasized the role of PN, if technically feasible, as the reference standard for surgical treatment of SRMs.[64]

THERMAL ABLATION

Thermal ablation (TA) includes cryoablation and radiofrequency ablation (RFA). These techniques have been endorsed as alternate minimally invasive nephron-sparing treatments for patients with renal masses less than 3.5 cm who are not candidates for surgery but who still desire or require treatment. Both techniques can be performed percutaneously under image guidance or laparoscopically under direct visual perspective.[65] The approach used largely depends on the location of the tumor. The percutaneous approach is optimally suited for posterior masses, whereas a laparoscopic approach is best if mobilization of adjacent structures is required to safely access the tumor. Cryoablation involves placement of probes within the tumor using CT scan or ultrasound guidance. The probes are then charged with argon to induce sequential freeze-thaw cycles to −20°C to destroy tumor tissue. Successful local control rates of 90% to 95% have been reported, although follow-up in most of these studies remains rather limited.[66,67] Matin and colleagues[66] reported cancer-specific survival rates at 5 and 10 years of 93% and 81%, respectively; and disease-free survival rates at 5 and 10 years of 78% and 51%, respectively—substantially lower than what would be expected with surgical excision.

RFA destroys tumor tissue by heating to temperatures above 50°C. Loss of enhancement within the lesion on cross-sectional imaging is used as an indicator of successful treatment. Local control rates of 80% to 90% have been reported, although follow-up is limited in most series.[68] At least one study has called into question the adequacy of radiologic follow-up and efficacy of treatment with RFA. Weight and colleagues[69] demonstrated that six patients (24%) with no enhancement on MRI had viable cancer cells on biopsies 6 months after RFA. Furthermore, a meta-analysis found that lesions treated with RFA had a higher rate of local tumor progression than those treated with cryoablation (12.3% vs 4.7%, $P<.0001$).[70] Long-term outcomes and treatment efficacy of TA have yet to be validated in a strict manner. Current studies have demonstrated that ablative therapies have higher local recurrent rates than extirpative treatment. Another factor to consider is that salvage therapy after ablative therapies can be associated with increased difficulty, and all options may no longer be available. Most patients with local recurrence after TA can undergo repeat ablation but 10% to 20% will require surgical salvage. In this setting, PN and minimally invasive approaches are often precluded due to the extensive fibrosis within the perinephric space. With continued refinement in technique, TA therapies will remain a viable treatment option in select patients who are not optimal candidates for PN.

AS

AS is a reasonable option for patients with significant comorbidities and limited life expectancy. It has been proposed that the relative benefit of treatment is diminished by competing causes of mortality in a subset of patients who are greater than or equal to 65 years old, and who have increased comorbidities and surgical risk. Lane and colleagues[10] demonstrated that RN and PN did not improve overall survival in patients greater than 75 years of age, and survival in this series was predominantly determined by age and comorbidities. Similarly, Hollingsworth and colleagues[8] observed that, despite surgical treatment, after 5 years, a third of patients greater than or equal to 70 years of age died from other causes. Kutikov and colleagues[71] recently published results from a competing risk analysis of 30,801 patients who were surgically treated for node-negative, localized RCC. Age and male gender were found to be closely associated with nononcologic mortality. Additionally, decreased tumor size was associated with an increase in nononcologic mortality, which indicated that treatment risk outweighed oncologic risk in a subset of patients. These data refer to general observations in elderly patient cohorts, but it should be emphasized that older patients with acceptable performance status and normal baseline kidney function can still benefit from extirpative surgery. Kutikov and colleagues[71] present a nomogram that may prove very useful for assessment of competing oncologic and nononcologic risks in these patients. Select, high-risk patients can be considered for an initial period of AS; only a minority will end up requiring active treatment.

At present there is no consensus regarding a uniform protocol for AS. Initial evaluation and staging should be conducted with contrast-enhanced CT scan or MRI, with strong consideration for RMB to rule out potentially aggressive features. Once the mass is confirmed as a cT1aN0M0 contrast-enhancing tumor, it can be monitored every 6 to 12 months. CT scan or MRI are reasonable ways to monitor tumor growth, but cost and radiation exposure can be decreased by use of renal ultrasound. Patients should be informed of the low, albeit real, risk of progression to incurable disease with AS.

There are also no uniform criteria for AS failure that signal the need to initiate delayed treatment. In some series, a tumor size cut-off of 3-4 cm is adopted. Others base the decision to intervene on interval tumor growth. The distinction between normal and abnormal growth rates are debatable, but most investigators assign tumors with growth rates less than 3 mm/y as low risk and those with greater than 3 mm/y as high risk. Additional studies are required to determine the association of liner growth rate and risk of metastatic progression.

CONTEMPORARY MANAGEMENT RECOMMENDATIONS

The 2009 AUA guidelines for the management of T1 renal masses outline recommendations for treatment of SRMs.[36] All patients with SRMs should be evaluated with a high-quality CT scan or MRI with and without contrast to assess tumor anatomy and enhancement features. Renal mass sampling should be conducted if the clinical scenario and imaging are suggestive of lymphoma, abscess, or metastases; or if it might change management. The patient should be counseled regarding the natural history of SRMs and the available management options (PN, RN, TA, and AS), and the potential risks and benefits of each. **Fig. 2** shows an algorithm for treatment of SRMs based upon patient health characteristics.

Management of SRMs in Healthy Patients

For healthy patients, PN is the reference standard. RN should be reserved as an alternate standard of care when tumor anatomy precludes a nephron-sparing approach. The relative risks of CKD and its associated comorbidities should be discussed. For the small minority of patients in whom RN is necessary, a laparoscopic approach should be considered due to its reduced morbidity and faster convalescence. TA is reserved as a less-invasive treatment option with an increased probability of local tumor recurrence in comparison to PN. Percutaneous renal mass core biopsy with or without FNA should be performed in all patients undergoing ablation therapy to define histology. Active surveillance with delayed intervention can be discussed as an option, but it must be stressed that it is associated with some degree of oncologic risk, particularly in patients with long life expectancy.

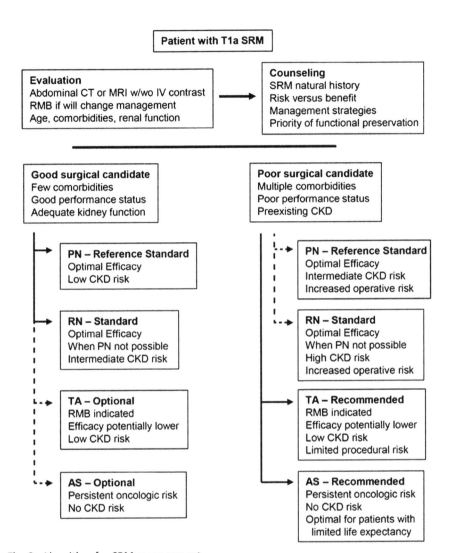

Fig. 2. Algorithm for SRM management.

Management of SRM in High-risk Patients

For high-risk patients with advanced age and significant comorbidities the same treatment options exist, but there should be increased consideration for alternative minimally invasive treatments or AS when appropriate. PN and RN are the standard of care when feasible, with a preference for PN when possible. RN is preferable to PN in certain situations due to its lower risk of operative blood loss and lower complication rate; as long as the contralateral kidney can provide adequate function. TA may be beneficial in high-risk patients who are not candidates for surgery, but who desire active treatment. Active surveillance should be discussed as a primary consideration in patients with decreased life expectancy or who are high-risk surgical candidates.

SUMMARY

SRMs are increasingly encountered in clinical practice and represent a challenging scenario with substantial risk of overtreatment, particularly in the elderly. Pathologic data demonstrate that only 20% to 25% of SRMs are likely to display aggressive clinical behavior. Surgical and CKD-related morbidity could potentially be minimized by improved targeting of therapy specifically to high-risk patients. Pathologic and radiologic tumor features, although limited, provide insight into the clinical behavior of SRMs. In the future, molecular biomarkers that can predict SRM behavior and metastatic potential with high reliability will be developed. This will dramatically increase the role of biopsy in the management of SRMs. Integration of RMB and biomarker analysis may lead to a shift from active treatment to surveillance or ablative therapies. The subset of patients with aggressive forms of RCC will be managed with extirpative surgery, whereas those with indolent disease may be followed using radiologic imaging and surveillance biopsy.

REFERENCES

1. Jemal A, Siegel R, Xu J, et al. Cancer statistics, 2010. CA Cancer J Clin 2010; 60(5):277–300.
2. Jayson M, Sanders H. Increased incidence of serendipitously discovered renal cell carcinoma. Urology 1998;51(2):203–5.
3. Rini BI, Campbell SC, Escudier B. Renal cell carcinoma. Lancet 2009;373(9669): 1119–32.
4. Cooperberg MR, Mallin K, Ritchey J, et al. Decreasing size at diagnosis of stage 1 renal cell carcinoma: analysis from the National Cancer Data Base, 1993 to 2004. J Urol 2008;179(6):2131–5.
5. Hollingsworth JM, Miller DC, Daignault S, et al. Rising incidence of small renal masses: a need to reassess treatment effect. J Natl Cancer Inst 2006;98(18):1331–4.
6. Hock LM, Lynch J, Balaji KC. Increasing incidence of all stages of kidney cancer in the last 2 decades in the United States: an analysis of surveillance, epidemiology and end results program data. J Urol 2002;167(1):57–60.
7. Sun M, Thuret R, Abdollah F, et al. Age-adjusted incidence, mortality, and survival rates of stage-specific renal cell carcinoma in North America: a trend analysis. Eur Urol 2011;59(1):135–41.
8. Hollingsworth JM, Miller DC, Daignault S, et al. Five-year survival after surgical treatment for kidney cancer: a population-based competing risk analysis. Cancer 2007;109(9):1763–8.
9. Huang WC. Impact of nephron sparing on kidney function and non-oncologic mortality. Urol Oncol 2010;28(5):568–74.
10. Lane BR, Abouassaly R, Gao T, et al. Active treatment of localized renal tumors may not impact overall survival in patients aged 75 years or older. Cancer 2010;116(13):3119–26.
11. Weight CJ, Larson BT, Fergany AF, et al. Nephrectomy induced chronic renal insufficiency is associated with increased risk of cardiovascular death and death from any cause in patients with localized cT1b renal masses. J Urol 2010;183(4): 1317–23.
12. Drucker BJ. Renal cell carcinoma: current status and future prospects. Cancer Treat Rev 2005;31(7):536–45.
13. Campbell SC, Novick AC, Belldegrun A, et al. Guideline for management of the clinical T1 renal mass. J Urol 2009;182(4):1271–9.

14. Huang WC, Levey AS, Serio AM, et al. Chronic kidney disease after nephrectomy in patients with renal cortical tumours: a retrospective cohort study. Lancet Oncol 2006;7(9):735–40.

15. Mues AC, Landman J. Small renal masses: current concepts regarding the natural history and reflections on the American Urological Association guidelines. Curr Opin Urol 2010;20(2):105–10.

16. Volpe A, Jewett MA. The natural history of small renal masses. Nat Clin Pract Urol 2005;2(8):384–90.

17. Waldert M, Haitel A, Marberger M, et al. Comparison of type I and II papillary renal cell carcinoma (RCC) and clear cell RCC. BJU Int 2008;102(10):1381–4.

18. Dalgliesh GL, Furge K, Greenman C, et al. Systematic sequencing of renal carcinoma reveals inactivation of histone modifying genes. Nature 2010;463(7279): 360–3.

19. Jones J, Otu H, Spentzos D, et al. Gene signatures of progression and metastasis in renal cell cancer. Clin Cancer Res 2005;11(16):5730–9.

20. Klatte T, Seligson DB, LaRochelle J, et al. Molecular signatures of localized clear cell renal cell carcinoma to predict disease-free survival after nephrectomy. Cancer Epidemiol Biomarkers Prev 2009;18(3):894–900.

21. Natalin RA, Prince MR, Grossman ME, et al. Contemporary applications and limitations of magnetic resonance imaging contrast materials. J Urol 2010;183(1): 27–33.

22. Lane BR, Babineau D, Kattan MW, et al. A preoperative prognostic nomogram for solid enhancing renal tumors 7 cm or less amenable to partial nephrectomy. J Urol 2007;178(2):429–34.

23. DeRoche T, Walker E, Magi-Galluzzi C, et al. Pathologic characteristics of solitary small renal masses: can they be predicted by preoperative clinical parameters? Am J Clin Pathol 2008;130(4):560–4.

24. Frank I, Blute ML, Cheville JC, et al. Solid renal tumors: an analysis of pathological features related to tumor size. J Urol 2003;170(6 Pt 1):2217–20.

25. Thompson RH, Kurta JM, Kaag M, et al. Tumor size is associated with malignant potential in renal cell carcinoma cases. J Urol 2009;181(5):2033–6.

26. Haramis G, Mues AC, Rosales JC, et al. Natural history of renal cortical neoplasms during active surveillance with follow-up longer than 5 years. Urology 2011;77(4):787–91.

27. Mues AC, Haramis G, Badani K, et al. Active surveillance for larger (cT1bN0M0 and cT2N0M0) renal cortical neoplasms. Urology 2010;76(3):620–3.

28. Bosniak MA, Birnbaum BA, Krinsky GA, et al. Small renal parenchymal neoplasms: further observations on growth. Radiology 1995;197(3):589–97.

29. Chawla SN, Crispen PL, Hanlon AL, et al. The natural history of observed enhancing renal masses: meta-analysis and review of the world literature. J Urol 2006;175(2):425–31.

30. Crispen PL, Wong YN, Greenberg RE, et al. Predicting growth of solid renal masses under active surveillance. Urol Oncol 2008;26(5):555–9.

31. Kunkle DA, Crispen PL, Chen DY, et al. Enhancing renal masses with zero net growth during active surveillance. J Urol 2007;177(3):849–53 [discussion: 853–4].

32. Kato M, Suzuki T, Suzuki Y, et al. Natural history of small renal cell carcinoma: evaluation of growth rate, histological grade, cell proliferation and apoptosis. J Urol 2004;172(3):863–6.

33. Birnbaum BA, Bosniak MA, Krinsky GA, et al. Renal cell carcinoma: correlation of CT findings with nuclear morphologic grading in 100 tumors. Abdom Imaging 1994;19(3):262–6.

34. Zhang J, Lefkowitz RA, Ishill NM, et al. Solid renal cortical tumors: differentiation with CT. Radiology 2007;244(2):494–504.
35. Alshumrani G, O'Malley M, Ghai S, et al. Small (< or = 4 cm) cortical renal tumors: characterization with multidetector CT. Abdom Imaging 2010;35(4):488–93.
36. Sun MR, Ngo L, Genega EM, et al. Renal cell carcinoma: dynamic contrast-enhanced MR imaging for differentiation of tumor subtypes—correlation with pathologic findings. Radiology 2009;250(3):793–802.
37. Pignot G, Elie C, Conquy S, et al. Survival analysis of 130 patients with papillary renal cell carcinoma: prognostic utility of type 1 and type 2 subclassification. Urology 2007;69(2):230–5.
38. Khan AA, Shergill IS, Quereshi S, et al. Percutaneous needle biopsy for indeterminate renal masses: a national survey of UK consultant urologists. BMC Urol 2007;7:10.
39. Campbell SC. The paradigm shift in renal mass biopsy. Clin Adv Hematol Oncol 2008;6(4):253–4, 8.
40. Wunderlich H, Hindermann W, Al Mustafa AM, et al. The accuracy of 250 fine needle biopsies of renal tumors. J Urol 2005;174(1):44–6.
41. Wood BJ, Khan MA, McGovern F, et al. Imaging guided biopsy of renal masses: indications, accuracy and impact on clinical management. J Urol 1999;161(5): 1470–4.
42. Volpe A, Mattar K, Finelli A, et al. Contemporary results of percutaneous biopsy of 100 small renal masses: a single center experience. J Urol 2008;180(6):2333–7.
43. Torp-Pedersen S, Juul N, Larsen T, et al. US-guided fine needle biopsy of solid renal masses–comparison of histology and cytology. Scand J Urol Nephrol Suppl 1991;137:41–3.
44. Dechet CB, Sebo T, Farrow G, et al. Prospective analysis of intraoperative frozen needle biopsy of solid renal masses in adults. J Urol 1999;162(4):1282–4 [discussion: 1284–5].
45. Richter F, Kasabian NG, Irwin RJ Jr, et al. Accuracy of diagnosis by guided biopsy of renal mass lesions classified indeterminate by imaging studies. Urology 2000;55(3):348–52.
46. Renshaw AA, Lee KR, Madge R, et al. Accuracy of fine needle aspiration in distinguishing subtypes of renal cell carcinoma. Acta Cytol 1997;41(4):987–94.
47. Blumenfeld AJ, Guru K, Fuchs GJ, et al. Percutaneous biopsy of renal cell carcinoma underestimates nuclear grade. Urology 2010;76(3):610–3.
48. Schmidbauer J, Remzi M, Memarsadeghi M, et al. Diagnostic accuracy of computed tomography-guided percutaneous biopsy of renal masses. Eur Urol 2008;53(5):1003–11.
49. Shannon BA, Cohen RJ, de Bruto H, et al. The value of preoperative needle core biopsy for diagnosing benign lesions among small, incidentally detected renal masses. J Urol 2008;180(4):1257–61 [discussion: 1261].
50. Neuzillet Y, Lechevallier E, Andre M, et al. Accuracy and clinical role of fine needle percutaneous biopsy with computerized tomography guidance of small (less than 4.0 cm) renal masses. J Urol 2004;171(5):1802–5.
51. Veltri A, Garetto I, Tosetti I, et al. Diagnostic accuracy and clinical impact of imaging-guided needle biopsy of renal masses. Retrospective analysis on 150 cases. Eur Radiol 2011;21(2):393–401.
52. Wang R, Wolf JS Jr, Wood DP Jr, et al. Accuracy of percutaneous core biopsy in management of small renal masses. Urology 2009;73(3):586–90 [discussion: 590–1].
53. Samplaski MK, Zhou M, Lane BR, et al. Renal mass sampling: an enlightened perspective. Int J Urol 2011;18(1):5–19.

54. Lechevallier E, Andre M, Barriol D, et al. Fine-needle percutaneous biopsy of renal masses with helical CT guidance. Radiology 2000;216(2):506–10.

55. Rybicki FJ, Shu KM, Cibas ES, et al. Percutaneous biopsy of renal masses: sensitivity and negative predictive value stratified by clinical setting and size of masses. AJR Am J Roentgenol 2003;180(5):1281–7.

56. Simmons MN, Brandina R, Hernandez AV, et al. Surgical management of bilateral synchronous kidney tumors: functional and oncological outcomes. J Urol 2010; 184(3):865–72 [quiz: 1235].

57. Go AS, Chertow GM, Fan D, et al. Chronic kidney disease and the risks of death, cardiovascular events, and hospitalization. N Engl J Med 2004;351(13): 1296–305.

58. Gill IS, Kavoussi LR, Lane BR, et al. Comparison of 1,800 laparoscopic and open partial nephrectomies for single renal tumors. J Urol 2007;178(1):41–6.

59. Thompson RH, Lane BR, Lohse CM, et al. Every minute counts when the renal hilum is clamped during partial nephrectomy. Eur Urol 2010;58(3):340–5.

60. Simmons MN, Schreiber MJ, Gill IS. Surgical renal ischemia: a contemporary overview. J Urol 2008;180(1):19–30.

61. Lane BR, Russo P, Uzzo RG, et al. Comparison of cold and warm ischemia during partial nephrectomy in 660 solitary kidneys reveals predominant role of nonmodifiable factors in determining ultimate renal function. J Urol 2011;185(2):421–7.

62. Simmons MN, Fergany AF, Campbell SC. Effect of parenchymal volume preservation on kidney function after partial nephrectomy. J Urol 2011, in press.

63. Miller DC, Hollingsworth JM, Hafez KS, et al. Partial nephrectomy for small renal masses: an emerging quality of care concern? J Urol 2006;175(3 Pt 1):853–7 [discussion: 858].

64. Campbell SC, Faraday M, Uzzo RG. Small renal mass. N Engl J Med 2010; 362(24):2334 [author reply: 2334–5].

65. Hinshaw JL, Shadid AM, Nakada SY, et al. Comparison of percutaneous and laparoscopic cryoablation for the treatment of solid renal masses. AJR Am J Roentgenol 2008;191(4):1159–68.

66. Matin SF, Ahrar K. Nephron-sparing probe ablative therapy: long-term outcomes. Curr Opin Urol 2008;18(2):150–6.

67. Berger A, Kamoi K, Gill IS, et al. Cryoablation for renal tumors: current status. Curr Opin Urol 2009;19(2):138–42.

68. Goldberg SN, Gazelle GS, Mueller PR. Thermal ablation therapy for focal malignancy: a unified approach to underlying principles, techniques, and diagnostic imaging guidance. AJR Am J Roentgenol 2000;174(2):323–31.

69. Weight CJ, Kaouk JH, Hegarty NJ, et al. Correlation of radiographic imaging and histopathology following cryoablation and radio frequency ablation for renal tumors. J Urol 2008;179(4):1277–81 [discussion: 1281–3].

70. Kunkle DA, Uzzo RG. Cryoablation or radiofrequency ablation of the small renal mass: a meta-analysis. Cancer 2008;113(10):2671–80.

71. Kutikov A, Egleston BL, Wong YN, et al. Evaluating overall survival and competing risks of death in patients with localized renal cell carcinoma using a comprehensive nomogram. J Clin Oncol 2010;28(2):311–7.

72. Remzi M, Ozsoy M, Klingler HC, et al. Are small renal tumors harmless? analysis of histopathological features according to tumors 4 cm or less in diameter. J Urol 2006;176(3):896–9.

73. Schlomer B, Figenshau RS, Yan Y, et al. Pathological features of renal neoplasms classified by size and symptomatology. J Urol 2006;176(4 Pt 1):1317–20 [discussion: 1320].

74. Pahernik S, Ziegler S, Roos F, et al. Small renal tumors: correlation of clinical and pathological features with tumor size. J Urol 2007;178(2):414–47 [discussion: 416–7].

75. Lamb GW, Bromwich EJ, Vasey P, et al. Management of renal masses in patients medically unsuitable for nephrectomy–natural history, complications, and outcome. Urology 2004;64(5):909–13.

76. Wehle MJ, Thiel DD, Petrou SP, et al. Conservative management of incidental contrast-enhancing renal masses as safe alternative to invasive therapy. Urology 2004;64(1):49–52.

77. Abouassaly R, Lane BR, Novick AC. Active surveillance of renal masses in elderly patients. J Urol 2008;180(2):505–8 [discussion: 508–9].

78. Kouba E, Smith A, McRackan D, et al. Watchful waiting for solid renal masses: insight into the natural history and results of delayed intervention. J Urol 2007; 177(2):466–70 [discussion: 470].

79. Abou Youssif T, Kassouf W, Steinberg J, et al. Active surveillance for selected patients with renal masses: updated results with long-term follow-up. Cancer 2007;110(5):1010–4.

80. Rosales JC, Haramis G, Moreno J, et al. Active surveillance for renal cortical neoplasms. J Urol 2010;183(5):1698–702.

81. Beland MD, Mayo-Smith WW, Dupuy DE, et al. Diagnostic yield of 58 consecutive imaging-guided biopsies of solid renal masses: should we biopsy all that are indeterminate? AJR Am J Roentgenol 2007;188(3):792–7.

82. Lebret T, Poulain JE, Molinie V, et al. Percutaneous core biopsy for renal masses: indications, accuracy and results. J Urol 2007;178(4 Pt 1):1184–8 [discussion: 1188].

83. Maturen KE, Nghiem HV, Caoili EM, et al. Renal mass core biopsy: accuracy and impact on clinical management. AJR Am J Roentgenol 2007;188(2):563–70.

84. Reichelt O, Gajda M, Chyhrai A, et al. Ultrasound-guided biopsy of homogenous solid renal masses. Eur Urol 2007;52(5):1421–6.

85. Somani BK, Nabi G, Thorpe P, et al. Image-guided biopsy-diagnosed renal cell carcinoma: critical appraisal of technique and long-term follow-up. Eur Urol 2007;51(5):1289–95 [discussion: 1296–7].

86. Masoom S, Venkataraman G, Jensen J, et al. Renal FNA-based typing of renal masses remains a useful adjunctive modality: evaluation of 31 renal masses with correlative histology. Cytopathology 2009;20(1):50–5.

The Role of Surgery in the Management of Early-Stage Renal Cancer

Paul Russo, MD

KEYWORDS

- Kidney cancer • Partial nephrectomy • Radical nephrectomy
- Renal tumors

There were an estimated 58,240 new cases and 13,040 deaths from kidney cancer in the United States in 2010.[1] Compared with 1971, this represents a fivefold increase in the incidence and twofold increase in the mortality of renal cancer. Associated risk factors for kidney cancer include hypertension, obesity, and African American race. Epidemiologic evidence suggests an increase in all stages of renal cancer, including the advanced and metastatic cases. It is now understood that renal cortical tumors (RCTs) are a family of distinct tumors with variable histology, cytogenetic defects, and metastatic potential.[2] Approximately 90% of the tumors that metastasize are the conventional clear cell carcinoma[3]; however, these account for only 54% of the resected tumors. Approximately 30% to 40% of patients with renal tumors will either present with or later develop metastatic disease. The widespread use of the modern abdominal imaging techniques (computed tomography [CT], magnetic resonance imaging [MRI], and ultrasound) over the past 2 decades, usually ordered to evaluate nonspecific abdominal and musculoskeletal complaints or during unrelated cancer care, has changed the profile of the typical patient with renal tumor from one with a massive, symptomatic tumor at presentation to one with a small, asymptomatic, renal mass (<4 cm) incidentally discovered in 70% of the cases.[4] A survival rate of 90% or greater, depending on the tumor histology, is expected for these small tumors whether partial (PN) or radical nephrectomy (RN) is performed.

RN was once considered the "gold standard" and used to treat all tumors, small and large, and even to solve diagnostic dilemmas when an uncertain renal mass was encountered. PN was used only in restricted conditions, such as tumor in a solitary kidney or in patients with conditions that compromised renal function. New concerns that RN could cause or worsen preexisting chronic kidney disease (CKD) has led to recommendations for more restricted use of RN, whether performed by open or

Urology Service, Department of Surgery, Memorial Sloan Kettering Cancer Center, Weill Medical College, Cornell University, 1275 York Avenue, New York, NY 10021, USA
E-mail address: RussoP@MSKCC.org

Hematol Oncol Clin N Am 25 (2011) 737–752
doi:10.1016/j.hoc.2011.04.009
0889-8588/11/$ – see front matter © 2011 Elsevier Inc. All rights reserved.

minimally invasive techniques, for the resection of large renal tumors, including those that destroy most of the kidney, invade the renal sinus, invade branched or main renal veins or extend into the inferior vena cava, and are associated with regional adenopathy or metastatic disease. The increased treatment and cure of small, incidentally discovered renal tumors, most of which are nonlethal in nature, has not offset the increased mortality caused by advanced and metastatic tumors. This "treatment disconnect" may result from unaccounted etiologic factors increasing the incidence of all RCTs and their virulence. In this article, the optimum approach to the surgical management of localized renal tumors and its impact on renal function are discussed.

RENAL CANCER SURGERY: HISTORICAL CONSIDERATIONS

Successful attempts to surgically cure renal tumors were reported widely after World War II, with surgical strategies designed to address the renal capsular and perinephric fat infiltration observed in up to 70% of the tumors.[5] Using a thoracoabdominal incision, Mortensen[6] reported the first radical nephrectomy in 1948, an operation that removed all of the contents of Gerota fascia. Radical nephrectomy was popularized in the 1960s by Robson,[7] who described the perifascial resection of the tumor-bearing kidney with its perirenal fat, regional lymph nodes, and ipsilateral adrenal gland. In 1969, Robson and colleagues[8] reported RN results in a series of 88 patients and described a 65% survival rate for tumors confined within Gerota fascia (Robson stage 1 and 2), but the finding of regional nodal metastases led to a less than 30% 5-year survival rate.

RN, ipsilateral adrenalectomy, and extensive regional lymphadenectomy, usually through large abdominal or transthoracic incisions, became the standard approach to renal tumors for the next 20 years as major centers began reporting favorable results.[9,10] In this era, the imaging studies used to diagnose a patient, who was usually symptomatic with a large renal tumor, was intravenous urograms, retrograde pyelograms, and arteriograms. These techniques were unable to detect small tumors and the incidental tumor detection rate was less than 5%. Despite this acceptance of RN by urologic surgeons, convincing data did not exist establishing the therapeutic impact of the component parts of the operation (ie, the need for adrenalectomy[11] or the need for and extent of lymph node dissection).[12,13] Historical series were subjected to selection biases, and the virtues of randomized trials in clinical investigation to address the many questions in kidney tumor surgery were not yet realized. Although a subsequent report with longer follow-up by Robson in 1982 projected declining long-term survival rates in the range of 40%,[14] there was no doubt that the surgical techniques associated with the safe removal of large renal tumors were established, well described, and reproducible, making RN the only effective treatment for RCTs. Today, at major centers with a commitment to renal tumor surgery, despite the previously described imaging induced stage and tumor size migration, RN is still required in approximately 20% to 30% of patients with renal tumors not amenable to kidney-sparing approaches.

In the past 20 years, surgical oncologists have increasingly used organ-sparing and limb-sparing approaches to treat malignancies, such as breast cancer and sarcoma, often with adjuvant chemotherapy or radiation therapy, with equivalent survival rates to their more radical predecessors. This approach was also applied to RCTs using PN, first for tumors of 4 cm or smaller and recently for tumors of 7 cm or smaller, with equivalent cancer-specific survival rates. Approximately 20% of resected renal tumors will be benign (ie, angiomyolipoma, oncocytoma, metanephric adenoma, or hemorrhagic cyst), 25% will be indolent (papillary, chromophobe carcinoma) with limited metastatic potential, and 55% will have the more potentially malignant conventional clear cell carcinoma that accounts for 90% of the metastatic renal tumors. Even for patients with T1 conventional clear cell carcinomas, a 90% long-term survival is anticipated. Using preoperative predictive nomograms coupled with the emerging view that preservation of renal function, particularly in elderly or comorbidly ill patients, is equally if not more important to the patient's long-term health than resection of a small renal mass, the use of active surveillance strategies is increasingly accepted.[15]

The introduction of laparoscopic RN by Clayman and colleagues[16,17] in 1991 began a new era of minimally invasive kidney surgery. McDougal and colleagues[18] investigated minimally invasive PN in the laboratory setting using a pig model, and in 1993 Winfield and colleagues[19] successfully performed the first laparoscopic partial nephrectomy (LPN). LPN is a technically demanding operation being increasingly used with success. Advances in minimally invasive instrumentation, including robotic assistance and dual-teaching counsels, coupled with sophisticated training simulators, may enhance the use of these techniques in the future.[20]

RENAL TUMOR SURGERY: PATIENT SELECTION AND PREOPERATIVE EVALUATION

To a large extent, the modern imaging studies of CT, ultrasound, and MRI that have been so effective in creating the era of the "incidentaloma" and the associated tumor size and stage migration, also provide the surgeon with an accurate description of the extent of disease before operation. At Memorial Sloan Kettering Cancer Center (MSKCC), tumors routinely selected for RN include those large and centrally localized tumors that have effectively replaced most of the normal renal parenchyma, often associated with regional adenopathy and renal vein extension.[21] In approximately 10% of patients with renal cell carcinoma, tumor involvement of major branched renal veins, the main renal vein, or extension into the inferior vena cava occurs. In the vast majority of these cases, preoperative imaging reveals the tumor thrombus and allows the surgical team to carefully plan its approach. In most cases, resection without venovenous bypass and cardiac bypass is possible with the prognosis directly related to the extent of disease. For patients with right atrial or ventricular renal tumor thrombus, open heart bypass with or without hypothermic arrest is required to complete the resection. Perioperative mortality can be up to 10% in those cases and completeness of the thrombectomy depends largely on whether the tumor thrombus is free floating in the caval lumen or has infiltrated the caval wall. For patients without regional nodal or distant metastatic disease, long-term survival is possible in 50% to 60% of patients, whereas the presence of either reduces survival to that of those patients undergoing cytoreductive nephrectomy.[22–25] In addition, RN is performed on patients with metastatic disease referred by medical oncology for cytoreductive nephrectomy before the initiation of systemic therapy.[26–28] Patients with extensive metastatic disease and a poor Karnofsky Performance Status are advised to undergo percutaneous needle biopsy of the primary tumor or a metastatic site and are subsequently referred for systemic therapy.

Although PN was initially restricted to patients with essential indications (tumor in an anatomic or functional solitary kidney, bilateral renal tumors, hereditary renal tumor syndromes), reports from the United States and abroad indicated that PN was not compromising the local tumor control or survival when compared with RN for patients with T1a renal tumors (4 cm or smaller) across all histologic subtypes with progression-free survival and metastasis-free survival the same whether PN or RN was performed.[15,29–31] The rationale for expanding the indications for PN to larger RCTs of 4 to 7 cm was articulated[32] and initial reports were met with similarly favorable results both in the United States and Europe.[33–35] A recently published report that combined the Mayo Clinic and MSKCC databases, evaluated 1159 patients with renal tumor between 4 and 7 cm treated with RN (n = 873, 75%) and PN (n = 286, 25%) and demonstrated no significant difference in survival between the groups.[36] We recently reported a series of even larger PN for T2 disease performed in 34 patients. Interestingly, 6 patients (16.2%) had benign and 12 patients (35%) had indolent (papillary or chromophobe) pathology. After 17 months of follow-up, 71% of patients with a malignant diagnosis are alive without evidence of disease. Although the resection of massive renal tumors (in this series up to 18 cm in diameter) is largely a function of favorable tumor location and careful case selection, this study indicates that local tumor control can be effectively achieved with results similar to those found in series of tumors of 7 cm or smaller.[37] Mayo Clinic investigators recently reported similar results in 276 patients with clinical stage higher than T2 treated with either PN (n = 69) or RN (n = 207).[38] These data indicate clearly that the ultimate oncological threat of a given tumor depends on biologic factors of the tumor, including histologic subtype, the presence or absence of symptoms, tumor grade, and tumor size with prognostic nomograms and algorithms available to predict outcomes with reasonable accuracy.[3,39] PN is clearly on firm oncological footing for T1 renal tumors. Over the past 3 years at our center, 1030 surgical nephrectomies have been performed with 21% RN and 79% PN, reflecting our center's commitment to kidney-sparing approaches whenever possible.

Before the operation, routine serum chemistries, coagulation profile, type and cross match (or autologous blood donation), and chest x-ray are obtained. Routine brain imaging and bone scanning are not performed unless site-specific abnormalities in the history, physical, or routine preoperative laboratory examination are discovered. For patients with significant comorbid conditions, particularly cardiac and pulmonary related, appropriate consultations are obtained with an effort made to optimize patients for operation whenever possible. Patients with significant coronary or carotid artery disease may require revascularization before operation. For patients with compromised pulmonary status, consultation with anesthesiology is requested for consideration of epidural postoperative analgesia.

OPEN RENAL TUMOR SURGERY: SURGICAL ANATOMY AND OPERATIVE CONSIDERATIONS

The kidneys are retroperitoneal organs located in the lumbar fossa. They are covered with a variable amount of perinephric fat and Gerota fascia and lay in proximity to the psoas major and quadratus lumborum muscles, and diaphragm. Depending on the patient's body habitus, the size of the tumor, and its relationship to adjacent organs such as the colon, duodenum, pancreas, and spleen, different surgical incisions can be used including subcostal, thoracoabdominal, 11th rib flank, and midline abdominal.[21] Transabdominal approaches are preferred for massive tumors with regional adenopathy and renal vein and inferior vena caval extension because access to major renal vessels and aorta and inferior vena cava can be optimized. Early ligation and division of the renal artery effectively decrease blood flow to the tumor-involved kidney, decompress fragile and engorged tumor parasitic vessels, and enhance the mobility of the kidney during its resection, all of which can facilitate the tumor resection and decrease intraoperative bleeding. This approach negates the need for preoperative renal artery embolization, which can be a painful and costly procedure. Before its division, the renal vein should be inspected and gently palpated to exclude a renal vein tumor thrombus. For smaller tumors requiring an RN and for all PNs, a "miniflank incision" has the advantage of speedy entry into the retroperitoneum and avoidance of the rib resection with a decreased likelihood (<5%) of subsequent atony of the flank muscles and bulge.[40]

Although the traditional RN described by Robson included ipsilateral adrenalectomy and regional lymph node dissection, no convincing evidence exists that these component parts offer a therapeutic advantage.[11–13,41] Contemporary survival data indicate that the presence of lymph node metastasis and/or adrenal metastasis has a similar negative prognostic impact to distant metastatic disease with median survival rates of less than 12 months. For patients undergoing RN for massive renal tumors, the rationale for ipsilateral adrenalectomy and regional node dissection is to maximize local tumor control and provide accurate pathologic staging information that may lead to entry into adjuvant systemic therapy clinical trials using the newly developed mTOR and tyrosine kinase inhibitors. It is our practice to perform ipsilateral adrenalectomy and regional node dissection to maximize local tumor control, decrease the chance of local recurrence if these tissues are harboring micrometastatic disease, and provide maximum pathologic staging to allow entry into ongoing adjuvant clinical trials.

Once the tumor resection is accomplished, postoperative nomograms are available that incorporate clinical presentation, tumor histologic subtype, size, and stage to provide a clinical prognosis. Results for our center indicate 5-year survival rates following resection of nonmetastatic tumors range from 30% to 98% depending on the previously mentioned clinical and pathologic features. These postoperative nomograms have been extremely useful in patient counseling, tailoring cost-effective follow-up strategies, and designing clinical trials.[3,39,42]

MINIMALLY INVASIVE APPROACHES TO EARLY-STAGE RENAL TUMOR

Following its introduction in 1991 by Clayman and colleagues,[16,17] laparoscopic radical nephrectomy (LRN) offered a minimally invasive alternative to the classical open RN with dividends of less wound pain and morbidity, decreased analgesic requirement, decreased hospitalization, more rapid convalescence, and faster return to normal activities. Survival rates were directly comparable with those achieved with open RN.[43–47] At the time of its introduction, RN in general was the preferred treatment for all renal masses and PN was largely reserved for only essential cases where RN would put a patient at risk for dialysis.

However, at centers with expertise in both open and minimally invasive renal surgical approaches, published experiences revealed inconsistencies in the management of small renal tumors. Open surgeons were more likely to perform PN, and laparoscopic surgeons were more likely to perform RN. These reports suggested that minimally invasive surgery learning curves were being conquered by RN applied to small renal tumors (<4 cm) despite the previously described clinical data that this was surgical overkill and deleterious to the patients' overall renal function.[48,49] Unique issues relative to minimally invasive renal surgery, such as the problem of tumor-bearing kidney retrieval (ie, morcellation vs an open extraction incision for removal) were debated in the literature. The case load required to extend the surgical limits for minimally invasive surgery was not known and the decision to perform open versus minimally invasive surgery kidney procedures more often depended on the relative surgical expertise of the individual surgeon rather than more clearly defined guidelines relating to tumor size and concerns about future renal function.

By 2000, because of the emerging literature supporting elective PN, several minimally invasive surgery groups began concerted efforts to develop laparoscopic PN techniques intending to closely simulate the open procedure, initially with smaller, exophytic renal tumors and, with time and increasing experience, to more complex centrally located or cystic renal tumors. Valiant attempts to duplicate the renal protective effects of cold ischemia, readily obtained in open PN, were reported and included cold renal arterial and ureteral perfusions, and recently, laparoscopic ice slush placement. Nonetheless, the vast majority of LPNs (many of which are complex) continue to be performed under warm ischemic conditions with the hope that rapid completion of the operation will limit any long-term ischemic effects on the kidney. Even for these expert surgeons, laparoscopic PN is currently described as a "complex" or "advanced" operation with published complication rates that are 3 to 4 times higher than for their open counterparts.[50,51] Interestingly, LPN teams report similar rates of resected benign lesions (20%–30%) and similar beneficial effects on overall renal function, as described previously in the open PN experience.

Investigators from the Mayo Clinic, Cleveland Clinic, and Johns Hopkins pooled their data on 1800 PNs of which 771 were LPNs and 1028 were open PNs for T1 tumors from 1998 to 2005. Even though the surgeons at these centers were experts in their respective laparoscopic and open operations, careful case selection was apparent. Patients who had open PN had larger tumors that were more likely centrally located and malignant, were at higher risk of perioperative complications as defined by their older age, increased comorbidities, decreased performance status, and decreased baseline renal function, all of which may have contributed to longer hospital stays for open PN (5.8 days) versus LPN (3.3 days). Patients in the LPN group were more likely to have elective indications rather than essential indications for PN, yet LPN was associated with longer ischemic time, more postoperative complications, particularly urologic, and increased number of subsequent procedures to treat complications. This comprehensive study leaves little doubt that the LPN is a technically challenging operation, even in the hands of such experts, where careful case selection may decrease the chance of surgical and urological complications.[52]

As minimally invasive surgeons gain more experience and instrumentation improves, coupled with further refinements in case selection, it is expected that complications related to LPN will decrease and larger tumors and those in the near the renal hilum will be increasingly resectable.[53,54] Surgeons are increasingly using robotic-assisted techniques to perform RN and PN with outcomes related to estimated blood loss and complications similar to classical laparoscopic techniques but, not surprisingly, with operating time and costs significantly greater in the robotic-assisted cases.[20,55–57] At this time, despite the published enthusiasm of many surgeons, little evidence exists that robotic techniques have a substantial advantage over standard laparoscopic techniques.

Renal tumor ablative modalities, including percutaneous and laparoscopic approaches to radiofrequency ablation (RFA) and cryoablation, are offered selectively to some patients with renal tumors that are exophytic and not encroaching upon renal hilar vessels or collecting system elements.[58] Patients considered by many as ideal candidates for ablation are often old or comorbidly ill individuals harboring small renal tumors, the very patients ideally suited for active surveillance.[59,60] Although the concept of nonsurgical ablation is appealing, the literature has serious deficiencies, including up to 40% of patients not having preablation confirmation of tumor owing to nondiagnostic or nonexistent biopsy, short overall follow-up, and high rates of tumor recurrence compared with PN ranging from 7.45-fold to 18.23-fold greater for RFA and cryotherapy respectively.[61] Additionally, because most studies lacked pathologic confirmation to confirm the completeness of the ablation, it is not known whether changes in radiological images after ablation represent complete or partial tumor destruction or simply a renal tumor, partially treated and not in active growth. The Cleveland Clinic experience reports difficult salvage operations after failed ablations, which usually lead to RN as the final outcome in a patient population initially candidates for either active surveillance or PN, an outcome that now must be viewed as unfavorable from both oncological and renal functional points of view.[62] Carefully designed "ablate and resect" clinical protocols need to be done, much like those done in the 1990s for cryotherapy in localized prostate cancer, to determine the true effectiveness of these approaches.

COMPLICATIONS OF RENAL TUMOR SURGERY

Complications of RN (n = 688) and PN (n = 361) were analyzed in a large MSKCC series using a graded 5-tiered scale based on the severity and the intensity of treatment required. For RN, there was a 3% complication rate directly related to the procedure, including adjacent organ damage, hemorrhage, and bowel obstruction with a surgical reintervention rate of 0.6%. There were 3 postoperative deaths attributable to myocardial infarction and pulmonary embolism. For PN, the commonest procedure-related complication was urinary fistula (9%), with reinterventions (2.5%) either by interventional radiology (percutaneous drainage) or endoscopy (stenting). Tumor location or elective or essential PN indications did not affect the complication rate.[63] Using the same 5-tiered complications grading scale, Cleveland Clinic minimally invasive surgeons evaluated 200 consecutive patients undergoing LPN using either transperitoneal or retroperitoneal approaches for cases performed between 2003 and 2005. A total of 35 patients (17%) experienced a complication. Of these, 29% and 42% were grade 1 and 2 respectively. Conversion to open radical (2 patients) and laparoscopic radical (1 patient) was an uncommon event.[64] Compared with their initial experience with LPN in 200 patients,[50] the investigators felt that their increased experience with laparoscopic techniques and ability to resect more complicated tumors based on size and location indicated that technical improvements in the operation were decreasing the overall complications by 44%, urological complications by 56%, and hemorrhagic complications by 53%.[65] A recent report refutes the notion that complications are more likely in elderly patients undergoing PN as opposed to RN and therefore surgeons should not deny PN to patients who by definition because of their age have a decreased renal reserve and would profit the most.[66]

RADICAL NEPHRECTOMY: ADVERSE RENAL MEDICAL IMPACT

A historical misconception exists that RN can cause a permanent rise in serum creatinine because of the sacrifice of normal renal parenchyma not involved by tumor, but will not cause serious long-term side effects as long as the patient has a normal contralateral kidney. The renal transplantation literature is cited as the clinical evidence to support this view because patients undergoing donor nephrectomy have not been reported to have higher rates of kidney failure requiring dialysis or death.[67] However, distinct differences between kidney donors and patients with kidney tumors exist. Donors tend to be carefully screened for medical comorbidities and are generally young (age 45 or younger).[68,69] In contrast, patients with renal tumors are not screened, are older (mean age 61 years), and many have significant comorbidities affecting baseline kidney function, including metabolic syndrome, hypertension, coronary artery disease, obesity, vascular disease, and diabetes. In addition, as patients age, particularly beyond 60 years, nephrons atrophy and glomerular filtration rate progressively decreases.[70] A study of 110 nephrectomy specimens in which the non–tumor-bearing kidney was examined demonstrated extensive and unsuspected underlying renal disease, including vascular sclerosis, diabetic nephropathy, glomerular hypertrophy, mesangial expansion, and diffuse glomerulosclerosis.[71] Only 10% of patients had completely normal renal tissue adjacent to the tumor.

Evidence that RN could cause a significant rise in the serum creatinine when compared with PN in patients with RCTs of 4 cm or smaller was published by investigators from the Mayo Clinic and MSKCC in 2000 and 2002, respectively. Patients who had RN were more likely to have elevated serum creatinine levels to higher than 2.0 ng/mL and proteinuria (Mayo Study),[72] a persistent finding even when study patients were carefully matched for associated risk factors (MSKCC study), including diabetes, smoking history, preoperative serum creatinine, and American Society of Anesthesiologists score.[73] In both studies, oncological outcomes were highly favorable (>90% survival rates) whether PN or RN was done.

CKD, defined as an estimated glomerular filtration rate (eGFR) of less than 60 mL/min/1.73 m^2, is increasingly viewed as a major public health problem in the United States and since 2003 is considered an independent cardiovascular risk factor.[74–78] An estimated 19 million adults in the United States have CKD and by the year 2030, 2 million will be in need of chronic dialysis or renal transplantation.[79] Traditional risk factors for CKD include age older than 60, hypertension, diabetes, cardiovascular disease, and family history of renal disease, factors also common in the population of patients who develop RCTs. A study involving 1,120,295 patients demonstrated a direct correlation between CKD and rates of hospitalization, cardiovascular events, and death, which occurred before overt renal failure requiring dialysis or renal transplantation.[80] As kidney function deteriorated, the percentage of patients with 2 associated cardiovascular risk factors increased from 34.7% (stage 1 and 2 CKD) to 83.6% (for stage 3) to 100% for stage 4 and 5 subjects. Patients with CKD are more likely to require medical interventions to treat cardiovascular disease than those with normal renal function. The low prevalence of patients with stage 4 or 5 CKD is attributable to their 5-year survival rates of only 30%.[81]

A concern that the overzealous use of RN, particularly in patients with small renal masses and common comorbidities that can affect renal function, could be causing or worsening preexisting CKD became a focus of intense research. MSKCC investigators used a widely available formula, the Modification in Diet and Renal Disease (MDRD) equation[82] (http://www.nephron.com/MDRD_GFR.cgi), to estimate the glomerular filtration rate (eGFR) in a retrospective cohort study of 662 patients with a normal serum creatinine and 2 healthy kidneys who underwent either elective PN or RN for an RCT 4 cm or smaller in diameter. To their surprise, 171 patients (26%) had preexisting CKD (GFR <60) before operation. Data were analyzed using 2 threshold definitions of CKD, a GFR lower than 60 mL/min/1.73 m^2 or a GFR lower than 45 mL/min/1.73 m^2. After surgery, the 3-year probability of freedom from new onset of GFR lower than 60 was 80% after PN but only 35% after RN. Corresponding values for 3-year probability of freedom from a GFR lower than 45, a more severe level of CKD, was 95% for PN and 64% for RN. Multivariable analysis indicated that RN was an independent risk factor for the development of new-onset CKD.[83] Mayo Clinic investigators identified 648 patients from 1989 to 2003 treated with RN or PN for a solitary renal tumor smaller than or equal to 4 cm with a normal contralateral kidney. In 327 patients younger than 65, it was found that RN was significantly associated with an increased risk of death, which persisted after adjusting for year of surgery, diabetes, Charlson-Romano index, and tumor histology.[84] Using the Surveillance, Epidemiology and End Results (SEER) cancer registry data linked with Medicare claims, MSKCC investigators studied 2991 patients older than 65 years for resected renal tumors of 4 cm or smaller from 1995 to 2002. A total of 254 patients (81%) underwent RN and

556 patients underwent PN. During a median follow-up of 4 years, 609 patients experienced a cardiovascular event and 892 patients died. After adjusting for preoperative demographic and comorbidity variables, RN was associated with a 1.38 times increased risk of overall mortality and a 1.40 times greater number of cardiovascular events.[85]

Similar results were reported in patients undergoing laparoscopic RN and PN.[86] Because of these reports, urologists are now increasingly aware that CKD status can be created or preexisting CKD significantly worsened by the liberal use of RN for the treatment of the small renal mass.[87] Short-term end points, including length of hospital stay, analgesic requirements, and cosmetic elements viewed by many as the reason to elect laparoscopic RN, must now be tempered by concerns that RN causes or worsens preexisting CKD and decreases overall patient survival. The most recent American Urologists Association guidelines for the management of the small renal tumor emphasize these points and strongly support the use of PN whenever technically feasible.[88]

RADICAL NEPHRECTOMY IS OVERUSED

Despite the well-described oncological and medical arguments in the contemporary literature supporting PN as an ideal treatment for small renal masses, the urological oncology community continues to use RN as the predominant treatment of the T1a renal mass. A cross-sectional view of clinical practice using the Nationwide Inpatient Sample revealed that only 7.5% of kidney tumor operations in the United States from 1988 to 2002 were PN.[89] Using the SEER database, investigators from the University of Michigan reported that from 2001, only 20% of all RCTs between 2 and 4 cm were treated by PN[90] and using the SEER database linked to Medicare claims, Huang and colleagues[85] from MSKCC reported a use rate of only 19% for T1a tumors (4 cm or smaller). Interestingly and for uncertain reasons, women and elderly patients are more likely to be treated with RN.[91] Many urologists believe a "quick" RN in an elderly patient would expose the patient to fewer postoperative complications than would a PN. However, MSKCC investigators, evaluating age and type of procedure performed in 1712 patients with kidney tumors, found the interactive term was not significant, indicating a lack of statistical evidence that the risk of complications associated with PN increased with advancing age. Furthermore, no evidence was reported linking age to estimated blood loss or operative time. Given the advantages of renal functional preservation, the investigators concluded that elderly patients should be perfectly eligible for PN.[66]

Although the urology literature has a great many articles written concerning the use of laparoscopic techniques to resect kidney tumors, the penetrance of laparoscopic RN according to the National Inpatient Sample from 1991 to 2003 was only 4.6%, with a peak incidence of 16.0% in 2003. These data indicate that the bulk of "kidney-wasting operations" are being done by traditional open surgical approaches.[92] In England, a similar under use of PN was reported in 2002 with only 108 (4%) PNs of 2671 nephrectomies performed.[93] Investigators at MSKCC tracked nephrectomy use in 1533 patients between 2000 and 2007, excluding patients with bilateral tumors and tumors in a solitary kidney and including only patients with an eGFR of greater than 45 mL/min/1.73 m[2]. Overall, 854 (56%) patients underwent PN and 679 (44%) underwent RN. In the 820 patients with a renal tumor of 4 cm or smaller, the frequency of PN increased from 69% in 2000 to 89% in 2007. In the 365 patients with a renal tumor from 4 to 7 cm, the frequency of PN increased from 20% in 2000 to 60% in 2007. Despite a commitment to kidney-sparing operations during this time frame by the MSKCC group, multivariate analysis indicated that PN was a significantly favored approach for males, younger patients, smaller tumors, and open surgeons.[94]

LONG-TERM FOLLOW-UP AFTER RESECTION OF LOCALIZED RENAL TUMORS

No uniform guidelines have been established for the follow-up of patients who have undergone surgical treatment of renal cell carcinoma.[95] Despite emerging evidence that some patients can benefit from aggressive surgical treatment of limited meta-static disease, different practices exist among urologic surgeons regarding the search for and management of recurrent disease. The intensity of follow-up and the tests ordered during follow-up also vary from center to center. In the absence of effective systemic therapy for metastatic disease, overly compulsive follow-up may diagnose asymptomatic metastatic disease earlier but not necessarily provide a therapeutic advantage. Excessive costs and patient anxiety may also occur unnecessarily during this follow-up. In addition, the previously described evidence that RN can have a dele-terious effect on renal function requires strict surveillance over renal function as well surveillance over the contralateral kidney that has a small (<5%) but real chance of developing an asynchronous RCT.[96]

Follow-up strategies were proposed from a nephrectomy series by Sandock and colleagues[97] after a detailed analysis of the pattern of metastatic disease progression, sites of metastatic failure, and the efficacy of tests required to diagnose recurrence. These investigators reviewed 137 patients with node-negative, nonmetastatic renal cell carcinoma who underwent radical nephrectomy between 1979 and 1993 at the Case Western–affiliated hospitals. Recurrence correlated closely with the clinical stage of the tumor at the time of diagnosis. Using the older American Joint Committee on Cancer classification (T1<2.5 cm), no patients with T1 disease relapsed, and 15% of patients with T2 and 53% of patients with T3 tumors relapsed. Of the 19 patients in whom pulmonary metastases developed, 14 (74%) had cough, dyspnea, pleuritic chest pain, or hemoptysis. In all patients with pulmonary metastases, the metastatic disease was diagnosed by a plain chest x-ray. Of the 13 patients in this series who developed intra-abdominal metastatic disease, 12 (92%) complained of abdominal symptoms or had abnormal liver function studies that led to the diagnosis. All 10 patients who developed bone metastases complained of new bone pain that directed the diagnosis by plain film and bone scan. Only one patient had an isolated brain metastasis, which was associated with central nervous system symptoms and was confirmed by brain CT. Two patients developed cutaneous metastases that were detected on physical examination. In this series, 85% of patients who experienced a recurrence of their disease did so during the first 3 years after nephrectomy, with the remaining relapses occurring between 3.4 and 11.4 years.

Levy and colleagues[98] from M.D. Anderson Cancer Center tracked the pattern of recurrence in 286 patients with P1-3N0 or Nx RCC operated on between 1985 and 1995. Perhaps reflecting the previously described stage migration that has occurred in RCC over the past 10 years, 59 (62%) of 92 patients diagnosed with metastatic disease were asymptomatic, including 32 detected by routine chest x-ray and 12 detected by routine blood work. Isolated asymptomatic intra-abdominal metastases were diagnosed by surveillance CT scan in only 6 patients (9%). As in the Sandock and colleagues'[97] study, as the P stage increased, the likelihood of recurrence increased from 7% for P1, 27% for P2, and 39% for P3, leading the investigatotrs to conclude that a stage-specific surveillance protocol would tailor the follow-up eval-uation intensity with the relative risk of recurrence.

At MSKCC, we use postoperative nomograms[3,39,42] that incorporate the tumor histologic subtype, tumor size, and mode of presentation with the P stage to fashion our follow-ups. Following the postoperative recovery, we generally see P1 (<7 cm) and P2 non–clear cell histology (papillary, chromophobe) patients back every 6 months with renal function studies and yearly with an imaging study of the remaining kidney (CT or renal ultrasound), chest x-ray, and renal function studies for a total of 3 years and then a yearly visit usually with CT chest/abdomen/pelvis or renal ultrasound and chest x-ray. For tumors higher than P2 (P3a-c, P4) particularly with conventional clear cell histology, we perform biannual chest x-ray and annual CT scan of the chest, abdomen, and pelvis coupled with renal function studies at each visit. Routine brain or bone scans are not performed unless the patient reports symptoms referable to those sites. Renal cell carcinoma is notorious for unusual, late, symptomatic, metastatic recurrences in organs such as the pancreas, thyroid, skin, duodenum, and adrenal glands. These recurrences are often mistaken for new primary tumors and aggressive surgical resection is undertaken and can be associated with long-term survival depending on patient age, the number of sites of metastases, and disease-free interval.[99,100] Whether such metastasectomy procedures are truly therapeutic or patient survival is within the confines of the often long and unpredictable natural history of renal cell carcinoma is not known.

SUMMARY

Modern imaging capabilities have created a renal tumor stage and size migration with approximately 70% of patients today detected incidentally with a median tumor size of 4 cm or smaller. In addition, our current understanding indicates that RCTs are a family of neoplasms with distinct histopathological and cytogenetic features and variable metastatic potential. The conventional clear cell tumor has a malignant potential and accounts for only 54% of the total RCTs but 90% of those that metastasize. RN nephrectomy, whether performed by open or minimally invasive surgical technique, plays an important role in the management of massive renal tumors that have replaced the normal renal parenchyma, invade the renal vein, and have associated regional lymphadenopathy or metastatic disease. For patients with smaller tumors amenable to PN, RN should not be performed because it is associated with the causation or worsening of preexisting CKD, which can cause an increased likelihood of cardiovascular morbidity and mortality. Despite a wealth of evidence supporting the more restricted indications for RN, strong evidence exists that it remains overused in the United States. Widespread education and training in kidney-preserving surgical strategies is essential going forward.

REFERENCES

1. Jemal A, Siegal R, Xu J, et al. Cancer statistics 2010. CA Cancer J Clin 2010;60: 277–300.
2. Linehan WM, Walther MM, Zbar B. The genetic basis of cancer of the kidney. J Urol 2003;170:2163–72.
3. Kattan MW, Reuter VE, Motzer RJ, et al. A postoperative prognostic nomogram for renal cell carcinoma. J Urol 2001;166:63–7, 2010.
4. Russo P. Renal cell carcinoma: presentation, staging, and surgical treatment. Semin Oncol 2000;27:160–76.
5. Beare JB, McDonald JR. Involvement of renal capsule in surgically removed hypernephroma: gross and histopathological study. J Urol 1949;61:857–61.
6. Mortensen H. Transthoracic nephrectomy. J Urol 1948;60:855.

7. Robson CJ. Radical nephrectomy for renal cell carcinoma. J Urol 1963;89:37.
8. Robson CJ, Churchill BM, Andersen W. The results of radical nephrectomy for renal cell carcinoma. J Urol 1969;101:297.
9. Skinner DG, Colvin RB, Vermillion CD, et al. Diagnosis and management of renal cell carcinoma: a clinical and pathological study of 309 cases. Cancer 1971;28: 1165–77.
10. Patel NP, Lavengood RW. Renal cell carcinoma: natural history and results of treatment. J Urol 1978;119:722.
11. Sagalowsky AI, Kadesky KT, Ewalt DM, et al. Factors influencing adrenal metastases in renal cell carcinoma. J Urol 1994;151:1181–4.
12. Herrlinger JA, Schrott KM, Schott G, et al. What are the benefits of extended dissection of the regional lymph nodes in the therapy of renal cell carcinoma? J Urol 1991;146:1224.
13. Ditonno P, Traficante A, Battaglia M, et al. Role of lymphadenectomy in renal cell carcinoma. Prog Clin Biol Res 1992;378:169.
14. Robson CJ. Results of radical thoraco-abdominal nephrectomy in the treatment of renal cell carcinoma. Prog Clin Biol Res 1982;100:481–8.
15. Russo P, Huang W. The medical and oncological rationale for partial nephrectomy for treatment of T1 renal cortical tumors. Urol Clin North Am 2008;35: 635–43.
16. Clayman RV, Kavoussi L, Soper NJ, et al. Laparoscopic nephrectomy. N Engl J Med 1991;324:1370–1.
17. Clayman RV, Kavoussi LR, Soper NJ. Laparoscopic nephrectomy: initial case report. J Urol 1991;146:278.
18. McDougall EM, Clayman RV, Chandhoke PJ, et al. Laparoscopic partial nephrectomy in the pig model. J Urol 1993;149:1633–6.
19. Winfield HN, Donovan JF, Clayman RV. Laparoscopic partial nephrectomy: initial case report for benign disease. J Endourol 1993;7:521–6.
20. Gettman MT, Blute ML, Chow GK. Robotic-assisted laparoscopic partial nephrectomy: initial experience. J Urol 2006;176:36.
21. Russo P. Open radical nephrectomy for localized renal cell carcinoma. In: Vogelzang NJ, editor. Genitourinary oncology. 3rd edition. Philadelphia: Lippincott Williams and Wilkins; 2006. p. 725–31.
22. Rabbani F, Hakimian P, Reuter VE, et al. Renal vein or inferior vena caval extension in patients with renal cortical tumors: impact of tumor histology. J Urol 2004; 171(3):1057–61.
23. Martinez-Salamanca JI, Millan I, Bertini R, et al, International Renal Cell Carcinoma-Venous Thrombus Consortium. Prognostic impact of the 2009 UICCA/AJCC TMN Staging system for renal cell carcinoma with venous extension. Eur Urol 2011;59(1):120–7.
24. Kaag MG, Toyen C, Russo P, et al. Radical nephrectomy with vena caval thrombectomy: a contemporary experience. BJU Int 2011;107:1386–93.
25. Feifer A, Savage C, Rayala H, et al. Prognostic impact of muscular venous branch invasion in localized renal cell carcinoma cases. J Urol 2011;185:37–42.
26. Flanigan RC, Salmon SE, Blumenstein BA, et al. Nephrectomy followed by interferon alfa-2b compared with interferon alfa-2b alone for metastatic renal-cell cancer. N Engl J Med 2001;23:1655–9.
27. Russo P, O'Brien MF. Surgical intervention in patients with metastatic renal cancer: metastasectomy and cytoreductive nephrectomy. Urol Clin North Am 2008;35:679–86.

28. Russo P. Multi-modal treatment for metastatic renal cancer—the role of surgery. World J Urol 2010;28:295–301.
29. Uzzo RG, Novick AC. Nephron sparing surgery for renal tumors: indications, techniques, and outcomes. J Urol 2001;166:6–18.
30. Lee CT, Katz J, Shi W, et al. Surgical management of renal tumors of 4 cm or less in a contemporary cohort. J Urol 2000;163:730–6.
31. Lessage K, Joniau S, Fransis K, et al. Comparison between open partial and radical nephrectomy for renal tumours: perioperative outcome and health-related quality of life. Eur Urol 2007;51:614.
32. Russo P, Goetzl M, Simmons R, et al. Partial nephrectomy: the rationale for expanding the indications. Ann Surg Oncol 2002;9:680–7.
33. Leibovich BC, Blute ML, Cheville JC, et al. Nephron sparing surgery for appropriately selected renal cell carcinoma between 4 and 7 cm resulting in outcome similar to radical nephrectomy. J Urol 2004;171:1066–70.
34. Dash A, Vickers AJ, Schachter LR, et al. Comparison of outcomes in elective partial vs. radical nephrectomy for clear cell renal cell carcinoma of 4–7 cm. BJU Int 2006;97:939–45.
35. Pahernik S, Roos F, Rohrig B, et al. Elective nephron sparing surgery for renal cell carcinoma larger than 4 cm. J Urol 2008;179:71–4.
36. Thompson HR, Siddiqui S, Lohse CM, et al. Evaluation of partial versus radical nephrectomy for renal cortical tumors 4–7 cm. J Urol 2009;182:2601–6.
37. Karellas ME, O'Brien MF, Jang TL, et al. Partial nephrectomy for selected renal cortical tumors greater than 7 centimeters. BJU Int 2010;106:1484–7.
38. Breau RH, Crispen PL, Jimenez RE, et al. Outcome of stage T2 or greater renal cell cancer treated with partial nephrectomy. J Urol 2010;183:903–8.
39. Lane BR, Kattan MW. Prognostic models and algorithms in renal cell carcinoma. Urol Clin North Am 2008;35:613–25.
40. Diblasio CJ, Snyder ME, Russo P. Mini flank supra-eleventh incision for open partial or radical nephrectomy. BJU Int 2006;97(1):149–56.
41. Vasselli JR, Yang JC, Linehan WM, et al. Lack of retroperitoneal lymphadenopathy predicts survival of patients with metastatic renal cell carcinoma. J Urol 2001;166:68.
42. Sorbellini M, Kattan MW, Snyder ME, et al. A postoperative prognostic nomogram predicting recurrence for patients with conventional clear cell renal cell carcinoma. J Urol 2005;173:48–51.
43. Dunn MD, Portis AJ, Shalhav AL, et al. Laparoscopic versus open radical nephrectomy: 9-year experience. J Urol 2000;164:1153–9.
44. Chan DY, Cadeddu JA, Jarrett TW, et al. Laparoscopic radical nephrectomy: cancer control for renal cell carcinoma. J Urol 2001;166:2095–100.
45. Makhoul B, De La Taille A, Vordos D, et al. Laparoscopic radical nephrectomy for T1 renal cancer: the gold standard? A comparison of laparoscopic vs. open nephrectomy. BJU Int 2004;93:67–70.
46. Matin S, Gill I, Worley S, et al. Outcome of laparoscopic radical nephrectomy for sporadic 4 cm or less renal tumor with a normal contra lateral kidney. J Urol 2002;168:1356–60.
47. Gill IS, Meraney AM, Schweizer DK, et al. Laparoscopic radical nephrectomy in 100 patients. Cancer 2001;92:1843–55.
48. Scherr DS, Ng C, Munver R, et al. Practice patterns among urologic surgeons treating localized renal cell carcinoma in the laparoscopic age: technology vs. oncology. Urology 2003;62:1007–11.

49. Russo P. Evolving strategies for renal tumor surgery: whether by open or by laparoscopic approaches, do the right operation! Urol Oncol 2005;23:456–7.

50. Ramani AP, Desai MM, Steinberg AP, et al. Complications of laparoscopic partial nephrectomy in 200 cases. J Urol 2005;173:42–7.

51. Kim FJ, Rha KH, Hernandez F, et al. Laparoscopic radical versus partial nephrectomy: assessment of complications. J Urol 2003;170:408–11.

52. Gill IS, Kavoussi LR, Lane BR, et al. Comparison of 1800 laparoscopic and open partial nephrectomies for single renal tumors. J Urol 2007;178:41–6.

53. Simmons MN, Weight CJ, Gill IS. Laparoscopic radical versus partial nephrectomy for tumors >4 cm: intermediate-term oncologic and functional outcomes. Urology 2009;73(5):1077–82.

54. Gill IS, Colombo JR, Frank I, et al. Laparoscopic partial nephrectomy for hilar tumors. J Urol 2005;174:850.

55. Aron M, Koenig P, Kaouk JH, et al. Robotic and laparoscopic partial nephrectomy: a matched pair comparison from a high volume centre. BJU Int 2008;102:86–92.

56. Roger M, Lucas SM, Popp SC, et al. Comparison of robotic assisted laparoscopic nephrectomy with laparoscopic and hand assisted laparoscopic nephrectomy. JSLS 2010;14:374–88.

57. Gupta GN, Boris R, Chung P, et al. Robot assisted laparoscopic partial nephrectomy for tumors greater than 4cm and high nephrometry score: feasibility, renal functional and oncological outcomes with minimum 1 year follow up. Urol Oncol Feb 1, 2011. [Epub ahead of print].

58. Gill IS, Remer EM, Hasan WA, et al. Renal cryoablation: outcome at 3 years. J Urol 2005;173:1903–7.

59. Wehle MJ, Thiel DD, Petrou SP, et al. Conservative management of incidental contrast-enhancing renal masses as safe alternative to invasive therapy. Urology 2004;64:49.

60. Volpe A, Jewett MA. The role of surveillance for small renal masses. Nat Clin Pract Urol 2007;4:2–3.

61. Kunkle DA, Egleston BL, Uzzo RG. Excise, ablate, or observe: the small renal mass dilemma—a meta-analysis and review. J Urol 2008;179:1277.

62. Nguyen CT, Lane BR, Kaouk JH, et al. Surgical salvage of renal cell carcinoma recurrence after thermal ablative therapy. J Urol 2008;180:104–9.

63. Stephanson A, Hakimian A, Snyder ME, et al. Complications of radical and partial nephrectomy in a large contemporary cohort. J Urol 2004;171:130–4.

64. Simmons MN, Gill IS. Decreased complications of contemporary laparoscopic partial nephrectomy: use of a standardized reporting system. J Urol 2007;177:2067–73.

65. Turna B, Frota R, Kamoi K, et al. Risk factor analysis of postoperative complications in laparoscopic partial nephrectomy. J Urol 2008;179:1289–95.

66. Lowrance WT, Yee DS, Savage C, et al. Complications after radical and partial nephrectomy as a function of age. J Urol 2010;183:1725–30.

67. Segev DL, Muzaale AD, Caffo BS, et al. Perioperative mortality and long-term survival following live kidney donation. JAMA 2010;503:959–66.

68. Fehrman-Ekholm I, Duner F, Brink B, et al. No evidence of loss of kidney function in living kidney donors from cross sectional follow up. Transplantation 2001;72:444–9.

69. Goldfarb DA, Matin SF, Braun WE, et al. Renal outcome 25 years after donor nephrectomy. J Urol 2001;166:2043.

70. Kaplan C, Pasternack B, Shah H, et al. Age-related incidence of sclerotic glomeruli in human kidneys. Am J Pathol 1975;80:227.
71. Bijol V, Mendez GP, Hurwitz S, et al. Evaluation of the nonneoplastic pathology in tumor nephrectomy specimens. Am J Surg Pathol 2006;30:575.
72. Lau WK, Blute ML, Weaver AL, et al. Matched comparison of radical nephrectomy vs. nephron-sparing surgery in patients with unilateral renal cell carcinoma and a normal contra lateral kidney. Mayo Clin Proc 2000;75:1236–42.
73. McKiernan J, Simmons R, Katz J, et al. Natural history of chronic renal insufficiency after partial and radical nephrectomy. Urology 2002;59:816–20.
74. Sarnak M, Levey AS, Schoolwerth AC, et al. Kidney disease as a risk factor for the development of cardiovascular disease: a statement from the American Heart Association Council on Kidney in Cardiovascular Disease. High Blood Pressure Research, Clinical Cardiology, and Epidemiology and Prevention. Circulation 2003;108:2154–69.
75. Chobanian AV, Bakris GL, Black HR, et al. The Seventh Report of the Joint National Committee on TN Prevention, detection, evaluation, and treatment of high blood pressure: the JNC 7 report. JAMA 2003;289:2560–72.
76. Kidney Disease Outcome Quality Imitative. K/DOQI clinical guideline for chronic kidney disease evaluation, classification, stratification. Am J Kidney Dis 2002; 39(2 Suppl 1):S1–266, 51:5246.
77. Ritz E, McClellan WW. Overview: increased cardiovascular risk in patients with minor renal dysfunction: an emerging issue with far-reaching consequences. J Am Soc Nephrol 2004;15:513–6.
78. Shlipak MG, Fried LF, Cushman M, et al. Cardiovascular mortality risk in chronic kidney disease. JAMA 2005;293:1737–45.
79. Coresh J, Selvin E, Stevens LA, et al. Prevalence of chronic kidney disease in the United States. JAMA 2007;298:2038–47.
80. Go AS, Chertow GM, Fan D, et al. Chronic kidney disease and the risks of death, cardiovascular events, and hospitalization. N Engl J Med 2004;351:1296.
81. Foley RN, Wang C, Collins AJ. Cardiovascular risk factor profiles and kidney function stage in the US general population: the NHANES 3 study. Mayo Clin Proc 2005;80:1270–7.
82. Stevens LA, Coresh J, Green T, et al. Assessing kidney function—measured and estimated glomerular filtration rate. N Engl J Med 2006;354:2473–83.
83. Huang WC, Levey AS, Serio AM, et al. Chronic kidney disease after nephrectomy in patients with renal cortical tumors: a retrospective cohort study. Lancet Oncol 2006;7:735–40.
84. Thompson HR, Boorjian SA, Lohse CM, et al. Radical nephrectomy for pT1a renal masses may be associated with decreased overall survival compared to partial nephrectomy. J Urol 2008;179:468–73.
85. Huang WC, Elkin EB, Levey AS, et al. Partial nephrectomy versus radical nephrectomy in patients with small renal tumors—is there a difference in mortality and cardiovascular outcomes. J Urol 2009;181:55–62.
86. Foyil KV, Ames CD, Ferguson GG, et al. Long-term changes in creatinine clearance after laparoscopic renal surgery. J Am Coll Surg 2008;206:511–5.
87. Lane BR, Poggio ED, Herts BR, et al. Renal function assessment in the era of chronic kidney disease: renewed emphasis on renal function centered patient care. J Urol 2009;182:436–44.
88. Campbell SC, Novick AC, Belldegrun A, et al. Guideline for management of the clinical T1 renal mass. J Urol 2009;182:1271–9.

89. Hollenback BK, Tash DA, Miller DC, et al. National utilization trends of partial nephrectomy for renal cell carcinoma: a case of underutilization? Urology 2006;67:254–9.
90. Miller DC, Hollingsworth JM, Hafez KS, et al. Partial nephrectomy for small renal masses. An emerging quality of care concern? J Urol 2006;175:853–7.
91. Dulabon LM, Lowrance WT, Russo P, et al. Trends in renal tumor surgery delivery within the United States. Cancer 2010;116:2316–21.
92. Miller DC, Taub DA, Dunn RL, et al. Laparoscopy for renal cell carcinoma: diffusion versus regionalization? J Urol 2006;176:1102–6.
93. Nuttail M, Cathcart P, van der Meulen J, et al. A description of radical nephrectomy practice and outcomes in England. 1995–2002. BJU Int 2005;96:58–61.
94. Thompson HR, Kaag M, Vickers A, et al. Contemporary use of partial nephrectomy at a tertiary care center in the United States. J Urol 2009;181:993–7.
95. Montie JE. Follow-up after partial or total nephrectomy for renal cell carcinoma. Urol Clin North Am 1994;21:589.
96. Patel MI, Simmons R, Kattan MW, et al. Long term follow up of bilateral sporadic renal tumors. Urology 2003;61:921–5.
97. Sandock DS, Seftel AD, Resnick MI. A new protocol for the follow-up of renal cell carcinoma based on pathological stage. J Urol 1995;154:28–31.
98. Levy DA, Slaton JW, Swanson DA, et al. Stage specific guidelines for surveillance after radical nephrectomy for local renal cell carcinoma. J Urol 1998;159:1163–7.
99. Kavolius JP, Mastorakos DP, Pavolvich C, et al. Resection of metastatic renal cell carcinoma. J Clin Oncol 1998;16:2261.
100. Adamy A, Chong KT, Chade D, et al. Clinical characteristics and outcomes in patients with recurrence 5 years after nephrectomy for localized renal cell carcinoma. J Urol 2011;185:433–8.

The Role of Surgery in Advanced Renal Cell Carcinoma: Cytoreductive Nephrectomy and Metastasectomy

Jose A. Karam, MD, Christopher G. Wood, MD*

KEYWORDS

- Advanced renal cell carcinoma • Metastasectomy
- Cytoreduction • Nephrectomy

Renal cell carcinoma (RCC) is considered a relatively rare malignancy worldwide, with 200,000 new cases of RCC diagnosed yearly and 100,000 patients dying of their disease.[1] Around a third of patients with RCC present with metastatic disease, and among those patients treated with nephrectomy with curative intent, more than one-third develop metastases during postoperative follow-up.[2] Due to the absence of curative medical treatments for metastatic RCC, surgery remains the mainstay of therapy. In this patient cohort, surgery plays a key role in two aspects: cytoreductive nephrectomy to remove the primary renal tumor in the presence of known metastatic disease, and metastasectomy to remove distant metastatic foci in patients with metastatic RCC.

PROGNOSTIC FACTORS

As many patients with metastatic RCC tend to have poor survival, several investigators have identified risk factors that are predictive of poor outcomes in patients with metastatic RCC. These risk stratification strategies are being used to stratify patients for entry into clinical trials, and to recommend the appropriate medical and surgical therapy. The risk groupings have been devised in two eras: the cytokine/chemotherapy era and, more recently, the targeted therapy era.

The most commonly used risk grouping in clinical practice today was reported by Motzer and colleagues[3] from the Memorial Sloan Kettering Cancer Center. After compiling data from 670 patients enrolled in 24 local clinical trials, 5 prognostic factors

Department of Urology, The University of Texas M.D. Anderson Cancer Center, 1515 Holcombe Boulevard, Unit 1373, Houston, TX 77030, USA
* Corresponding author.
E-mail address: cgwood@mdanderson.org

Hematol Oncol Clin N Am 25 (2011) 753–764
doi:10.1016/j.hoc.2011.05.002
0889-8588/11/$ – see front matter © 2011 Elsevier Inc. All rights reserved.

indicative of poor outcomes were discovered: low Karnofsky performance status, low hemoglobin, high lactate dehydrogenase, high corrected serum calcium, and lack of prior nephrectomy. Based on these factors, 3 risk groups were identified: good risk (0 factors), intermediate risk (1–2 factors), and poor risk (3–5 factors). Median survival was 20 months, 10 months, and 4 months, respectively for each of the groups.

Other risk groupings have been devised but are less commonly used. Using patients treated with interleukin-2, Fallick and colleagues[4] identified the following as benefiting the most from up-front cytoreductive nephrectomy clear-cell histology; ECOG performance status of 0 or 1; absence of bone, liver, and central nervous system lesions; adequate cardiac and pulmonary function; and where debulking more than 75% of tumor burden is achievable. Similarly, Leibovich and colleagues[5] reported 5 prognostic factors associated with patient survival: lymph node status, constitutional symptoms, location of metastases, sarcomatoid histology, and thyroid-stimulating hormone level. Based on these factors, patients were stratified into 3 risk groups, where the good-risk group had a 92% 1-year survival rate and the poor-risk group had a 1% 1-year survival rate. Using data from the SWOG 8949 randomized clinical trial, Lara and colleagues[6] identified ECOG performance status of 0, normal alkaline phosphatase, and presence of lung-only metastases to be factors associated with improved outcomes.

Unlike the prior risk groupings that studied patients treated with chemotherapy or immunotherapy, Heng and colleagues[7] recently studied patients treated with targeted therapies (bevacizumab, sunitinib, or sorafenib). Their study identified 6 prognostic factors associated with poor outcomes using retrospective data from patients treated with: Karnofsky performance status less than 80%; time from current diagnosis to current treatment less than 1 year; hemoglobin counts under the lower limit of normal; and corrected calcium, platelet, or neutrophil counts over the upper limit of normal. This study constituted a validation of their original pilot study,[8] and is probably more relevant in the design and conduct of future trials using targeted therapies. Nonetheless, risk grouping based on clinical and simple laboratory criteria alone does not accurately identify true risk, and future genomic studies should help in further refining risk stratification.

CYTOREDUCTIVE NEPHRECTOMY
Immunotherapy Era

In 2001, two randomized phase 3 clinical trials[9,10] and their combined meta-analysis[11] clearly identified cytoreductive nephrectomy as the standard of care in selected patients with metastatic RCC prior to starting interferon therapy (**Table 1**). The primary end point of both studies was overall survival, with the secondary end point being response rate.

Flanigan and colleagues[9] randomized 241 patients to either cytoreductive nephrectomy followed by interferon-α2b or interferon-α2b alone (SWOG 8949). Patients were stratified by SWOG performance status (0 vs 1), presence or absence of lung metastases only, and presence or absence of at least one measurable metastatic lesion. Interferon was started at a median of 19.9 days after cytoreductive nephrectomy. Severe complications were noted in 10 patients in the nephrectomy plus interferon group, and in 13 patients in the interferon-only group. Median survival was 11.1 months in the surgery plus interferon group and 8.1 months in the interferon-only group. Response rates were similar between the two groups.

Mickisch and colleagues[10] randomized 85 patients to receive either cytoreductive nephrectomy followed by interferon-α2b or interferon-α2b alone (EORTC GU 30947). Patients were stratified by treating institution, World Health Organization performance

Table 1
Studies investigating the role of cytoreductive nephrectomy in the immunotherapy era

Study	Study Type	No. of Patients	Objective Response Rate (%)		Survival (Months)	
			Nephrectomy	No Nephrectomy	Nephrectomy	No Nephrectomy
Flanigan et al[9]	Prospective phase 3 trial	221	4.2	2.5	11.1 (OS)	8.1 (OS)
Mickisch et al[10]	Prospective phase 3 trial	85	19	11.6	5 (PFS)	3 (PFS)
					17 (OS)	7 (OS)
Flanigan et al[11]	Meta-analysis	331	6.9	5.7	13.6 (OS)	7.8 (OS)

Abbreviations: NR, not reported; OS, overall survival; PFS, progression-free survival.

status, presence of lung metastases only, and presence of measurable metastatic lesions. Six patients experienced postoperative complications. Five surgical patients and one interferon-only patient had a complete response. Median survival was 17 months in the surgery plus interferon group and 7 months in the interferon-only group. Response rates were similar (19% vs 12%, respectively).

These two randomized studies constitute the basis on which cytoreductive nephrectomy has been used in patients with metastatic RCC, and have continued to do so in the beginning of the targeted therapy era.

A meta-analysis of these two randomized trials[11] showed that overall median survival was longer in the nephrectomy plus interferon group (13.6 vs 7.8 months, hazard ratio 0.69). One-year overall survival in the nephrectomy plus interferon group was 51.9% versus 37.1% in the interferon-only group. Patients with a zero performance status had significantly longer survival. On the other hand, the site of metastases and amount of measurable disease did not affect overall survival.

Further support of these two randomized studies comes from the Surveillance, Epidemiology, and End Results (SEER) database, where Zini and colleagues[12] compared 2447 patients with metastatic RCC who underwent cytoreductive nephrectomy with 2925 patients who did not. Treatment type (nephrectomy vs no nephrectomy), tumor size, and patient age were independent predictors of survival on multivariate analyses. The 1-, 2-, 5-, and 10-year overall survival rate of the patients treated with cytoreductive nephrectomy was 53.6%, 36.3%, 19.4%, and 12.7% compared with 18.5%, 7.4%, 2.3%, and 1.2% for patients who did not undergo surgery, respectively. Patients who underwent cytoreductive nephrectomy had a significant 2.5-fold lower risk of overall and cancer-specific mortality compared with patients who did not receive surgical intervention.

Targeted Therapy Era

Most randomized phase 3 trials of targeted therapies in patients with metastatic RCC enrolled patients with good and intermediate risk, where 85% to 100% of those patients had undergone prior cytoreductive nephrectomy.[13–17] The only exception is the temsirolimus trial, where patients with poor risk were enrolled, and as such only 67% of those patients had a prior nephrectomy.[18]

There are no data at present to directly show the benefit (or lack thereof) of cytoreductive nephrectomy in the targeted therapy era. This surgery is still being done in selected patients based on data from randomized trials in the cytokine era, as well as retrospective data from the current targeted therapy era (**Table 2**). Choueiri and colleagues[19] studied 314 patients treated with targeted therapy, and compared 201 patients who underwent cytoreductive nephrectomy with 113 patients who did not. In multivariable analysis, cytoreductive nephrectomy was associated with improved overall survival in the general cohort (19.8 months in patients who underwent nephrectomy vs 9.4 months in those who did not, hazard ratio 0.68), but on subanalysis it was noted that patients with poor risk features derived marginal benefit from surgery, further strengthening the concept of careful selection of patients who should undergo cytoreductive nephrectomy.

Two ongoing trials are currently being conducted to answer this question in a prospective manner. The CARMENA trial in Europe[20] (NCT00930033) is actively enrolling patients and aims to enroll 576 patients with clear-cell metastatic RCC. This trial is a randomized phase 3 noninferiority trial designed to compare overall survival in patients treated with sunitinib alone with cytoreductive nephrectomy followed by sunitinib. The EORTC has designed a phase 3 randomized trial[21] aiming to investigate the optimal timing of cytoreductive nephrectomy in 440 patients. To

Table 2
Studies investigating the role of cytoreductive nephrectomy in the targeted therapy era

Study	Study Type	No. of Patients	Objective Response Rate (%)		Survival (Months)	
			Nephrectomy	No Nephrectomy	Nephrectomy	No Nephrectomy
Choueiri et al[19]	Retrospective analysis	314	26.3	11.5	8.1 (PFS) 19.8 (OS)	5.5 (PFS) 9.4 (OS)
CARMENA[20]	Prospective phase 3 trial	576 (planned)	Pending			
EORTC[21]	Prospective phase 3 trial	440 (planned)	Pending			

Abbreviations: OS, overall survival; PFS, progression-free survival.

achieve this goal, progression-free survival will be compared in patients treated with cytoreductive nephrectomy followed by sunitinib versus sunitinib followed by surgery.

Recently, the authors investigated the effect of targeted systemic therapy on renal tumor response in patients with the primary tumor in place.[22] One hundred and sixty-eight patients with a median follow-up of 15 months were evaluated, and were noted to experience a median maximum decrease of renal tumor size of only 7.1%, at a median time of 62 days. The authors found that patients who experienced a greater than 10% decrease in renal tumor size in the first 60 days of treatment had a more pronounced eventual objective response, as compared with those who did not achieve this milestone (objective response 24.5% vs 7.2%, respectively). However, due to the relatively small number of patients with greater than 10% decrease in renal tumor size (**Fig. 1**), the authors do not recommend presurgical targeted therapy in patients who are otherwise candidates for up-front cytoreductive nephrectomy, except as part of controlled clinical trials.

Selection Criteria for Cytoreductive Nephrectomy

As the biology and natural history of metastatic RCC is diverse, there are some patients who do not benefit from cytoreductive nephrectomy when routine selection criteria are used. In this patient subset, the risk of surgery and its potential comorbidities is felt to outweigh any benefit that these patients might derive. With this concept in mind, the authors retrospectively studied 556 patients with metastatic RCC treated with cytoreductive nephrectomy, and compared them with 110 patients treated with systemic therapy alone.[23] Seven independent preoperative clinical, laboratory, and radiological variables that were associated with worse overall survival were identified: symptoms related to metastatic disease, low albumin level, high lactate dehydrogenase level, clinical T3 or T4 disease, retroperitoneal adenopathy, and supradiaphragmatic adenopathy. Not surprisingly, patients with 4 risk factors or more who underwent cytoreductive nephrectomy experienced lower overall survival (median 12.2 months), similar to patients treated with medical therapy alone (9.6 months), whereas those with 3 risk factors or less experienced a median overall survival of 22.7 months (**Fig. 2**).

ALTERNATIVES TO OPEN CYTOREDUCTIVE NEPHRECTOMY

As open cytoreductive nephrectomy could lead to significant morbidity in selected patients, alternatives to this radical approach have been sought and then reported

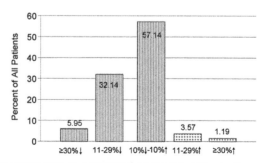

Fig. 1. Primary tumor response to a targeted agent according to the amount of response. Most patients show minimal response or tumor stability during treatment. (*Adapted from* Abel EJ, Culp SH, Tannir NM, et al. Primary tumor response to targeted agents in patients with metastatic renal cell carcinoma. Eur Urol 2011;59:10; with permission.)

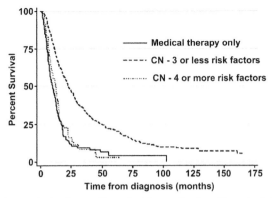

Fig. 2. Kaplan-Meier analysis of overall survival for patients with metastatic renal cell carcinoma who underwent cytoreductive nephrectomy (CN) based on the number of preoperative risk factors (1–3 vs 4–7; P<.001). The solid line represents patients with metastatic RCC who underwent medical therapy alone (reference line). (*Adapted from* Culp SH, Tannir NM, Abel EJ, et al. Can we better select patients with metastatic renal cell carcinoma for cytoreductive nephrectomy? Cancer 2010;116:3378; with permission.)

in the literature. These studies all have in common a small number of patients treated, which reflect very careful selection criteria prior to offering such therapies.

Partial Nephrectomy

Krambeck and colleagues[24] reported on 16 patients from the Mayo Clinic treated with partial nephrectomy in the setting of metastatic RCC. These patients had imperative indications for nephron sparing, such as chronic kidney disease or solitary renal unit. Eleven patients died of their disease at a median of 18 months. One-year, 3-year, and 5-year cancer-specific survival was 81.3%, 49.2%, and 49.2%, respectively. Hutterer and colleagues[25] studied 45 patients from 16 institutions who underwent partial nephrectomy, and noted that the 1-, 2-, and 3-year cancer-specific survival was 86.6%, 86.6%, and 75%, respectively. Finally, Capitanio and colleagues[26] used the SEER database and identified 46 patients who underwent partial nephrectomy in the metastatic setting, and reported that their 1-, 2-, 5-, and 10-year cancer-specific survival was 79.4%, 61.1%, 40.3%, and 40.3%, respectively. Overall, these 3 retrospective studies show the feasibility of partial nephrectomy in the metastatic setting, in carefully selected patients with imperative indications for nephron sparing.

Laparoscopic Nephrectomy

In attempts to decrease the surgical morbidity resulting from open cytoreductive nephrectomy, Walther and colleagues[27] initially reported on the use of laparoscopic radical nephrectomy in 11 patients and showed the feasibility of this approach, which was also shown in other subsequent studies.[28,29] The authors recently reported on 38 patients treated with laparoscopic radical nephrectomy and compared them with a cohort of patients who underwent open nephrectomy.[30] Three patients had an elective conversion to open cytoreductive nephrectomy. Patients who underwent laparoscopic nephrectomy had shorter hospital stay and lower blood loss. There was no difference in complication rate or time to start of systemic therapy. The authors believe that ideal candidates for this laparoscopic approach are patients with tumors less than

15 cm, with no evidence of bulky adenopathy, inferior vena cava thrombus, or locoregional invasion, who are otherwise good surgical candidates with a good performance status.

Radiofrequency Ablation

Recently, the authors studied 15 carefully selected patients whose primary renal tumor was treated with percutaneous radiofrequency ablation.[31] Before or at radiofrequency ablation, metastases were present in the lung in 10 patients, bone in 5, adrenal gland in 4, and liver/perihepatic nodules in 3. Metastasis to the brain, pancreas, soft tissue, pleura, retroperitoneal nodes, and paraesophageal nodes was present in 1 patient each. Eight patients had a solitary metastasis. Four patients had major complications. Three patients with a solitary kidney developed hematuria with ureteral clot occlusion, and subsequently underwent temporary ureteral stent placement until hematuria and acute kidney injury resolved. Two patients experienced acute hypertension after the procedure, and were medically treated with no sequelae. One patient developed a perinephric hematoma that was managed conservatively. None of these patients required renal angiography, and no cardiopulmonary complications or deaths occurred within 30 days of treatment. Four patients were in complete remission with no evidence of disease at a median follow-up of 25.5 months. Four patients had no evidence of local recurrence but had evidence of distant disease at a median follow-up of 45 months. The remaining 7 patients died of disease at a median follow-up of 10 months.

METASTASECTOMY

In selected patients with metastatic RCC, surgical resection of metastatic foci, known as metastasectomy, is a treatment option that can yield long-term disease-free survival. Eggener and colleagues[32] reported that patients who underwent a complete metastasectomy derived a clinical benefit across all 3 MSKCC risk groups, but most significantly in the good-risk and intermediate-risk groups. More recently, Alt and colleagues[33] reported on the benefit of complete metastasectomy, even in the presence of multiple sites of metastases, with median cancer-specific survival of 4.8 years with complete resection versus 1.3 years with incomplete resection. Of interest, this benefit was noted in both the synchronous and metachronous metastatic settings.

Recently, the authors reported a feasibility study including 22 patients who received targeted therapy prior to metastasectomy.[34] Three patients experienced postoperative chylous ascites, and one patient experienced chylous ascites, atrial fibrillation, and ileus, all of which resolved without long-term sequelae. No postoperative bleeding, thromboembolic events, or wound complications were noted within 3 months after surgery. Eleven patients were free of disease 10 months after metastasectomy, while another 11 recurred at a median of 10 months after surgery. Twenty-one patients were alive at a median of 2 years after metastasectomy. This study consisted of a cohort of highly selected patients with limited tumor burden after targeted therapy, and provides preliminary evidence that consolidative metastasectomy is feasible, with acceptable morbidity in this setting.

Bone

Bone metastasectomy can be performed in patients with no symptoms but who are at risk of impending pathologic fracture based on imaging, and in patients who are symptomatic due to severe pain or neurologic functional compromise. In general, survival is poor in patients with bony metastases, with reported 5-year survival rates of around 15%.[35,36] Nevertheless, certain subgroups of patients do have a fairly good outcome.

Patients with solitary bone lesions diagnosed more than 1 year after nephrectomy and treated with curative intent have a 54% 5-year survival.[35] Similarly, patients with a solitary lesion, prior nephrectomy, and wide resection margins achieved 100% disease-specific survival.[37] From a symptomatic standpoint, surgery can result in a high rate of improvement of neurologic symptoms as well as pain relief.[36] In addition, preoperative adjunctive therapies (systemic therapy, radiotherapy, or embolization) are frequently used before surgical resection, to maximize therapeutic benefit as well as to decrease operative morbidity.[36]

Brain

Brain lesions have been traditionally treated with surgical resection, whole brain irradiation, or stereotactic radiosurgery. Median survival from time of treatment of brain metastases is 12 to 13 months,[38,39] with a 5-year survival rate of 12%.[40] Patients with a solitary brain metastasis have longer recurrence-free survival compared with those with more than one brain lesion (13 months vs 4 months).[40] Other good prognostic factors for patients undergoing brain metastasectomy include prior resection of pulmonary metastases, supratentorial brain lesion, and lack of preoperative neurologic deficit.[39] In older series postoperative mortality can be as high as 10%[39] whereas the complication rate in more recent series is 12%, with no reported mortalities.[38]

Liver

Few series report on surgical resection of RCC metastases to the liver. Stief and colleagues[41] reported on 17 patients with solitary liver metastases, 11 of whom underwent complete resection. Four patients died postoperatively. Mean survival was 16 months. Large tumors, high alkaline phosphatase level, and high γ-glutamyltranspeptidase levels were associated with poor outcomes.[41] More recently, Alves and colleagues[42] reported on 10 patients with RCC metastases to the liver and did not record any postoperative deaths. The 2-year survival was 56%. Factors associated with better outcome after liver resection included curative intent, interval of more than 24 months from RCC diagnosis to development of liver metastases, tumor size less than 5 cm, and feasibility of repeat hepatectomy if necessary.[42]

Lung

Several series reported on metastasectomy for lung lesion, with the lung being a common site of RCC metastasis. Median 5-year overall survival ranges between 31% and 37%, and median survival is from 33 to 61 months.[43–48] Predictors of good outcome include completeness of resection, disease-free interval of more than 2 years, presence of less than 7 pulmonary metastases, and absence of pulmonary and mediastinal lymphatic metastases.[47] Complete resection of lung-only metastases is associated with a marked improved survival when completely resected, as compared with incomplete resection (5-year cancer-specific survival 73.6% vs 19%, respectively).[33]

Pancreas

A recent review[49] of 321 patients who underwent resection of RCC metastases to the pancreas revealed that more than half of the resected patients were symptomatic, and two-thirds had solitary pancreatic metastases. Two-year and 5-year disease-free survival was 76% and 57%, and 2- and 5-year overall survival was 80.6% and 72.6%, respectively. Postoperative in-hospital mortality associated with pancreatic resection was 2.8%. The presence of extrapancreatic RCC metastases was associated with worse disease-free survival, while symptomatic metastases were associated with worse overall survival. Surprisingly, the size of largest tumor resected, number of pancreatic metastases, type of pancreatic resection, and interval from diagnosis of RCC to pancreatic metastasis were not predictive of survival.[49]

Thyroid

Iesalnieks and colleagues[50] studied 45 patients with RCC metastasis to the thyroid gland, and noted a 51% 5-year survival rate. Poor prognostic indicators were patient age greater than 70 years, and prior nephrectomy for contralateral renal metastases. The investigators concluded that general condition of the patient and performance status dictated outcome in this subgroup, rather than the thyroid metastases per se.

SUMMARY

Cytoreductive nephrectomy has been shown to improve patient survival in prospective studies in the immunotherapy era, and in retrospective studies in the targeted therapy era. Metastasectomy in selected patients offers long-term cure and palliation, and its role is being redefined in the targeted therapy era. At present, surgical therapy in the form of cytoreductive nephrectomy and/or metastasectomy remains the mainstay of treatment for many patients with metastatic RCC, and the only chance for cure.

REFERENCES

1. Parkin DM, Bray F, Ferlay J, et al. Global cancer statistics, 2002. CA Cancer J Clin 2005;55:74.
2. Motzer RJ, Bander NH, Nanus DM. Renal-cell carcinoma. N Engl J Med 1996; 335:865.
3. Motzer RJ, Mazumdar M, Bacik J, et al. Survival and prognostic stratification of 670 patients with advanced renal cell carcinoma. J Clin Oncol 1999;17:2530.
4. Fallick ML, McDermott DF, LaRock D, et al. Nephrectomy before interleukin-2 therapy for patients with metastatic renal cell carcinoma. J Urol 1997;158: 1691.
5. Leibovich BC, Han KR, Bui MH, et al. Scoring algorithm to predict survival after nephrectomy and immunotherapy in patients with metastatic renal cell carcinoma: a stratification tool for prospective clinical trials. Cancer 2003;98:2566.
6. Lara PN Jr, Tangen CM, Conlon SJ, et al. Predictors of survival of advanced renal cell carcinoma: long-term results from Southwest Oncology Group Trial S8949. J Urol 2009;181:512.
7. Heng DY, Xie W, Regan MM, et al. Prognostic factors for overall survival in patients with metastatic renal cell carcinoma treated with vascular endothelial growth factor-targeted agents: results from a large, multicenter study. J Clin Oncol 2009;27:5794.
8. Choueiri TK, Garcia JA, Elson P, et al. Clinical factors associated with outcome in patients with metastatic clear-cell renal cell carcinoma treated with vascular endothelial growth factor-targeted therapy. Cancer 2007;110:543.
9. Flanigan RC, Salmon SE, Blumenstein BA, et al. Nephrectomy followed by interferon alfa-2b compared with interferon alfa-2b alone for metastatic renal-cell cancer. N Engl J Med 2001;345:1655.
10. Mickisch GH, Garin A, van Poppel H, et al. Radical nephrectomy plus interferon-alfa-based immunotherapy compared with interferon alfa alone in metastatic renal-cell carcinoma: a randomised trial. Lancet 2001;358:966.

11. Flanigan RC, Mickisch G, Sylvester R, et al. Cytoreductive nephrectomy in patients with metastatic renal cancer: a combined analysis. J Urol 2004;171:1071.

12. Zini L, Capitanio U, Perrotte P, et al. Population-based assessment of survival after cytoreductive nephrectomy versus no surgery in patients with metastatic renal cell carcinoma. Urology 2009;73:342e6.

13. Escudier B, Eisen T, Stadler WM, et al. Sorafenib in advanced clear-cell renal-cell carcinoma. N Engl J Med 2007;356:125.

14. Escudier B, Pluzanska A, Koralewski P, et al. Bevacizumab plus interferon alfa-2a for treatment of metastatic renal cell carcinoma: a randomised, double-blind phase III trial. Lancet 2007;370:2103.

15. Motzer RJ, Escudier B, Oudard S, et al. Efficacy of everolimus in advanced renal cell carcinoma: a double-blind, randomised, placebo-controlled phase III trial. Lancet 2008;372:449.

16. Motzer RJ, Hutson TE, Tomczak P, et al. Sunitinib versus interferon alfa in metastatic renal-cell carcinoma. N Engl J Med 2007;356:115.

17. Rini BI, Halabi S, Rosenberg JE, et al. Bevacizumab plus interferon alfa compared with interferon alfa monotherapy in patients with metastatic renal cell carcinoma: CALGB 90206. J Clin Oncol 2008;26:5422.

18. Hudes G, Carducci M, Tomczak P, et al. Temsirolimus, interferon alfa, or both for advanced renal-cell carcinoma. N Engl J Med 2007;356:2271.

19. Choueiri TK, Xie W, Kollmannsberger C, et al. The impact of cytoreductive nephrectomy on survival of patients with metastatic renal cell carcinoma receiving vascular endothelial growth factor targeted therapy. J Urol 2011;185:60.

20. Bellmunt J. Future developments in renal cell carcinoma. Ann Oncol 2009; 20(Suppl 1):i13.

21. Biswas S, Kelly J, Eisen T. Cytoreductive nephrectomy in metastatic clear-cell renal cell carcinoma: perspectives in the tyrosine kinase inhibitor era. Oncologist 2009;14:52.

22. Abel EJ, Culp SH, Tannir NM, et al. Primary tumor response to targeted agents in patients with metastatic renal cell carcinoma. Eur Urol 2011;59:10.

23. Culp SH, Tannir NM, Abel EJ, et al. Can we better select patients with metastatic renal cell carcinoma for cytoreductive nephrectomy? Cancer 2010;116:3378.

24. Krambeck AE, Leibovich BC, Lohse CM, et al. The role of nephron sparing surgery for metastatic (pM1) renal cell carcinoma. J Urol 2006;176:1990.

25. Hutterer GC, Patard JJ, Colombel M, et al. Cytoreductive nephron-sparing surgery does not appear to undermine disease-specific survival in patients with metastatic renal cell carcinoma. Cancer 2007;110:2428.

26. Capitanio U, Zini L, Perrotte P, et al. Cytoreductive partial nephrectomy does not undermine cancer control in metastatic renal cell carcinoma: a population-based study. Urology 2008;72(5):1090–5.

27. Walther MM, Lyne JC, Libutti SK, et al. Laparoscopic cytoreductive nephrectomy as preparation for administration of systemic interleukin-2 in the treatment of metastatic renal cell carcinoma: a pilot study. Urology 1999;53:496.

28. Eisenberg MS, Meng MV, Master VA, et al. Laparoscopic versus open cytoreductive nephrectomy in advanced renal-cell carcinoma. J Endourol 2006;20:504.

29. Finelli A, Kaouk JH, Fergany AF, et al. Laparoscopic cytoreductive nephrectomy for metastatic renal cell carcinoma. BJU Int 2004;94:291.

30. Matin SF, Madsen LT, Wood CG. Laparoscopic cytoreductive nephrectomy: the M. D. Anderson Cancer Center experience. Urology 2006;68:528.

31. Karam JA, Ahrar K, Wood CG, et al. Radio frequency ablation of renal tumors in patients with metastatic renal cell carcinoma. J Urol 2010;184:1882.

32. Eggener SE, Yossepowitch O, Kundu S, et al. Risk score and metastasectomy independently impact prognosis of patients with recurrent renal cell carcinoma. J Urol 2008;180:873.
33. Alt AL, Boorjian SA, Lohse CM, et al. Survival after complete surgical resection of multiple metastases from renal cell carcinoma. Cancer 2011. [Epub ahead of print].
34. Karam JA, Rini BI, Varella L, et al. Metastasectomy after targeted therapy in patients with advanced renal cell carcinoma. J Urol 2011;185:439.
35. Durr HR, Maier M, Pfahler M, et al. Surgical treatment of osseous metastases in patients with renal cell carcinoma. Clin Orthop Relat Res 1999;(367):283.
36. Jackson RJ, Loh SC, Gokaslan ZL. Metastatic renal cell carcinoma of the spine: surgical treatment and results. J Neurosurg 2001;94:18.
37. Jung ST, Ghert MA, Harrelson JM, et al. Treatment of osseous metastases in patients with renal cell carcinoma. Clin Orthop Relat Res 2003;(409):223.
38. Vecil GG, Lang FF. Surgical resection of metastatic intraventricular tumors. Neurosurg Clin N Am 2003;14:593.
39. Wronski M, Arbit E, Russo P, et al. Surgical resection of brain metastases from renal cell carcinoma in 50 patients. Urology 1996;47:187.
40. Shuch B, La Rochelle JC, Klatte T, et al. Brain metastasis from renal cell carcinoma: presentation, recurrence, and survival. Cancer 2008;113:1641.
41. Stief CG, Jahne J, Hagemann JH, et al. Surgery for metachronous solitary liver metastases of renal cell carcinoma. J Urol 1997;158:375.
42. Alves A, Adam R, Majno P, et al. Hepatic resection for metastatic renal tumors: is it worthwhile? Ann Surg Oncol 2003;10:705.
43. Assouad J, Petkova B, Berna P, et al. Renal cell carcinoma lung metastases surgery: pathologic findings and prognostic factors. Ann Thorac Surg 2007;84:1114.
44. Cerfolio RJ, Allen MS, Deschamps C, et al. Pulmonary resection of metastatic renal cell carcinoma. Ann Thorac Surg 1994;57:339.
45. Hofmann HS, Neef H, Krohe K, et al. Prognostic factors and survival after pulmonary resection of metastatic renal cell carcinoma. Eur Urol 2005;48:77.
46. Murthy SC, Kim K, Rice TW, et al. Can we predict long-term survival after pulmonary metastasectomy for renal cell carcinoma? Ann Thorac Surg 2005;79:996.
47. Pfannschmidt J, Hoffmann H, Muley T, et al. Prognostic factors for survival after pulmonary resection of metastatic renal cell carcinoma. Ann Thorac Surg 2002;74:1653.
48. Piltz S, Meimarakis G, Wichmann MW, et al. Long-term results after pulmonary resection of renal cell carcinoma metastases. Ann Thorac Surg 2002;73:1082.
49. Tanis PJ, van der Gaag NA, Busch OR, et al. Systematic review of pancreatic surgery for metastatic renal cell carcinoma. Br J Surg 2009;96:579.
50. Iesalnieks I, Winter H, Bareck E, et al. Thyroid metastases of renal cell carcinoma: clinical course in 45 patients undergoing surgery. Assessment of factors affecting patients' survival. Thyroid 2008;18:615.

Adjuvant and Neoadjuvant Therapies in High-Risk Renal Cell Carcinoma

Marc C. Smaldone, MD[a], Chunkit Fung, MD[b],
Robert G. Uzzo, MD[a],[*],[1], Naomi B. Haas, MD[b],[1]

KEYWORDS

- Renal cell carcinoma • Prognosis • Targeted therapy
- Neoadjuvant • Adjuvant

Kidney cancer, predominantly renal cell carcinoma (RCC), represents the most lethal of all urologic malignancies. In 2010, approximately 58,240 men and women will be diagnosed with cancer of the kidney or renal pelvis, and 13,040 (22.4%) will ultimately succumb to their disease.[1] Because of the increased use of cross-sectional abdominal imaging over the past several decades,[2,3] a stage and size migration toward the detection of small localized renal tumors (<4 cm) has been observed, and incidental detection of asymptomatic lesions now accounts for greater than 50% of all renal masses discovered.[4] Traditionally, clinically localized renal masses have been managed with surgical excision, and 5-year cancer-specific survival (CSS) rates of 97% and 87% following radical nephrectomy have been reported for pT1a and pT1b tumors, respectively.[5] Concern that radical nephrectomy may predispose patients to the sequelae of chronic kidney disease,[6,7] including increased

This publication was supported in party by grant number P30 CA006927 from the National Cancer Institute. Its contents are solely the responsibility of the authors and do not necessarily represent the official views of the National Cancer Institute or the National Institutes of Health. Additional funds were provided by Fox Chase Cancer via institutional support of the Kidney Cancer Keystone Program.

[a] Division of Urologic Oncology, Department of Surgery, Fox Chase Cancer Center, 333 Cottman Avenue, Philadelphia, PA 19111, USA
[b] Division of Hematology/Oncology, Department of Medicine, Abramson Cancer Center, University of Pennsylvania, 12 Penn Tower, 3400 Spruce Street, Philadelphia, PA 19104, USA
[1] Contributed equally to this work.
* Corresponding author.
E-mail address: R_Uzzo@fccc.edu

Hematol Oncol Clin N Am 25 (2011) 765–791
doi:10.1016/j.hoc.2011.06.002
0889-8588/11/$ – see front matter © 2011 Elsevier Inc. All rights reserved.

cardiovascular risk and shortened overall survival,[8–10] has led to the increased use of nephron sparing techniques[11]; and 5- and 10-year CSS rates of 96% and 90% have been reported following partial nephrectomy for tumors less than 4 cm.[12]

Although the rates of renal surgery have also risen in conjunction with increased tumor detection, mortality rates have also paradoxically risen.[3] This observation can be explained largely by the substantial proportion of patients still presenting with either locally advanced (20%) or metastatic (22%) RCC.[1] In comparison to the high CSS associated with localized disease, 5-year survival rates for patients with regional nodal metastases range from 11% to 35%, and cure rates are low, even with aggressive multimodal therapy.[13] Despite a demonstrated survival benefit,[14] cytoreductive nephrectomy for metastatic disease (mRCC) results in poor CSS outcomes, with reported median survivals ranging from 12 to 24 months.[15–17] The contemporary era of targeted therapy for RCC has focused on inhibition of the angiogenesis pathway implicated in RCC tumorigenesis and led to several Food and Drug Administration (FDA)-approved agents for mRCC. These agents target the vascular endothelial growth factor (VEGF) or the mammalian target of rapamycin inhibitor (mTOR). Prospective randomized trials with these agents have demonstrated that a proportion of patients with mRCC treated with tyrosine kinase inhibitors (TKIs) exhibit an objective primary tumor response (10%–31%), whereas a larger proportion demonstrate disease stabilization (26%–74%) and increased progression-free survival when compared with placebo and immunotherapeutic agents.[18–22] These findings have resulted in the increased interest in the use of targeted therapy in the adjuvant setting for primary tumors with high-risk pathologic features following extirpative surgery and, in the neoadjuvant setting, to reduce tumor burden, treat micrometastatic disease, and help select patients that may best respond to surgical therapy.

RCC is a heterogeneous disease, and a gradation of risk exists between the extremes of incidental localized and mRCC. Approximately one-third of patients undergoing surgical resection for clinically localized RCC progress to recurrence,[5,13,23,24] suggesting that there are some individuals in whom surgical excision is necessary but insufficient because of the presence of micrometastatic disease.[25] In these patients, the development of effective adjuvant strategies is imperative, but to date trials have been limited because of ineffective systemic therapies for mRCC, the high toxicity profile for existing immunomodulatory agents, and difficulty recruiting to multi-institutional and cooperative group adjuvant trials.[25] In this review, the authors summarize prognostic variables and clinical algorithms currently used to identify patients at high risk for disease recurrence following surgical resection of RCC, outcomes of contemporary adjuvant systemic therapy trials, and the rationale supporting the use of neoadjuvant therapy.

DEFINING RISK IN RCC
Patterns of Disease Recurrence

Integral to designing appropriate adjuvant or neoadjuvant strategies is a basic understanding of which patient and tumor characteristics are associated with the risk of local or systemic recurrence. For patients with local or locally advanced RCC, the risk of recurrence following partial or radical nephrectomy largely depends on tumor size, stage, grade, histology, completeness of resection, presence of symptoms, and performance status, and ranges from 15% to 27% at 5 years.[26–29] Local or contralateral recurrence following surgical resection is rare, but it is more common following partial nephrectomy.[30] The most frequent sites of distant recurrence include the lung, lymph nodes, liver, bone, and brain; prognosis for patients with mRCC is very poor, with a 5-year survival of less than 10%.[31] Although the majority of recurrences are discovered during routine radiographic surveillance,[32] most patients who relapse have distant metastases and are rarely cured. Although patients are at a lifelong risk, the greatest recurrence risk is in the first 3 to 5 years following surgery, with approximately 10% recurring after 5 years.[33,34] Patients with a higher tumor grade and stage at initial presentation seem to be at a higher risk for early recurrence, whereas recurrent lesions detected at delayed intervals are more likely to be incidentally diagnosed, have primary tumors with less aggressive features, and are associated with improved overall survival.[33] Because targeted therapy rarely results in complete tumor response,[35] surgical resection (metastasectomy) has been proposed as the only potentially curable therapy in appropriately selected patients, with the exception of the extremely uncommon durable complete responses following high-does interleukin (IL)-2.[36] Five-year survival rates ranging from 30% to 45% have been reported following metastasectomy for patients with isolated renal fossa recurrences or lung metastases.[37,38] Currently, the role of systemic therapy in a neoadjuvant or adjuvant setting to metastasectomy remains unclear.

Prognostic Variables

Characteristics that have associated with cancer-specific outcomes following surgical resection include presence of clinical symptoms, laboratory values, anatomic variables, histologic subtype, and molecular features (**Table 1**). Patients presenting with clinical symptoms at presentation attributable to the primary tumor, including pain, hematuria, hematuria, cachexia, or paraneoplastic symptoms, appear to have a significantly worse prognosis than those presenting with incidentally diagnosed lesions.[13] Interestingly, as a greater number of clinically localized lesions are diagnosed incidentally, these prognostic differences become less apparent when controlling for pathologic stage because far fewer patients are now diagnosed from imaging prompted by clinical symptoms.[39] Overall health status, quantitated by scoring systems designed to assess competing medical risk and performance status, including the Karnofsky scale,[40] the Eastern Cooperative Oncology Group performance status (ECOG-PS),[41] and the Charlson comorbidity index,[42] have been closely correlated with survival in patients with RCC and have been integrated into the inclusion criteria for contemporary clinical trials. Likewise, laboratory parameters indicating systemic disease involvement, including anemia, elevated liver function tests, thrombocytosis, elevated C-reactive protein, hypercalcemia, and elevated erythrocyte sedimentation rate, have been investigated in large institutional series that have demonstrated an association with poor disease-specific and overall survival.[43–45]

Currently, pathologic tumor stage is the single most important prognostic indicator in resected RCC, which incorporates important anatomic variables, including tumor size; local tumor extension; adrenal, venous, or lymphatic involvement; and distant metastases. Originally developed in 1997, the American Joint Committee on Cancer tumor, nodes, metastases (TNM) staging system was modified in 2002 and again in 2010 to improve predictive accuracy. Recent adaptations include the stratification of pT1 tumors by tumor size (<4, 4–7 cm) and pT3 disease by venous involvement above or below the diaphragm.[5] Estimated disease-specific survival by 2002 TNM classification is 97% (pT1a), 87% (pT1b), 71% (pT2), 53% (pT3a), 44% (pT3b), 37% (pT3c), and 20% (pT4), respectively.[5] In 2010, the TNM system was again revised, reclassifying pT2 disease by tumor size ($\geq$7–<10 cm, $\geq$10 cm) and recategorizing adrenal involvement to pT4 disease. T3 disease was reclassified as renal vein involvement or involving Gerota fascia (pT3a), inferior vena cava (IVC) involvement below the

Table 1
Clinical and pathologic characteristics associated with cancer-specific prognosis in patients with localized RCC

Clinical Factors	Measures of Performance Status	Laboratory Values	Anatomic Variables (Staging)	Histologic Features	Molecular Features
Localized symptoms/pain	Karnofsky score	Thrombocytosis	Tumor size	Nuclear grade	*Hypoxia Inducible:* CA IX, CA XII, VEGF, IGF-1, CXCR4, HIF-1α
Cachexia	ECOG-PS	Anemia	Tumor extension into perisinuous or perinephric fat	Histologic subtype	*Proliferation:* Ki-67, PCNA, Ag-NORs
Hematuria	Charlson comorbidity index	Hypercalcemia	Adrenal involvement	Sarcomatoid features	*Cell-cycle regulation:* p53, PTEN, Bcl-2, Cyclin A, p27
Obesity		Elevated alkaline phosphatase	Vascular involvement	Necrosis (microscopic or macroscopic)	*Cell Adhesion:* EpCAM, EMA (MUC1), E-cadherin, α-Catenin, Cadherin-6
Paraneoplastic symptoms		Elevated C-reactive protein	Invasion of adjacent organs	Microvascular invasion	*Cytogenetics:* Aberrant DNA methylation, loss of VHL, c-myc expression Loss of 3p, 9p, and trisomy 17 (papillary); loss or polysomy 3p (clear cell) *Miscellaneous:* Gelsolin, Vimentin, CA-125, CD44, Androgen receptors, Caveolin-1, TGF-β
		Elevated erythrocyte sedimentation rate	Regional lymph node involvement		
		Elevated serum erythropoietin	Distant metastasis		

Abbreviations: AgNORs, argyrophilic nucleolar organizer regions; CA IX, carbonic anhydrase IX; CA XII, carbonic anhydrase XII; ECOG-PS, Eastern Cooperative Oncology Group performance status; EMA, epithelial membrane antigen; EpCAM, epithelial cell adhesion molecule; HIF-1α, hypoxia-inducible factor-1α; IGF, insulinlike growth factor; MUC1, Mucin 1; PCNA, proliferating cell nuclear antigen; PTEN, phosphatase and tensin homolog; TGF-β, transforming growth factor-β; VEGFR, vascular endothelial growth factor receptor; VHL, von Hippel-Lindau tumor suppressor.

Adapted from Kunkle DA, Haas NB, Uzzo RG. Adjuvant therapy for high risk renal cell carcinoma patients. Curr Urol Rep 2007;8(1):19–30; and Current Medicine Group, LLC.

level of the diaphragm (pT3b), and tumor thrombus growing into the chest or invading the wall of the IVC (pT3c).[46]

To explain disparities in survival among stages, additional histologic characteristics have been investigated. Fuhrman nuclear grade, histologic subtype, and presence of sarcomatoid or necrotic features have been associated with increased risk of disease progression and poor cancer-specific survival.[25] Large series have demonstrated a significant correlation between tumor grade and disease-specific survival that is independent of tumor stage.[23] Likewise, biologic aggressiveness varies by histologic classification,[47] with chromophobe and papillary type I tumors often demonstrating indolent clinical courses, whereas papillary type II and clear cell RCCs or more uncommon variants, such as collecting duct carcinomas that demonstrate more aggressive behavior, and are associated with a worse prognosis.[13,23,44] Specific features regardless of cell type that have been associated with the increased likelihood of cancer-specific death include tumor necrosis[48] and sarcomatoid features.[49] Prognostic value appears to be related to percent involvement rather than simply the presence or absence of a given feature.[49,50] It is important to note that interobserver and intraobserver variation in nuclear grading for RCC has been demonstrated, and the presence/absence or percent involvement of sarcomatoid features and tumor necrosis is not universally mentioned in pathology reports.[51]

The treatment of advanced RCC has evolved significantly following the identification of the von Hippel-Lindau (VHL) gene and increasing delineation of its tumor suppressor function and role in angiogenesis. Inactivation of the VHL gene leads to the failure of proteolytic regulation of the α subunits of hypoxia-inducible factor (HIF) and constitutive upregulation of the HIF complex. The resulting overexpression of HIF target genes, including VEGF and platelet-derived growth factor (PDGF), has been implicated in tumorigenesis and has provided novel targets for molecular directed targeted therapy in advanced RCC.[52] With the development of effective targeted agents, molecular markers are being actively sought to both assess risk (predict response to therapy) and to identify other novel molecular pathways worthy of targeting.[53] Although the description of mechanisms and accumulation of scientific evidence for each marker currently being studied is beyond the scope of this review, the breadth of molecular markers under investigation is described in **Table 1**. Carbonic anhydrase (CA) IX is a transmembrane enzyme that is thought to play a role in the adaptation of tumors to hypoxic conditions by regulating the pH of the intracellular and extracellular compartment, facilitating the proliferation of malignant cells and tumor metastasis.[54] Overexpressed in greater than 95% of clear cell RCC tumors and rarely expressed in non–clear cell variants, fetal tissues, or adult benign kidney specimens, the degree of CA IX expression has been inversely correlated with survival in patients with high-risk clinically localized and mRCC.[55] The specificity of CA IX for clear cell RCC makes it an excellent candidate for use as a prognostic marker as well as therapeutic applications, and a monoclonal antibody (Girentuximab or G250) targeting CA IX is currently under clinical trial investigation as a primary therapy and in the adjuvant setting for advanced RCC.[56] In a novel histologic-specific diagnostic application with important implications for guiding management decisions, G250 labeled with 124-iodine (immuno-positron emission tomography)[57] was able to discriminate clear cell renal cell carcinoma (ccRCC) from non-ccRCC with a specificity of 86% and a positive predictive value of 95% in a recent phase III trial (REDECT, Munich, Germany) of 202 patients with solid renal masses undergoing planned surgical excision.[58]

Other biomarkers that have been linked to prognosis in RCC include p53, gelsolin, Ki67, vimentin, phosphatase and tensin homolog (PTEN), epithelial cell adhesion molecule (EpCAM), and CA XII.[25] Increased p53 (cell cycle regulator), gelsolin (cell motility), Ki67 (proliferation marker), and vimentin (eukaryotic cell structural filament) expression and decreased staining of PTEN (regulator of cellular migration, proliferation, and apoptosis), EpCAM (epithelial cell adhesion molecule), and CA XII have been shown to correlate with poor prognosis.[59–62] Likewise, an association between CA IX, vimentin, and p53 expression and RCC-specific survival has been demonstrated independent of the pathologic stage, presence of metastasis, performance status, and histologic grade.[13] Assessment of hypermethylation of CpG islands in the promoter regions of genes has been associated with transcriptional silencing and has been documented in several malignancies.[63] Quantitative gene methylation profiling has been used to identify unique patterns of gene methylation among RCC histologic subtypes and lesions of differing pathologic stages.[64,65] In future investigations, the degree of aberrant methylation present may show utility in determining the risk of recurrence or the response to targeted therapy. Currently, contemporary biomarker studies offer insight into molecular tumor biology and malignant potential. However, the strength of current evidence is not sufficiently robust to guide clinical decision making in patients with RCC. As our understanding of the genetics and molecular pathways driving renal cell carcinoma grows, it is hoped that future clinical decisions will be made on an individual patient basis tailored by molecular phenotype.[66]

STRATIFICATION OF RISK USING PROGNOSTIC ALGORITHMS

A variety of prognostic algorithms designed to predict overall and cancer-specific survival for patients with RCC have been constructed using a combination of clinical variables, histopathologic features, and laboratory values (**Table 2**). Nomograms consist of graphic depictions of prediction models that account for multiple prognostic variables simultaneously and provide unbiased predictions based on objective data. The concordance index (CI) is a measure of the predictive accuracy of prognostic algorithms. An accuracy of 100% is determined by a value of 1.0, whereas random chance is depicted by a value of 0.5. When using contemporary renal cell prognostic algorithms, it is important to consider that each of the described tools has a CI less than 1.0, indicating less than 100% accuracy and the need for continued evaluation and improvement.[67] Despite these limitations, determination of the risk of recurrence in patients with and without evidence of metastasis is valuable for patient counseling, individualizing surveillance imaging, and identifying patients with the greatest likelihood of benefiting from adjuvant treatment.[25]

Preoperative Algorithms for Stratifying Risk in Patients with Suspected Renal Malignancies

Preoperative nomograms have been developed to predict the likelihood of benign or malignant pathology, high- versus low-grade disease, overall survival, and recurrence-free survival. Using a large institutional cohort, Lane and colleagues[68] constructed a nomogram based on the findings that gender, tumor size, and smoking history were predictive of malignant versus benign disease. However, although the CI of this model was 0.64, additional efforts to differentiate indolent from aggressive cancers were less successful (CI 0.56). Utilizing a multi-institutional dataset, Jeldres and colleagues[69] developed a tool to accurately predict high-grade (Fuhrman grade III–IV) features at nephrectomy using 4 covariates (age at diagnosis, gender, tumor size, and symptom classification). Of these factors, only tumor size was significantly associated with high-grade disease on univariate analysis, and their most accurate multivariate nomogram for high-grade disease prediction was only 58.3%. Using a large prospectively maintained institutional cohort, Kutikov and colleagues[70] evaluated the relationship between nephrometry score (a reproducible standardized classification system designed to quantitate the salient anatomy of renal masses) and malignant or high-grade pathologic features at the time of surgical resection. They found that the total nephrometry score and all individual anatomic descriptor components significantly differed between tumor histology groups with the exception of the anterior/posterior designation. Based on these data, predictive nomograms integrating anatomic tumor attributes with patients' age and gender were constructed for the preoperative prediction of tumor malignant histology (area under the curve [AUC] 0.76) and high-grade features (AUC 0.73).[71] This model represents the most accurate preoperative predictive model for tumor grade or malignant features to date, with accuracy rates that rival the results of contemporary percutaneous core biopsy series.[72] In an effort to develop a clinical tool to stratify the competing risks of comorbidity and tumor malignant potential, Kutikov and colleagues[73] developed a comprehensive nomogram to predict the 5-year risk of kidney cancer death, death from other malignancy, and non–cancer death using select preoperative clinical and demographic variables. This nomogram is currently being refined to incorporate comorbidity assessment stratified by the Charlson comorbidity index.[74] Although the preoperative determination of aggressive tumor features and competing risks of death may ultimately provide useful data in identifying candidates for neoadjuvant protocols, the predictive information gleaned from these nomograms is currently more applicable in determining the need for initial treatment versus active surveillance in patients with significant competing risks.

In the first model using purely clinical variables to assess postoperative prognosis in RCC, Yaycioglu and colleagues[75] developed a preoperative scoring system incorporating clinical presentation and tumor size, using recurrence-free survival as an end point. Using this system, the investigators were able to demonstrate a significant difference in the 5-year disease-free survival (92% vs 57%, $P<.001$) when patients were stratified into low-risk ($R_{rec} \leq 3$) and high-risk ($R_{rec} > 3$) groups. Similarly, Cindolo and colleagues[76] constructed a recurrence risk formula (RRF) using tumor size and clinical presentation. From this series of 660 patients, 2- and 5-year survival was 96% and 93% for patients with a calculated RRF of less than or equal to 1.2, compared with 83% and 68% with a calculated RRF of greater than 1.2. In a multi-institutional dataset of 2517 patients undergoing surgical resection, Raj and colleagues[77] developed an accurate nomogram (CI 0.80) predicting freedom from metastatic recurrence at 12 years incorporating gender, mode of presentation, evidence of lymphadenopathy or necrosis on imaging, and tumor size. Although encouraging initial data has been reported, the clinical utility of these nomograms remains undefined because no individual preoperative nomogram has been developed that performs as well as algorithms incorporating pathologic data obtained at the time of surgical resection.[67]

Postoperative Algorithms for the Prediction of Disease Recurrence

The first nomogram designed to predict freedom from recurrence after surgical resection for RCC was developed by investigators from the Memorial Sloan Kettering Cancer Center. From a cohort of 601 patients with localized RCC, their algorithm incorporating pathologic tumor stage, tumor size, histologic subtype, and symptoms at the time of presentation. The 5-year probability of freedom from failure in this cohort was 86% (95% confidence interval 82%–89%), and their model was able to accurately predict disease recurrence with an AUC of 0.74.[78] This nomogram was subsequently updated in 2005 in a cohort of 833 patients with localized conventional ccRCC undergoing resection, using stage, Fuhrman grade, tumor size, necrosis, vascular invasion

Table 2
Prognostic staging systems for risk stratification of patients with localized and locally advanced RCC

Study	Prognostic Information	Extent of Disease	Histologic Subtype	Prognostic Variables	Presentation (Accuracy)
Preoperative Assessment					
Lane et al[68]	Malignancy	Localized (<7 cm)	All	Age, gender, tumor size, symptoms, smoking history	Nomogram; Malignancy (c-index 0.64)
Jeldres et al[69]	Grade	Localized (cT1a)	All	Age, gender, tumor size, symptoms	Nomogram (AUC 0.58)
Kutikov et al[71]	Malignancy grade	Localized	All	Age, gender, anatomic attributes[a]	Nomogram; Malignancy (AUC 0.76), grade (AUC 0.73)
Kutikov et al[73]	OS, CSS	Localized	All	Age, gender, tumor size, race	Nomogram
Yaycioglu et al[75]	RFS	Localized	All	Symptoms, tumor size	Algorithm
Cindolo et al[76]	RFS	Localized	All	Symptoms, tumor size	Algorithm
Raj et al[77]	Metastases	Nonmetastatic	All	Gender, presentation, lymphadenopathy/necrosis on imaging, tumor size	Nomogram (c-index 0.80)
Postoperative Assessment					
Kattan et al[78]	RFS	Localized	All	TNM stage, tumor size, histology, symptoms	Nomogram (c-index 0.74)
Sorbellini et al[79]	RFS	Localized	ccRCC	TNM stage, tumor size, nuclear grade, necrosis, microvascular invasion, symptoms	Nomogram (c-index 0.82)

Study	Endpoint	Disease state	Histology	Variables	Model
Frank et al[80]	RFS	Localized	All	TNM stage, tumor size, nuclear grade, necrosis	Algorithm (c-index 0.84)
Leibovich et al[82]	Metastases	Nonmetastatic	ccRCC	TNM stage, lymph node status, tumor size,[b] nuclear grade, necrosis	Algorithm (c-index 0.82)
Zisman et al[84]	OS	Localized, metastatic	All	TNM stage, nuclear grade, performance status[c]	Algorithm
Zisman et al[85]	OS	Localized, metastatic	All	TNM stage, nuclear grade, performance status[c]	Algorithm
Leibovich et al[86]	OS	Metastatic	All	Lymph node status, symptoms, metastasis location, histology, TSH	Algorithm
Motzer et al[87]	OS	Metastatic	All	hemoglobin, LDH, corrected calcium, performance status,[d] interval to treatment	Algorithm
Motzer et al[40]	OS	Metastatic	All	hemoglobin, corrected calcium, performance status[d]	Algorithm

Abbreviations: AUC, area under the curve; LDH, lactate dehydrogenase; OS, overall survival; RFS, recurrence-free survival; TSH, thyroid stimulating hormone.

[a] Quantitated by nephrometry score.
[b] Tumor size <10 or ≥10 cm.
[c] Eastern Cooperative Oncology Group performance status.
[d] Karnofsky score.

and clinical presentation. The 5-year probability of freedom from failure in this cohort was 80.9% (95% confidence interval 75.7%–85.1%), and the accuracy of their model improved evidenced by a CI of 0.82.[79] Also using cancer-specific survival as their primary outcome, investigators from the Mayo Clinic devised the state, size, grade, and necrosis (SSIGN) score from a cohort of 1801 patients with ccRCC. Using this system, points are assigned based on 1997 TNM stage, tumor size, nuclear grade, and presence of histologic necrosis, which are then used to estimate CSS at 1-, 5-, and 10-year intervals (CI 0.84).[80] This scoring algorithm has recently been externally validated with a high degree of prognostic accuracy in an Italian series of 388 patients (CI 0.88).[81] From the same institution, a separate scoring algorithm was developed to predict progression to metastatic disease in patients with clinically localized ccRCC. From a cohort of 1671 patients undergoing surgical resection, this novel system is based on points assigned to pathologic tumor stage, regional lymph node status, tumor size ($\geq$10, <10 cm), nuclear grade, and presence of histologic necrosis. With good predictive accuracy (CI 0.82), patients further stratified as high risk ($\geq$6) had a 42% and 63% chance of developing progressive disease at 1 and 3 years, respectively.[82]

Postoperative Nomograms for the Prediction of Survival

Several algorithms using pathologic features and specific laboratory parameters have been designed to predict overall survival in patients with mRCC before or following systemic therapy, including the University of California Los Angeles Integrated Staging System (UISS),[83–85] the Survival after Nephrectomy and Immunotherapy,[86] and the Memorial Sloan Kettering Cancer Center Motzer criteria.[40,87] Although specific discussion regarding these algorithms are deferred to chapters discussing metastatic disease, the pertinent details are summarized in **Table 2**. A significant limitation of these algorithms is that they do not predict the probability of an adverse event on an individual basis but instead place patients into risk-stratified groups. Although useful for stratifying patients for clinical protocols, this has less clinical applicability on the individual patient level. Other limitations include significant variety in patient selection criteria and lack of internal or external validation.[67] The discriminating ability of 4 prognostic algorithms[75,76,78,84] was compared using an independent multi-institutional dataset of 2404 patients with nonmetastatic RCC. Calculations of CIs and 95% bootstrap confidence intervals for overall survival, cancer-specific survival, and recurrence-free survival at 5 years consistently revealed that postoperative algorithms performed with higher accuracy than preoperative models. Of the 4 algorithms, the Kattan model was consistently found to be the most accurate (CI 0.71), although the UISS model was only slightly less well performing (CI 0.68).[88] Further comparative evaluation and validation of existing prognostic algorithms is necessary before any contemporary models can be rigorously employed.

ADJUVANT THERAPY FOR ADVANCED RENAL CELL CARCINOMA
Completed RCC Adjuvant Trials

Radiotherapy, hormonal therapy, cytotoxic chemotherapy, immunotherapy, and recently antiangiogenic therapies have been studied in the adjuvant setting for high-risk RCC (**Table 3**). Adjuvant radiotherapy, hormonal therapy, and cytotoxic chemotherapy for high-risk RCC both have showed no measurable survival benefit. An early study randomizing patients to surgery alone to surgery plus radiation reported improved survival for patients treated with surgery alone.[89] In a prospective trial evaluating radiotherapy after nephrectomy for stage II and III RCC, no differences in

Table 3
Completed randomized trials of adjuvant therapy for high-risk RCC

Treatment	References	Year	(N)	Median Follow-Up (Mo)	Outcomes	P Value
Cytotoxic Agents, Hormonal Agents, and Radiotherapy						
Radiation + surgery vs radiation	Finney[89]	1973	N/A	N/A	No differences in recurrence or survival	NS
Radiation vs observation	Kjaer et al[90]	1987	72	N/A	OS at 26 mo: 50% vs 62%	NS
Megace vs observation	Pizzocaro et al[91]	1987	136	60.0	Relapse rate: 32.7% vs 33.9%	NS
UFT vs observation	Naito et al[92]	1997	71	112.9	Nonrecurrence rate: 80.5% vs 77.1%	NS
Immunotherapeutic Agents						
Tumor cells + BCG vs observation	Galligioni et al[95]	1996	120	61.0	5-yr DFS: 63% vs 72%	NS
IFN vs observation	Pizzocaro et al[97]	2001	247	N/A	5-yr OS: 66.5% vs 66.0%	NS
IFN vs observation	Messing et al[96]	2003	283	124.0	Median OS: 5.1 vs 7.4 years	NS
High-dose IL-2 vs observation	Clark et al[94]	2003	69	N/A	Median DFS: 19.5 vs 36.0 mo	NS
Tumor cell vaccine vs observation	Jocham et al[100]	2004	558	N/A	5-yr PFS: 77.4% vs 67.8%	.02
IL-2 +IFN+FU vs observation	Atzpodien et al[98]	2005	203	51.0	8-yr RFS: 39% vs 49%	NS
HSPPC-96 vs observation	Wood et al[102]	2006	818	21.0	1.9-yr RFS: 62.3% vs 60.2%	NS
IL-2 +IFN+FU vs observation	NCT00053807	2006	550	N/A	Phase III completed, results pending	N/A
Thalidomide vs observation	Margulis et al[99]	2006	46	43.9 mo	3-yr RFS: 28.7% vs 69.3%	.02
Targeted/Antiangiogenic Agents						
Sunitinib vs sorafenib vs observation	NCT00326898	2010	1923	N/A	Phase III completed, results pending	N/A
Girentuximab vs observation	NCT00087022	2008	864	N/A	Phase III completed, results pending	N/A

Abbreviations: BCG, Bacillus Calmette-Guerin; DFS, disease-free survival; FU, fluorouracil; HSP, heat shock protein; IFN, interferon; IL, interleukin; NS, not significant; N/A, not applicable; OS, overall survival; PFS, progression-free survival; RFS, recurrence-free survival; UFT, tegafur and uracil.

relapse or survival rates were demonstrated between the radiotherapy and observation groups.[90] Medroxyprogesterone acetate, which has been shown to block glucocorticoid receptors on some RCC cells, also failed to demonstrate efficacy for high-risk RCC in the adjuvant setting.[91] Similarly, comparison of 71 patients randomized to adjuvant tegafur and uracil (UFT) revealed no significant differences in recurrence rates in patients with low-grade (Robson I and II) tumors.[92]

Although immunotherapy agents have demonstrated improved survival in patients with mRCC,[14,16,93] to date they have shown no benefit in the adjuvant setting for high-risk RCC.[94–97] A multicenter, randomized, controlled study was conducted to evaluate use of adjuvant interferon (IFN) in 247 patients with stage II and III RCC.[97] No significant differences for overall survival probabilities ($P = .86$) and event-free survival probabilities ($P = .11$) were demonstrated between the treatment and observation groups. Similarly, a prospective, randomized, controlled, phase III adjuvant trial using high-dose IL-2 also showed no benefit in patients with high-risk RCC. This trial was closed early when an interim analysis determined that the 30% improvement in 2-year disease-free survival could not be achieved despite complete accrual. There were no differences seen in disease-free survival between the treatment and control arms (19.5 vs 36.0 months, $P = .43$), and although no serious adverse events or treatment-related deaths were observed in the treatment arm, many suffered from hypotension (52%), nausea/vomiting (27%), and electrolyte abnormalities (27%).[94] Other investigators have studied the effectiveness of combining subcutaneous cytokine therapy with chemotherapeutic agents, such as 5-fluorouracil (5FU), in the adjuvant setting. A prospective trial from the German Cooperative Renal Carcinoma Chemoimmunotherapy Group investigating a combination of IL-2, IFN, and 5-FU in the adjuvant setting for high-risk RCC demonstrated a significantly worse 8-year overall survival rate for the treatment group (58%) when compared with the observation group (66%; $P = .03$). However, they observed no difference in 8-year relapse survival rates between the two groups.[98] Thalidomide, which possesses both immunomodulatory and antiangiogenic properties, was studied in an adjuvant, randomized trial for high-risk RCC following surgical resection. After enrollment of 46 patients, this trial was terminated early at a median follow-up of 43.9 months when the 2- and 3-year probabilities of relapse-free survival for the treatment group were found to be inferior to controls (47.8% vs 69.3% and 28.7% vs 69.3%, respectively; $P = .02$).[99]

Adjuvant vaccine trials continue to be an area of focused interest because of their finite treatment course and low toxicity. In the only adjuvant study to date to demonstrate a significant progression-free survival benefit, use of an autologous RCC vaccine (randomized, controlled, phase III trial) resulted in improved 5-year progression-free survival in patients with stage II and III RCC when compared with observation alone (77.4% vs 67.8%, $P = .02$). This trial suffers from several limitations, including the number of patients lost after the randomization step (32%), the imbalance of this loss between study arms, and the absence of overall survival reporting, which have led to challenging the clinical validity of these findings.[100] However, a recently reported updated 10-year survival analysis did reveal an overall survival difference between both groups, particularly in patients with pT3 disease.[101] Another recent adjuvant vaccine trial investigating the use of a heat-shock protein (glycoprotein 96) peptide complex derived from autologous RCC (HSPPC-96) in patients with high-risk RCC did not demonstrate the same benefit. With a median follow-up of 1.9 years, disease recurrence was similar in both the treatment and observation groups (37.7% vs 39.8%, $P = .50$).[102]

Girentuximab (WX-G250, Rencarex, Wilex Pharmaceuticals) is a targeted agent currently being evaluated in the adjuvant setting for high-risk RCC.[56,103] G250 is a monoclonal IgG1 antibody that binds to the CA IX antigen, which is expressed by 95% of clear cell RCC cells. Binding to this antigen may recruit effector cells or activate complement to result in the death of RCC cells.[54] A phase III trial, Adjuvant Rencarex Immunotherapy trial to Study Efficacy in nonmetastatic RCC, completed accrual in 2008. A total of 864 patients were enrolled and treated for 6 months with a once-weekly infusion of girentuximab or placebo. As of January 2011, 340 recurrences have been reported and the interim analysis of efficacy of adjuvant c-G250 has been initiated (NCT00087022, www.clinicaltrials.gov).

The use of antiangiogenic therapy in the adjuvant setting for high-risk RCC is another current area of intense interest. Both VEGF neutralizing antibodies and tyrosine kinase inhibitors, which block the receptors of VEGF, have been shown to improve outcomes in mRCC.[18,20,22,104] A randomized, controlled, phase III adjuvant sorafenib or sunitinib for unfavorable renal carcinoma (ASSURE) trial evaluating sorafenib and sunitinib for high-risk RCC in the adjuvant setting was recently completed in September 2010 after accrual of 1944 patients (NCT00326898). The primary endpoint of this study is disease free survival (DFS), with a 20% reduction in adverse events hypothesized for each experimental arm compared with placebo. When 842 DFS events have been observed, the primary efficacy analysis will be conducted. The ASSURE trial is also designed to assess multiple correlative endpoints to address several unresolved questions, including optimal duration of adjuvant targeted therapy and the benefit of sunitinib or sorafenib for non–clear cell histologies.

Ongoing Adjuvant RCC Trials

Based on activity demonstrated in advanced and mRCC, several multi-targeted vascular endothelial growth factor receptor (VEGFR) inhibitors and mTOR inhibitors are currently being investigated in the adjuvant setting. Five multi-targeting TKIs are currently commercially approved for development in advanced RCC, including sunitinib,[19] sorafenib,[21] pazopanib,[105] axitinib,[106,107] and tivozanib.[108] Currently, there are 4 trials investigating adjuvant targeted therapy for advanced RCC actively accruing patients (**Table 4**). Three trials (sorafenib versus placebo in patients with resected primary renal cell carcinoma [SORCE], sunitinib treatment of renal adjuvant cancer [S-TRAC], and pazopanib as adjuvant therapy in localized/locally advanced RCC after nephrectomy [PROTECT]) compare a VEGFR inhibitor against placebo, whereas the fourth everolimus for renal cancer ensuing therapy (EVEREST), is designed to compare everolimus with placebo. These trials are similarly designed regarding high-risk patient selection, collection of tissue for biomarker investigation, and central pathology review. The benefits of comparing similar patient populations cannot be overstated, and ultimately these trials will provide data for analysis of thousands of patients with advanced RCC. To address the role of targeted therapies in non–clear cell histologies, SORCE and EVEREST include patients with both clear cell and non–clear cell histologic types, whereas S-TRAC and PROTECT exclude non–clear cell tumors. To evaluate the optimal length of adjuvant treatment, the 3-arm SORCE trial will compare patients completing 1- and 3-year periods of sorafenib postoperatively to placebo.

Adjuvant Trials in Consideration of Development

The development of new agents active in RCC will undoubtedly lead to their application in the adjuvant setting. For instance, although bevacizumab, an anti-VEGF antibody, has shown efficacy in prolonging progression-free survival of patients with metastatic RCC,[22] there are currently no ongoing clinical trials evaluating its role in the adjuvant setting. Furthermore, if the second-generation VEGFR inhibitors (with

Table 4
Ongoing randomized trials of adjuvant therapy for high-risk RCC

	EVEREST (NCT01120249)	SORCE (NCT00492258)	S-TRAC (NCT00375674)	PROTECT (NCT01235962)
Sponsor	SWOG	Medical Research Council	Pfizer	GSK
Study design	Phase III, randomized, double blind, placebo controlled	Phase III, 3 arm, double blind, placebo controlled	Phase III, randomized, double blind, placebo controlled	Phase III, randomized, double blind, placebo controlled
Intervention	Everolimus x 54 wk	Sorafenib x 1 y or 2 y	Sunitinib x 1 y	Pazopanib x 1 y
Accrual #	1218	1656	500	1500
Inclusion criteria	Clear cell or papillary High-grade (G3/4) T1b or T2–4; any N if positive nodes are fully resected; and M0 Partial or radical nephrectomy No history of isolated or distant metastases Performance status 0 or 1 Enrollment ≥4 wk and ≤12 wk after surgery	Clear or non–clear cell Intermediate or high-risk disease Partial or radical nephrectomy No evidence of residual disease after resection with Leibovich score 3–11 Performance status 0 or 1 Enrollment ≥4 wk and ≤3 mo after surgery	Predominant clear cell High-risk disease per modified UISS criteria Partial or radical nephrectomy No evidence of residual disease after resection Performance status 0–2 Have had surgery at least 4 wk but no more than 12 wk before treatment start date	Predominant clear cell High-risk disease per Mayo Clinic SSIGN score M0 disease with pT2, Grade 3/4, N0, pT3–4, any G, N0, pTx, any G, N1 Partial or radical nephrectomy No evidence of residual disease after resection KPS ≥80 Have had surgery at least 4 wk but no more than 12 wk before treatment start date
Exclusion criteria	Histologically medullary or collecting duct carcinoma Positive surgical margins Positive renal vein margins are eligible but not positive renal vein wall margin Prior anticancer therapy other than nephrectomy	Diagnosis of second malignancy Prior anticancer treatment other than nephrectomy	Histologically undifferentiated carcinoma, predominant (>50%) sarcomatoid feature, collecting duct carcinoma, lymphoma, or sarcoma Diagnosis of second malignancy ≤5 y Prior anticancer treatment other than nephrectomy	Histologically predominant non–clear cell Diagnosis of second malignancy ≤5 y Prior anticancer treatment other than nephrectomy

Abbreviations: GSK, GlaxoSmithKline; SWOG, Southwest Oncology Group.

higher affinity), such as axitinib and tivozanib, show efficacy in patients with advanced or metastatic RCC, trials may be considered to study their role after resection of high-risk RCC in the adjuvant setting. The mTOR inhibitor, everolimus (Novartis Pharmaceuticals Corporation, East Hanover, NJ,) was approved by the FDA for the treatment of patients with advanced RCC after failure of treatment with sunitinib or sorafenib, after a phase III trial demonstrated improvement in progression-free survival of 4.9 and 1.9 months in the everolimus and placebo arms, respectively.[109] As previously mentioned, everolimus is to be imminently tested in the adjuvant setting. Similarly, novel immunotherapy, such as PD-1, and modified TKIs that have both fibroblast growth factor and VEGF activities may also be attractive for future applications in the adjuvant setting.

Still, many questions remain about the strategy that should be employed to further investigate adjuvant administration. Should duration of therapy be longer than 1 year? Are current doses used in metastatic disease suitable in the adjuvant setting? Should only the extremely high risk for recurrence populations be evaluated given drug tolerability? Should the pace of investigation and design of such trials slow down and wait for the availability of reliable biomarkers that can be used as screening eligibility criteria?

NEOADJUVANT STRATEGIES FOR LOCALIZED AND METASTATIC RENAL CELL CARCINOMA

In the absence of level I data, the administration of systemic therapy for RCC before surgical resection remains controversial. However, there are distinct advantages unique to neoadjuvant strategies. Recurrence rates following resection of high-risk tumors remain high primarily because of the existence of micrometastatic disease.[25] Neoadjuvant systemic therapy offers the potential to treat micrometastatic disease and reduce recurrence risk outside the surgical field. In addition, treatment before surgery affords the ability to assess resected tissue for treatment effect and guide future biomarker investigations. Additional potential benefits include the reduction of primary tumor burden to optimize surgical cure rates, ensure clear surgical margins, and facilitate minimally invasive or nephron sparing techniques in select cases.[110,111] This has led to the speculation that neoadjuvant therapy may be beneficial across a wide variety of applications, including debulking of unresectable disease, down staging tumor thrombi, treatment of local recurrence before metastasectomy, or identification of patients with rapidly progressive mRCC who would not benefit from cytoreductive nephrectomy.[112] These benefits must be balanced against the risks that preoperative systemic therapy may lead to increased perioperative morbidity and may even delay the timing of surgery.[113] Finally, inherent toxicities of some therapies may be incompatible with multimodality treatment strategies, including increased risks of bleeding, deficiencies in wound healing, and anesthesia complications.[114]

Neoadjuvant studies for kidney cancer have been limited during the cytokine era because of the poor responses in the primary tumor and the significant toxicity associated with treatment.[115] Results from a nonrandomized, controlled, phase II trial of patients treated with perioperative subcutaneous IL-2 before nephrectomy demonstrated small but significant improvements in cancer-specific and progression-free survival but has yet to be validated in phase III trials.[116] Preoperative tumor embolization has also been retrospectively investigated with a suggestion of a survival benefit but to date has not been prospectively evaluated.[117] However, in comparison to immunomodulatory agents, targeted TKI therapies have more demonstrable radiographic primary and metastatic tumor response rates as well as a more favorable safety profile.[112] Extrapolated from clinical trial data in mRCC, sunitinib has demonstrated the most dramatic partial response rate using response evaluation criteria in solid tumors criteria (31%),[19] compared with sorafenib which shows a response rate closer to 10%.[21] As a corollary, predictable growth characteristics make RCC amenable to neoadjuvant strategies. Recent evidence suggests that localized renal tumors can grow very large without acquiring metastatic potential.[118] Historically, slow growth kinetics, even for some metastatic tumors, affords the ability to delay surgical resection for the administration of systemic therapy for up to several weeks with minimal risk for disease progression in select patients. However, variables, including optimum duration of therapy and interval before surgery, are dependent on systemic agent half-life and have yet to be well defined (**Table 5**). Although targeted therapy often results in disease stabilization and necrosis rather than tumor regression,[35] retrospective clinical experiences using TKI therapy have demonstrated that the greatest degree of tumor reduction occurs within the first few cycles of therapy followed by disease stability,[119] which implies that a short highly defined treatment period immediately preceding surgical therapy may be most effective for neoadjuvant strategies.

Contemporary Clinical Experiences with Neoadjuvant Targeted Therapy

Although prospective clinical trial experience is limited, contemporary institutional experiences with neoadjuvant sunitinib, sorafenib, and bevacizumab have demonstrated no significant differences in surgery complexity, estimated blood loss, hospital stay, or perioperative morbidity across a wide variety of applications.[120–122] In a small case series of 4 patients, Shuch[112] demonstrated tumor response with preoperative TKI therapy for tumor thrombus, nodal involvement, renal fossa recurrence, and lymph node metastases, demonstrating tumor effects not previously seen with use of immunomodulation based therapies. In the first reported series of 9 patients receiving either sorafenib or sunitinib preoperatively for locally advanced or mRCC, Amin and colleagues[119] reported a mean tumor response rate of 12.9% with no significant

Table 5
Mechanism of action and duration of systemic longevity of contemporary targeted therapy agents for surgical considerations

Agent	Mechanism of Inhibition	Half-Life	Proposed Interval to Surgery (5 Half-Lives) (d)
Sunitinib	PDGFR-α,β, VEGFR-1,2,3, KIT, FLT3, RET	40–60 h	8–12
Sorafenib	PDGFR- β, VEGFR-2,3, KIT, FLT-3, Raf kinase	25–48 h	5–10
Pazopanib	VEGFR-1,2,3	35 h	7–8
Axitinib	VEGFR-1,2,3	2–5 h	1–2
Tivozanib	VEGFR-1,2,3	5 d	25
Bevacizumab	Anti-VEGF monoclonal antibody	20 d	100[a]
Temsirolimus	mTOR	17 h	4–5
Everolimus	mTOR	28 h	5–6

Abbreviations: FLT, Fms-like tyrosine kinase; KIT, stem cell factor receptor; PDGFR, platelet-derived growth factor receptor; RET, glial cell-line derived neurotrophic factor receptor; TOR, mammalian target of rapamycin; VEGFR, vascular endothelial growth factor receptor.
[a] Current neoadjuvant trials report a washout period of 1 month before surgical resection.

intraoperative or postoperative complications attributed to TKI therapy. In a single-arm, phase II trial, 50 patients with resectable metastatic ccRCC were treated with bevacizumab plus erlotinib (n = 23) or bevacizumab alone (n = 27) followed by restaging imaging. Ultimately, 42 patients underwent cytoreductive surgery, with median progression-free and overall survival rates of 11.0 and 25.4 months, respectively. Two perioperative deaths occurred that were not attributed to the study drugs, but wound dehiscences resulted in treatment discontinuation for 3 patients and treatment delays for 2 others.[123] Chapin and colleagues[124] recently reviewed the MD Anderson experience of patients with mRCC undergoing cytoreductive nephrectomy, and identified 67 patients who underwent neoadjuvant targeted therapy before surgery. They observed that complications occurred in 64% (30% with greater than or equal to a Clavien grade III) of patients within 1 year following nephrectomy. Of these, the most common occurrences were superficial wound dehiscence (25%) and wound infection (15%).

In an effort to evaluate the use of neoadjuvant therapy to downstage unresectable disease for consolidative surgery, investigators from the Cleveland Clinic reported results in 19 patients with locally advanced RCC treated with 1 cycle of sunitinib before surgery. They observed a partial response rate of 11%, with 37% of patients demonstrating stable disease and 53% showing signs of disease progression, and concluded that neoadjuvant administration of sunitinib is feasible with acceptable toxicity and can lead to a reduction in tumor burden that may facilitate surgical resection. At a median follow-up of 6 months, 21% of patients underwent surgical resection and 26% patients had died of disease progression.[125] In a prospective single-arm, open-label trial of 20 patients with biopsy proven localized or metastatic ccRCC receiving 3 months of neoadjuvant sunitinib therapy, Hellenthal and colleagues[126] reported a reduction in mean tumor diameter in 17 of 20 patients (85%). Of these patients, 8 patients ultimately underwent laparoscopic partial nephrectomy, and the investigators concluded that preoperative sunitinib may facilitate nephron sparing surgery and decrease the risk of recurrence in patients with localized RCC with high-risk features. In the largest prospective neoadjuvant experience to date, 30 patients with greater than or equal to stage II RCC underwent preoperative treatment with sorafenib before resection (median 33 days). All patients were able to proceed to nephrectomy with no perioperative complications related to drug administration reported. No patient demonstrated progression of disease before therapy, whereas reported partial response and disease stabilization rates were 7.1% and 92.9%, respectively.[127] In a recent report, Salem and colleagues[128] compared before and after sunitinib treatment imaging before surgical intervention, observing significantly decreased radiographic size/attenuation and increased necrosis before surgery. Post-therapy, 88% of the tumors had decreased long diameter (median 32% decrease, $P<.001$ vs baseline), 88% decreased attenuation (median 30 hounsfield units reduction, $P = .006$), and 69% increased necrosis ($P = .001$).

To summarize these findings, there is now a growing body of evidence to suggest a role for neoadjuvant targeted therapy in the treatment of advanced RCC in a variety of settings. Although concerns still exist regarding wound healing, neoadjuvant treatment appears to be well tolerated and safe, with no demonstrable increase in surgical perioperative or postoperative morbidity. Use of neoadjuvant targeted therapy (sunitinib, sorafenib, everolimus, axitinib) for locally advanced and mRCC is currently being evaluated in phase II clinical trials, (**Table 6**) but significant questions remain unanswered regarding the need and timing for cytoreductive nephrectomy in patients that show a complete or dramatic response to upfront targeted therapies, as well as the necessity of neoadjuvant administration in patients with metastatic but indolent

Table 6
Contemporary clinical trials investigating the use of neoadjuvant targeted therapy in advanced or metastatic RCC

Center	Drug	Target	Design	Activity	Duration	Accrual Goal	Primary Outcome
MD Anderson NCT00126659	Sorafenib	mRCC (cc)	II, 3 arms[a]	Closed	10 wk	45	Safety, response
MD Anderson NCT00113217	Bevacizumab	mRCC (cc)	II, single arm	Not recruiting	1 cycle	50	Safety, time to progression
University of North Carolina NCT00405366	Sorafenib	Advanced, mRCC	II, single arm	Not recruiting	1 cycle, 4–8 wk	30	Safety, biomarkers
University of Toronto NCT00480935	Sunitinib	Localized RCC (cc)	II, single arm	Active	2 cycles[a]	30	Safety, biomarkers
Orchid Clinical Trials Group, London NCT01024205	Sunitinib	mRCC (cc)	II, single arm	Active	3 cycles	43	Response
Roswell Park Cancer Institute NCT00849186	Sunitinib	Advanced or mRCC	II, single arm	Active	3 mo	20	Safety, safety of surgery
Northwestern University NCT00727532	Sorafenib	Advanced or mRCC (cc)	II, single arm	Active	1 cycle	10	response, time to progression
Medical University of South Carolina NCT00747305	Sunitinib	mRCC (cc)	II, single arm	Active	1 cycle	28	Biomarkers, response

Gruppo Italiano Carcinoma Renale NCT00626509	Sunitinib	mRCC	II, 2 arms[b]	Active	2 cycles	110	Safety, response
University of Pennsylvania NCT00717587	Sunitinib	mRCC	II, single arm	Active	1 cycle	20	Response, biomarkers
Korean Urological Oncology Society NCT01069770	Sunitinib	mRCC (cc)	II, single arm	Active	2 cycles	32	Safety, response
St Josephs, Ontario NCT01107509	Everolimus	Advanced or mRCC	II, single arm	Active	12 wk	20	Response, biomarkers
University of California, Los Angeles NCT01070186	Sunitinib	Localized RCC	II, single arm	Active	1 cycle	30	Time to recurrence, biomarkers
Baylor College of Medicine NCT00831480	Everolimus	Advanced or mRCC	II, single arm	Not yet recruiting	3–5 wk	27	Progression
MD Anderson NCT01263769	Axitinib	Advanced RCC (cc)	II, single arm	Not yet recruiting	12 wk	24	Response

Abbreviation: cc, clear cell.

[a] Arm I: immediate cytoreductive nephrectomy followed by 10 weeks adjuvant sorafenib; Arm II: 1 week sorafenib followed by cytoreductive nephrectomy and 9 additional weeks of sorafenib; Arm III: 4 weeks sorafenib followed by cytoreductive nephrectomy and 6 additional weeks of sorafenib (sequential assignment, nonrandomized).

[b] Arm I: immediate cytoreductive nephrectomy then adjuvant sunitinib for up to 1 year; Arm II: 2 cycles of neoadjuvant sunitinib followed by cytoreductive nephrectomy (randomized).

disease at presentation.[114] A phase II randomized trial comparing neoadjuvant and adjuvant sunitinib in patients with mRCC undergoing cytoreductive nephrectomy is currently nearing accrual completion, and an European Organization for the Research and Treatment of Cancer trial randomizing patients with mRCC to 3 cycles of neoadjuvant sunitinib (with nonprogressors proceeding to cytoreductive nephrectomy) or adjuvant treatment following resection to assess progression-free survival is in the early planning phases. Additional questions currently under investigation are the use of targeted therapy for non–clear cell tumors,[129] and the role of targeted therapy for locally recurrent lesions amenable to metastatectomy.[130] It is the authors' hope that these ongoing clinical trials and biomarker investigations will ultimately provide insight into which patients will benefit from up-front targeted therapy, surgical resection, or a combination of both.

SUMMARY

The standard of care for clinically localized RCC remains surgical resection because of the favorable prognosis associated with surgery and the relative ineffectiveness of systemic therapy alone. Prognostic variables have been integrated into predictive algorithms to better identify patients at high risk for disease recurrence and guide future clinical trial development. Molecular and genetic markers of prognosis are currently under investigation and may improve the predictive power of these risk-stratification instruments. Although adjuvant cytotoxic agents, immunotherapy and radiation therapies for advanced and mRCC have not yet been shown to be effective, a better understanding of the molecular and cellular biology of RCC has led to the development of promising systemic targeted agents that have demonstrated efficacy in clinical trials of patients with unresected mRCC. Simple administration and low systemic toxicity of these targeted agents has led to considerable interest for use in the adjuvant setting for patients at high risk for recurrence, which is currently being evaluated prospectively with initial results expected soon. The timing and role of neoadjuvant therapy before cytoreductive surgery to downstage bulky disease and eradicate micrometastatic disease is currently controversial and is under investigation in phase II clinical trials. Further investigation of molecular and genetic tumor biology may help to identify additional cellular targets for future adjuvant or neoadjuvant therapies for advanced RCC.

REFERENCES

1. Jemal A, Siegel R, Xu J, et al. Cancer statistics, 2010. CA Cancer J Clin 2010;60: 277.
2. Chow WH, Devesa SS, Warren JL, et al. Rising incidence of renal cell cancer in the United States. JAMA 1999;281:1628.
3. Hollingsworth JM, Miller DC, Daignault S, et al. Rising incidence of small renal masses: a need to reassess treatment effect. J Natl Cancer Inst 2006;98:1331.
4. Jayson M, Sanders H. Increased incidence of serendipitously discovered renal cell carcinoma. Urology 1998;51:203.
5. Frank I, Blute ML, Leibovich BC, et al. Independent validation of the 2002 American Joint Committee on cancer primary tumor classification for renal cell carcinoma using a large, single institution cohort. J Urol 2005;173:1889.
6. Huang WC, Levey AS, Serio AM, et al. Chronic kidney disease after nephrectomy in patients with renal cortical tumours: a retrospective cohort study. Lancet Oncol 2006;7:735.

7. McKiernan J, Simmons R, Katz J, et al. Natural history of chronic renal insufficiency after partial and radical nephrectomy. Urology 2002;59:816.
8. Go AS, Chertow GM, Fan D, et al. Chronic kidney disease and the risks of death, cardiovascular events, and hospitalization. N Engl J Med 2004;351:1296.
9. Huang WC, Elkin EB, Levey AS, et al. Partial nephrectomy versus radical nephrectomy in patients with small renal tumors–is there a difference in mortality and cardiovascular outcomes? J Urol 2009;181:55.
10. Thompson RH, Boorjian SA, Lohse CM, et al. Radical nephrectomy for pT1a renal masses may be associated with decreased overall survival compared with partial nephrectomy. J Urol 2008;179:468.
11. Gill IS, Kavoussi LR, Lane BR, et al. Comparison of 1,800 laparoscopic and open partial nephrectomies for single renal tumors. J Urol 2007;178:41.
12. Hafez KS, Fergany AF, Novick AC. Nephron sparing surgery for localized renal cell carcinoma: impact of tumor size on patient survival, tumor recurrence and TNM staging. J Urol 1999;162:1930.
13. Lam JS, Shvarts O, Leppert JT, et al. Renal cell carcinoma 2005: new frontiers in staging, prognostication and targeted molecular therapy. J Urol 2005;173:1853.
14. Flanigan RC, Salmon SE, Blumenstein BA, et al. Nephrectomy followed by interferon alfa-2b compared with interferon alfa-2b alone for metastatic renal-cell cancer. N Engl J Med 2001;345:1655.
15. Fallick ML, McDermott DF, LaRock D, et al. Nephrectomy before interleukin-2 therapy for patients with metastatic renal cell carcinoma. J Urol 1997;158:1691.
16. Mickisch GH, Garin A, van Poppel H, et al. Radical nephrectomy plus interferon-alfa-based immunotherapy compared with interferon alfa alone in metastatic renal-cell carcinoma: a randomised trial. Lancet 2001;358:966.
17. Wolf JS Jr, Aronson FR, Small EJ, et al. Nephrectomy for metastatic renal cell carcinoma: a component of systemic treatment regimens. J Surg Oncol 1994;55:7.
18. Escudier B, Eisen T, Stadler WM, et al. Sorafenib in advanced clear-cell renal-cell carcinoma. N Engl J Med 2007;356:125.
19. Motzer RJ, Hutson TE, Tomczak P, et al. Sunitinib versus interferon alfa in metastatic renal-cell carcinoma. N Engl J Med 2007;356:115.
20. Motzer RJ, Rini BI, Bukowski RM, et al. Sunitinib in patients with metastatic renal cell carcinoma. JAMA 2006;295:2516.
21. Ratain MJ, Eisen T, Stadler WM, et al. Phase II placebo-controlled randomized discontinuation trial of sorafenib in patients with metastatic renal cell carcinoma. J Clin Oncol 2006;24:2505.
22. Escudier B, Pluzanska A, Koralewski P, et al. Bevacizumab plus interferon alfa-2a for treatment of metastatic renal cell carcinoma: a randomised, double-blind phase III trial. Lancet 2007;370:2103.
23. Tsui KH, Shvarts O, Smith RB, et al. Prognostic indicators for renal cell carcinoma: a multivariate analysis of 643 patients using the revised 1997 TNM staging criteria. J Urol 2000;163:1090.
24. Lam JS, Shvarts O, Leppert JT, et al. Postoperative surveillance protocol for patients with localized and locally advanced renal cell carcinoma based on a validated prognostic nomogram and risk group stratification system. J Urol 2005;174:466.
25. Kunkle DA, Haas NB, Uzzo RG. Adjuvant therapy for high-risk renal cell carcinoma patients. Curr Urol Rep 2007;8:19.
26. Eggener SE, Yossepowitch O, Pettus JA, et al. Renal cell carcinoma recurrence after nephrectomy for localized disease: predicting survival from time of recurrence. J Clin Oncol 2006;24:3101.

27. Levy DA, Slaton JW, Swanson DA, et al. Stage specific guidelines for surveillance after radical nephrectomy for local renal cell carcinoma. J Urol 1998; 159:1163.

28. Sandock DS, Seftel AD, Resnick MI. A new protocol for the follow-up of renal cell carcinoma based on pathological stage. J Urol 1995;154:28.

29. Stephenson AJ, Chetner MP, Rourke K, et al. Guidelines for the surveillance of localized renal cell carcinoma based on the patterns of relapse after nephrectomy. J Urol 2004;172:58.

30. Hafez KS, Novick AC, Campbell SC. Patterns of tumor recurrence and guidelines for follow-up after nephron sparing surgery for sporadic renal cell carcinoma. J Urol 1997;157:2067.

31. Pantuck AJ, Zisman A, Belldegrun AS. The changing natural history of renal cell carcinoma. J Urol 2001;166:1611.

32. Janzen NK, Kim HL, Figlin RA, et al. Surveillance after radical or partial nephrectomy for localized renal cell carcinoma and management of recurrent disease. Urol Clin North Am 2003;30:843.

33. Adamy A, Chong KT, Chade D, et al. Clinical characteristics and outcomes of patients with recurrence 5 years after nephrectomy for localized renal cell carcinoma. J Urol 2011;185:433.

34. Ljungberg B, Alamdari FI, Rasmuson T, et al. Follow-up guidelines for nonmetastatic renal cell carcinoma based on the occurrence of metastases after radical nephrectomy. BJU Int 1999;84:405.

35. Motzer RJ, Bukowski RM. Targeted therapy for metastatic renal cell carcinoma. J Clin Oncol 2006;24:5601.

36. Fyfe G, Fisher RI, Rosenberg SA, et al. Results of treatment of 255 patients with metastatic renal cell carcinoma who received high-dose recombinant interleukin-2 therapy. J Clin Oncol 1995;13:688.

37. Boorjian SA, Crispen PL, Lohse CM, et al. Surgical resection of isolated retroperitoneal lymph node recurrence of renal cell carcinoma following nephrectomy. J Urol 2008;180:99.

38. Russo P, Synder M, Vickers A, et al. Cytoreductive nephrectomy and nephrectomy/complete metastasectomy for metastatic renal cancer. ScientificWorldJournal 2007;7:768.

39. Lane BR, Kattan MW, Novick AC. Prediction models of renal cell carcinoma. AUA Update Series 25. American Urological Association; 2006. p. 57.

40. Motzer RJ, Bacik J, Schwartz LH, et al. Prognostic factors for survival in previously treated patients with metastatic renal cell carcinoma. J Clin Oncol 2004;22:454.

41. Shuch B, La Rochelle JC, Wu J, et al. Performance status and cytoreductive nephrectomy: redefining management in patients with poor performance. Cancer 2008;113:1324.

42. Santos Arrontes D, Fernandez Acenero MJ, Garcia Gonzalez JI, et al. Survival analysis of clear cell renal carcinoma according to the Charlson comorbidity index. J Urol 2008;179:857.

43. Kim HL, Belldegrun AS, Freitas DG, et al. Paraneoplastic signs and symptoms of renal cell carcinoma: implications for prognosis. J Urol 2003;170:1742.

44. Kontak JA, Campbell SC. Prognostic factors in renal cell carcinoma. Urol Clin North Am 2003;30:467.

45. Johnson TV, Abbasi A, Owen-Smith A, et al. Absolute preoperative C-reactive protein predicts metastasis and mortality in the first year following potentially curative nephrectomy for clear cell renal cell carcinoma. J Urol 2010; 183:480.

46. Edge SB, Byrd DR, Compton CC, et al, editors. AJCC: kidney. 7th edition. (AJCC Cancer Staging Manual). New York: Springer; 2010. p. 479.
47. Leibovich BC, Lohse CM, Crispen PL, et al. Histological subtype is an independent predictor of outcome for patients with renal cell carcinoma. J Urol 2010; 183:1309.
48. Katz MD, Serrano MF, Grubb RL 3rd, et al. Percent microscopic tumor necrosis and survival after curative surgery for renal cell carcinoma. J Urol 2010;183:909.
49. Cangiano T, Liao J, Naitoh J, et al. Sarcomatoid renal cell carcinoma: biologic behavior, prognosis, and response to combined surgical resection and immunotherapy. J Clin Oncol 1999;17:523.
50. Klatte T, Said JW, de Martino M, et al. Presence of tumor necrosis is not a significant predictor of survival in clear cell renal cell carcinoma: higher prognostic accuracy of extent based rather than presence/absence classification. J Urol 2009;181:1558.
51. Ficarra V, Martignoni G, Maffei N, et al. Original and reviewed nuclear grading according to the Fuhrman system: a multivariate analysis of 388 patients with conventional renal cell carcinoma. Cancer 2005;103:68.
52. Smaldone MC, Maranchie JK. Clinical implications of hypoxia inducible factor in renal cell carcinoma. Urol Oncol 2009;27:238.
53. Wood CG. Molecular markers of prognosis in renal cell carcinoma: insight into tumor biology helps define risk and provides targets for therapy. J Surg Oncol 2006;94:264.
54. Atkins M, Regan M, McDermott D, et al. Carbonic anhydrase IX expression predicts outcome of interleukin 2 therapy for renal cancer. Clin Cancer Res 2005;11:3714.
55. Bui MH, Seligson D, Han KR, et al. Carbonic anhydrase IX is an independent predictor of survival in advanced renal clear cell carcinoma: implications for prognosis and therapy. Clin Cancer Res 2003;9:802.
56. Davis ID, Wiseman GA, Lee FT, et al. A phase I multiple dose, dose escalation study of cG250 monoclonal antibody in patients with advanced renal cell carcinoma. Cancer Immun 2007;7:13.
57. Divgi CR, Pandit-Taskar N, Jungbluth AA, et al. Preoperative characterisation of clear-cell renal carcinoma using iodine-124-labelled antibody chimeric G250 (124I-cG250) and PET in patients with renal masses: a phase I trial. Lancet Oncol 2007;8:304.
58. Uzzo RG, Russo P, Chen D, et al. The multicenter phase III redect trial: a comparative study of 124 I-girentuximab-PET/CT versus diagnostic CT for the preoperative diagnosis of clear cell Renal Cell Carcinoma (ccRCC). late breaking abstract. San Francisco (CA): AUA; 2010.
59. Bui MH, Visapaa H, Seligson D, et al. Prognostic value of carbonic anhydrase IX and KI67 as predictors of survival for renal clear cell carcinoma. J Urol 2004; 171:2461.
60. Kim HL, Seligson D, Liu X, et al. Using tumor markers to predict the survival of patients with metastatic renal cell carcinoma. J Urol 2005;173:1496.
61. Kim HL, Seligson D, Liu X, et al. Using protein expressions to predict survival in clear cell renal carcinoma. Clin Cancer Res 2004;10:5464.
62. Lam JS, Leppert JT, Figlin RA, et al. Role of molecular markers in the diagnosis and therapy of renal cell carcinoma. Urology 2005;66:1.
63. Jones PA, Baylin SB. The fundamental role of epigenetic events in cancer. Nat Rev Genet 2002;3:415.

64. Gonzalgo ML, Yegnasubramanian S, Yan G, et al. Molecular profiling and classification of sporadic renal cell carcinoma by quantitative methylation analysis. Clin Cancer Res 2004;10:7276.
65. Dulaimi E, Ibanez de Caceres I, Uzzo RG, et al. Promoter hypermethylation profile of kidney cancer. Clin Cancer Res 2004;10:3972.
66. Uzzo RG. Renal masses–to treat or not to treat? If that is the question are contemporary biomarkers the answer? J Urol 2008;180:433.
67. Lane BR, Kattan MW. Prognostic models and algorithms in renal cell carcinoma. Urol Clin North Am 2008;35:613.
68. Lane BR, Babineau D, Kattan MW, et al. A preoperative prognostic nomogram for solid enhancing renal tumors 7 cm or less amenable to partial nephrectomy. J Urol 2007;178:429.
69. Jeldres C, Sun M, Liberman D, et al. Can renal mass biopsy assessment of tumor grade be safely substituted for by a predictive model? J Urol 2009;182:2585.
70. Kutikov A, Uzzo RG. The R.E.N.A.L. nephrometry score: a comprehensive standardized system for quantitating renal tumor size, location and depth. J Urol 2009;182:844.
71. Kutikov A, Manley BJ, Canter DJ, et al. Anatomical features of enhancing renal masses predict histology and grade - an analysis using nephrometry (AUA abstract no. 1238). J Urol 2010;183:e479.
72. Lane BR, Samplaski MK, Herts BR, et al. Renal mass biopsy–a renaissance? J Urol 2008;179:20.
73. Kutikov A, Egleston BL, Wong YN, et al. Evaluating overall survival and competing risks of death in patients with localized renal cell carcinoma using a comprehensive nomogram. J Clin Oncol 2010;28:311.
74. Kutikov A, Egleston BL, Smaldone MC, et al. Quantification of competing risks of death with localized renal cell carcinoma (RCC): a comprehensive nomogram incorporating co-morbidities Podium presentation; American Urologic Association meeting. Washington, May, 2011.
75. Yaycioglu O, Roberts WW, Chan T, et al. Prognostic assessment of nonmetastatic renal cell carcinoma: a clinically based model. Urology 2001;58:141.
76. Cindolo L, de la Taille A, Messina G, et al. A preoperative clinical prognostic model for non-metastatic renal cell carcinoma. BJU Int 2003;92:901.
77. Raj GV, Thompson RH, Leibovich BC, et al. Preoperative nomogram predicting 12-year probability of metastatic renal cancer. J Urol 2008;179:2146.
78. Kattan MW, Reuter V, Motzer RJ, et al. A postoperative prognostic nomogram for renal cell carcinoma. J Urol 2001;166:63.
79. Sorbellini M, Kattan MW, Snyder ME, et al. A postoperative prognostic nomogram predicting recurrence for patients with conventional clear cell renal cell carcinoma. J Urol 2005;173:48.
80. Frank I, Blute ML, Cheville JC, et al. An outcome prediction model for patients with clear cell renal cell carcinoma treated with radical nephrectomy based on tumor stage, size, grade and necrosis: the SSIGN score. J Urol 2002;168:2395.
81. Ficarra V, Martignoni G, Lohse C, et al. External validation of the Mayo Clinic Stage, Size, Grade and Necrosis (SSIGN) score to predict cancer specific survival using a European series of conventional renal cell carcinoma. J Urol 2006;175:1235.
82. Leibovich BC, Blute ML, Cheville JC, et al. Prediction of progression after radical nephrectomy for patients with clear cell renal cell carcinoma: a stratification tool for prospective clinical trials. Cancer 2003;97:1663.

83. Patard JJ, Kim HL, Lam JS, et al. Use of the University of California Los Angeles integrated staging system to predict survival in renal cell carcinoma: an international multicenter study. J Clin Oncol 2004;22:3316.

84. Zisman A, Pantuck AJ, Dorey F, et al. Improved prognostication of renal cell carcinoma using an integrated staging system. J Clin Oncol 2001;19:1649.

85. Zisman A, Pantuck AJ, Wieder J, et al. Risk group assessment and clinical outcome algorithm to predict the natural history of patients with surgically resected renal cell carcinoma. J Clin Oncol 2002;20:4559.

86. Leibovich BC, Han KR, Bui MH, et al. Scoring algorithm to predict survival after nephrectomy and immunotherapy in patients with metastatic renal cell carcinoma: a stratification tool for prospective clinical trials. Cancer 2003;98:2566.

87. Motzer RJ, Bacik J, Murphy BA, et al. Interferon-alfa as a comparative treatment for clinical trials of new therapies against advanced renal cell carcinoma. J Clin Oncol 2002;20:289.

88. Cindolo L, Patard JJ, Chiodini P, et al. Comparison of predictive accuracy of four prognostic models for nonmetastatic renal cell carcinoma after nephrectomy: a multicenter European study. Cancer 2005;104:1362.

89. Finney R. The value of radiotherapy in the treatment of hypernephroma–a clinical trial. Br J Urol 1973;45:258.

90. Kjaer M, Frederiksen PL, Engelholm SA. Postoperative radiotherapy in stage II and III renal adenocarcinoma. A randomized trial by the Copenhagen Renal Cancer Study Group. Int J Radiat Oncol Biol Phys 1987;13:665.

91. Pizzocaro G, Piva L, Di Fronzo G, et al. Adjuvant medroxyprogesterone acetate to radical nephrectomy in renal cancer: 5-year results of a prospective randomized study. J Urol 1987;138:1379.

92. Naito S, Kumazawa J, Omoto T, et al. Postoperative UFT adjuvant and the risk factors for recurrence in renal cell carcinoma: a long-term follow-up study. Kyushu University Urological Oncology Group. Int J Urol 1997;4:8.

93. Yang JC, Sherry RM, Steinberg SM, et al. Randomized study of high-dose and low-dose interleukin-2 in patients with metastatic renal cancer. J Clin Oncol 2003;21:3127.

94. Clark JI, Atkins MB, Urba WJ, et al. Adjuvant high-dose bolus interleukin-2 for patients with high-risk renal cell carcinoma: a cytokine working group randomized trial. J Clin Oncol 2003;21:3133.

95. Galligioni E, Quaia M, Merlo A, et al. Adjuvant immunotherapy treatment of renal carcinoma patients with autologous tumor cells and bacillus Calmette-Guerin: five-year results of a prospective randomized study. Cancer 1996;77:2560.

96. Messing EM, Manola J, Wilding G, et al. Phase III study of interferon alfa-NL as adjuvant treatment for resectable renal cell carcinoma: an Eastern Cooperative Oncology Group/Intergroup trial. J Clin Oncol 2003;21:1214.

97. Pizzocaro G, Piva L, Colavita M, et al. Interferon adjuvant to radical nephrectomy in Robson stages II and III renal cell carcinoma: a multicentric randomized study. J Clin Oncol 2001;19:425.

98. Atzpodien J, Schmitt E, Gertenbach U, et al. Adjuvant treatment with interleukin-2- and interferon-alpha2a-based chemoimmunotherapy in renal cell carcinoma post tumour nephrectomy: results of a prospectively randomised trial of the German Cooperative Renal Carcinoma Chemoimmunotherapy Group (DGCIN). Br J Cancer 2005;92:843.

99. Margulis V, Matin SF, Tannir N, et al. Randomized trial of adjuvant thalidomide versus observation in patients with completely resected high-risk renal cell carcinoma. Urology 2009;73:337.

100. Jocham D, Richter A, Hoffmann L, et al. Adjuvant autologous renal tumour cell vaccine and risk of tumour progression in patients with renal-cell carcinoma after radical nephrectomy: phase III, randomised controlled trial. Lancet 2004;363:594.

101. May M, Brookman-May S, Hoschke B, et al. Ten-year survival analysis for renal carcinoma patients treated with an autologous tumour lysate vaccine in an adjuvant setting. Cancer Immunol Immunother 2010;59:687.

102. Wood C, Srivastava P, Bukowski R, et al. An adjuvant autologous therapeutic vaccine (HSPPC-96; vitespen) versus observation alone for patients at high risk of recurrence after nephrectomy for renal cell carcinoma: a multicentre, open-label, randomised phase III trial. Lancet 2008;372:145.

103. Davis ID, Liu Z, Saunders W, et al. A pilot study of monoclonal antibody cG250 and low dose subcutaneous IL-2 in patients with advanced renal cell carcinoma. Cancer Immun 2007;7:14.

104. Motzer RJ, Michaelson MD, Redman BG, et al. Activity of SU11248, a multitargeted inhibitor of vascular endothelial growth factor receptor and platelet-derived growth factor receptor, in patients with metastatic renal cell carcinoma. J Clin Oncol 2006;24:16.

105. Sternberg CN, Davis ID, Mardiak J, et al. Pazopanib in locally advanced or metastatic renal cell carcinoma: results of a randomized phase III trial. J Clin Oncol 2010;28:1061.

106. Rini BI, Wilding G, Hudes G, et al. Phase II study of axitinib in sorafenib-refractory metastatic renal cell carcinoma. J Clin Oncol 2009;27:4462.

107. Rixe O, Bukowski RM, Michaelson MD, et al. Axitinib treatment in patients with cytokine-refractory metastatic renal-cell cancer: a phase II study. Lancet Oncol 2007;8:975.

108. Bhargava P, Esteves B, Al-Adhami M, et al. Activity of tivozanib (AV-951) in patients with renal cell carcinoma (RCC): subgroup analysis from a phase II randomized discontinuation trial (RDT). J Clin Oncol 2010;28:15 [abstract: 4599].

109. Motzer RJ, Escudier B, Oudard S, et al. Efficacy of everolimus in advanced renal cell carcinoma: a double-blind, randomised, placebo-controlled phase III trial. Lancet 2008;372:449.

110. Rabets JC, Kaouk J, Fergany A, et al. Laparoscopic versus open cytoreductive nephrectomy for metastatic renal cell carcinoma. Urology 2004;64:930.

111. Krambeck AE, Leibovich BC, Lohse CM, et al. The role of nephron sparing surgery for metastatic (pM1) renal cell carcinoma. J Urol 2006;176:1990.

112. Shuch B, Riggs SB, LaRochelle JC, et al. Neoadjuvant targeted therapy and advanced kidney cancer: observations and implications for a new treatment paradigm. BJU Int 2008;102:692.

113. Wood CG. Multimodal approaches in the management of locally advanced and metastatic renal cell carcinoma: combining surgery and systemic therapies to improve patient outcome. Clin Cancer Res 2007;13:697s.

114. Rathmell WK, Pruthi R, Wallen E. Neoadjuvant treatment of renal cell carcinoma. Urol Oncol 2010;28:69.

115. Wagner JR, Walther MM, Linehan WM, et al. Interleukin-2 based immunotherapy for metastatic renal cell carcinoma with the kidney in place. J Urol 1999;162:43.

116. Klatte T, Ittenson A, Rohl FW, et al. Perioperative immunomodulation with interleukin-2 in patients with renal cell carcinoma: results of a controlled phase II trial. Br J Cancer 2006;95:1167.

117. Zielinski H, Szmigielski S, Petrovich Z. Comparison of preoperative embolization followed by radical nephrectomy with radical nephrectomy alone for renal cell carcinoma. Am J Clin Oncol 2000;23:6.

118. Rothman J, Egleston B, Wong YN, et al. Histopathological characteristics of localized renal cell carcinoma correlate with tumor size: a SEER analysis. J Urol 2009;181:29.
119. Amin C, Wallen E, Pruthi RS, et al. Preoperative tyrosine kinase inhibition as an adjunct to debulking nephrectomy. Urology 2008;72:864.
120. Margulis V, Matin SF, Tannir N, et al. Surgical morbidity associated with administration of targeted molecular therapies before cytoreductive nephrectomy or resection of locally recurrent renal cell carcinoma. J Urol 2008;180:94.
121. Thomas AA, Rini BI, Stephenson AJ, et al. Surgical resection of renal cell carcinoma after targeted therapy. J Urol 2009;182:881.
122. Wood CG, Margulis V. Neoadjuvant (presurgical) therapy for renal cell carcinoma: a new treatment paradigm for locally advanced and metastatic disease. Cancer 2009;115:2355.
123. Jonasch E, Wood CG, Matin SF, et al. Phase II presurgical feasibility study of bevacizumab in untreated patients with metastatic renal cell carcinoma. J Clin Oncol 2009;27:4076.
124. Chapin BF, Delacroix SE Jr, Culp SH, et al. Postoperative complications from cytoreductive nephrectomy after neoadjuvant targeted therapy for metastatic renal cell carcinoma. J Clin Oncol 2011;29:7 [abstract: 300].
125. Thomas AA, Rini BI, Lane BR, et al. Response of the primary tumor to neoadjuvant sunitinib in patients with advanced renal cell carcinoma. J Urol 2009;181:518.
126. Hellenthal NJ, Underwood W, Penetrante R, et al. Prospective clinical trial of preoperative sunitinib in patients with renal cell carcinoma. J Urol 2010;184:859.
127. Cowey CL, Amin C, Pruthi RS, et al. Neoadjuvant clinical trial with sorafenib for patients with stage II or higher renal cell carcinoma. J Clin Oncol 2010;28:1502.
128. Salem M, Shah SN, Wood LS, et al. Contrast enhanced CT (CE-CT) changes and nephrometry down-scoring of unresectable primary renal cell carcinoma (RCC) tumors in patients (Pts) treated with neoadjuvant sunitinib. J Clin Oncol 2011;29:7 [abstract: 299].
129. Rodriguez Faba O, Breda A, Rosales A, et al. Neoadjuvant temsirolimus effectiveness in downstaging advanced non-clear cell renal cell carcinoma. Eur Urol 2010;58:307.
130. Karam JA, Rini BI, Varella L, et al. Metastasectomy after targeted therapy in patients with advanced renal cell carcinoma. J Urol 2011;185:439.

Immunotherapy for Renal Cell Carcinoma

Jacalyn Rosenblatt, MD, David F. McDermott, MD*

KEYWORDS

• Renal cell carcinoma • PD-1 blockade • Immunotherapy

The ability of some renal tumors to evoke an immune response and the lack of benefit seen with standard chemotherapy and radiation led to the application of immunotherapy for patients with metastatic renal cell carcinoma (RCC).[1,2] In an attempt to reproduce or accentuate this response, various immunotherapeutic strategies have been used, including adoptive immunotherapy, the induction of a graft-versus-tumor response via allogeneic hematopoietic stem cell transplantation, and the administration of partially purified or recombinant cytokines.[3–7]

Although several cytokines have shown antitumor activity in RCC, the most consistent results have been reported with interleukin-2 (IL-2) and interferon-α (IFN-α). In contrast to the results seen with molecularly targeted therapies (eg, sunitinib), the administration of high-dose bolus IL-2 (HD IL-2) has consistently produced durable responses in a small percentage of patients with advanced renal cell cancer.[8] However, the substantial toxicity and limited efficacy that is associated with HD IL-2 limits its application to highly selected patients treated at specialized centers.[9]

Once the standard of care, the advent of novel therapies that target angiogenesis and signal transduction pathways has produced significant clinical benefits and prompted a reassessment of the role of immunotherapy for metastatic RCC.[10–13] Recent insights into how the immune response to a tumor is regulated holds the promise of allowing patients to obtain a durable response to immunotherapy, perhaps without the significant toxicity associated with conventional approaches. This review describes how improvements in patient selection, combination therapy, and investigational agents might expand and better define the role of IL-2 in metastatic RCC.

CYTOKINE THERAPY

Although several cytokines have shown antitumor activity in RCC, the most consistent results have been reported with IL-2 and IFN-α. In contrast to the results seen with molecularly targeted therapies (eg, sorafenib, sunitinib), which lead to tumor shrinkage

Disclosure: Supported in part by the DF/HCC Renal Cancer SPORE: P50 CA101942-01.
Department of Medicine, Beth Israel Deaconess Medical Center, Harvard Medical School, 330 Brookline Avenue, Boston, MA 02215, USA
* Corresponding author.
E-mail address: dmcdermo@bidmc.harvard.edu

in most treated patients but do not produce remissions of cancer when therapy is discontinued, the administration of HD IL-2 has consistently produced durable responses in a small percentage of patients with advanced RCC.[8,14,15] However, the substantial toxicity and limited efficacy that are associated with IL-2 have narrowed its application to highly selected patients treated at specialized centers.[9,16] Although IFN-α has produced modest benefits in unselected patients, randomized clinical trials have revealed a small survival benefit with manageable toxic effects when compared with non–IFN-α control arms.[17–23] As it became the de facto standard of care worldwide, regulatory agencies have supported the use of IFN-α as the control arm for randomized trials with targeted therapies that are described elsewhere in this issue.[10–13] The results of these investigations have, in general, established the superiority of targeted agents in previously untreated patients, thereby narrowing the future use of IFN-α as a single agent in this setting.

In recent years, the relative merits of these low-dose and high-dose cytokine regimens have been clarified by the results of 4 randomized trials (**Table 1**).[24–27] In the most consequential trial, the French Immunotherapy Group randomized patients with an intermediate likelihood of response to IL-2 and IFN-α to receive medroxyprogesterone (control group), subcutaneous IFN-α, subcutaneous IL-2, or the combination of IFN-α and IL-2.[27] Although significant toxicity was more common in the IL-2 and IFN-α arm, median overall survival did not differ between the arms. The investigators concluded that subcutaneous IFN-α and IL-2 should no longer be recommended in patients with metastatic RCC and intermediate prognosis.

Taken together, these studies suggest that high-dose intravenous (IV) bolus IL-2 is superior in terms of response rate and possibly response quality to regimens that involve low-dose IL-2 and IFN-α, intermediate-dose or low-dose IL-2 alone, or low-dose IFN-α alone. Consequently, although low-dose single cytokine therapy has a limited role in patients with metastatic RCC, high-dose IV IL-2 remains a reasonable option for appropriately selected patients with access to such therapy. More significantly, correlative biomarker investigations associated with these trials suggest

Table 1
Select randomized trials of cytokine therapy in metastatic renal cell cancer

Trial	Treatment Regimens	N	Response Rate (%)	Durable Complete Response (%)	Overall Survival (mo)[a]
French	CIV IL-2	138	6.5	1	12
Immunotherapy	LD SC IFN-α	147	7.5	2	13
Group[24]	CIV IL-2 + IFN-α	140	18.6	5	17
	MPA	123	2.5	1	14.9
French Immunotherapy	LD SC IFN-α	122	4.4	3	15.2
Group[27]	LD SC IL-2	125	4.1	0	15.3
	SC IL-2 + IFN	122	10.9	0	16.8
National Cancer	HD IV IL-2	156	21	8	NR
Institute	LD IV IL-2	150	13	3	NR
Surgery Branch[24]	HD IV IL-2	95	23	7	17.5
CWG[26]	LD SC IL-2/ IFN-α	91	10	NR	13
	HD IV IL-2	95	23	NR	17.5

Abbreviations: CIV, continuous IV infusion; CR, complete response; HD, high dose; LD, low dose; MPA, medroxyprogesterone acetate; NR, not reported; RR, response rate; SC, subcutaneous.
[a] The overall survival difference was not statistically significant in all cases.

that the potential exists for identifying predictors of response (or resistance) and limiting IL-2 therapy to those most likely to benefit.

PATHOLOGIC AND MOLECULAR PREDICTORS OF RESPONSE TO IL-2
Influence of Histologic Subtype

Responses to immunotherapy are most frequently seen in patients with clear cell RCC.[28–30] This observation was detailed in a retrospective analysis of pathology specimens obtained from 231 patients (163 primary and 68 metastatic tumor specimens) who had received IL-2 therapy in Cytokine Working Group (CWG) clinical trials.[30] For patients with primary tumor specimens available for review, the response rate to IL-2 was 21% (30 of 146) for patients with clear cell histologic primary tumors compared with 6% for patients with nonclear cell histologic tumors (1 responder in 17 patients). Among the patients with clear cell carcinoma, response to IL-2 was also associated with the presence of good predictive features (eg, more than 50% alveolar and no granular or papillary features) and the absence of poor predictive features (eg, more than 50% granular or any papillary features). As a result of these data, it may be appropriate for patients whose primary tumor is of nonclear cell histologic type or of clear cell histologic type but with poor predictive features to forgo IL-2–based treatment altogether.

Immunohistochemical Markers

Carbonic anhydrase IX (CAIX) has been identified as an immunohistochemical marker that might predict the outcomes of patients with RCC. In an analysis by Bui and colleagues,[31] CAIX expression in more than 85% of tumor cells (high CAIX expression) has been associated with improved survival and a higher objective response rate in IL-2–treated patients. Building on this work, Atkins and colleagues[32] developed a 2-component model that combined pathology analysis and immunohistochemical staining for CAIX. In a retrospective analysis, this model was able to identify a good risk group that contained 26 (96%) of 27 responders to IL-2 compared with only 18 (46%) of 39 nonresponders (odds ratio, 30; P<.01). A significant survival benefit was also seen for this group (P<.01).

Molecular Markers

Through gene expression profiling of tumor specimens, Pantuck and colleagues[33] were able to identify a set of 73 genes the expression of which distinguished complete responders from nonresponders after IL-2 therapy. In their hands, complete responders to IL-2 have a signature gene and protein expression pattern that includes CAIX, PTEN, and CXCR4. A similar analysis identified loss of chromosome 4, 9, and 17p as possible predictors of IL-2 nonresponse.[34] Further investigation into these regions may improve our understanding of the molecular basis of an effective immune response in RCC. Although this approach requires prospective validation, it may become a powerful aid for clinicians in selecting appropriate treatment options.

CURRENT INVESTIGATION IN PATIENT SELECTION

The CWG conducted the high-dose IL-2 Select trial to determine, in a prospective fashion, if the predictive model proposed by Atkins and colleagues[32] can identify a group of patients with advanced RCC who are significantly more likely to respond to high-dose IL-2–based therapy (good risk) than a historical, unselected patient population. The preliminary clinical results of this trial revealed a response rate (28%) that was significantly higher that the historical experience with high-dose IL-2.[35] However, analysis of proposed tumor biomarkers (eg, central pathology review and staining for CAIX) was unable to confirm hypotheses generated in retrospective studies and limit the application of HD IL-2. Efforts to confirm other proposed biomarkers (eg, CAIX SNPs, B7-H1 expression) are ongoing to understand tumor and host factors that predict for remissions after IL-2 therapy. An improved model for IL-2 patient selection will likely emerge from these efforts and improve its therapeutic index. Lessons from this work should guide the development of targeted immunotherapies (eg, CTLA-4, PD-1 antibodies) in solid tumors. As the list of effective therapies for metastatic RCC grows, improvements in patient selection will be necessary to ensure that patients who might attain a durable remission with immunotherapy do not miss this opportunity.

COMBINATION OF IMMUNOTHERAPY AND TARGETED/ANTIANGIOGENIC THERAPY

Although the role of low-dose single-agent cytokines is limited, combinations of immunotherapy with vascular endothelial growth factor (VEGF) targeted therapy may have merit. Two recently completed, large phase III trials of IFN plus bevacizumab versus IFN alone have shown superior efficacy with the combination regimen compared with cytokine monotherapy and suggest the potential of an additive effect.

Soon after bevacizumab became the first VEGF targeted agent to show efficacy as monotherapy in metastatic RCC, investigators explored the value of combining it with the de facto standard of care, IFN.[36] Two phase III trials of IFN plus bevacizumab versus IFN (AVOREN and CALGB 90,206) were initiated in Europe and the United States for first-line treatment of patients with metastatic RCC.[13,37] In both trials, patients were randomized bevacizumab plus IFN versus IFN alone. Unlike the CALGB trial, AVOREN (N = 649) was placebo-controlled, double-blind, and mandated previous nephrectomy. Compared with IFN alone, the combination arm in the AVOREN trial showed significantly better median progression-free survival (PFS) (10.4 vs 5.5 months; $P = .0001$), overall response rate (ORR) (31% vs 13%; $P = .0001$), and median time to progression (10.2 vs 5.5 months; $P = .0001$).[13] The overall survival data analysis was subsequently published in 2010 and showed no significant survival difference between 2 arms (23.3 vs 21.3 months; $P = .1291$).[38]

Further confirmation of the superiority of bevacizumab plus IFN to IFN alone came from the CALGB 90,206 trial. Unlike AVOREN, CALGB 90,206 was an open-labeled study and did not require previous nephrectomy. Relative to IFN alone, therapy with bevacizumab plus IFN significantly improved ORR (25.5% vs 13.1%, $P<.0001$) and median PFS (8.4 vs 4.9 months, $P<.0001$.) On the other hand, overall survival was similar in both arms: 18.3 months in the combination arm and 17.4 months in the IFN-only arm ($P = .097$). Although the AVOREN and CALGB trials led to the regulatory approval of this combination of VEGF pathway inhibition with immunotherapy in patients with RCC, clarification of the relative contribution of IFN to this regimen requires a randomized trial comparing the combination with bevacizumab alone.

Bevacizumab has also been combined with high-dose IL-2 in a CWG phase II trial. Investigators reported a response rate of 28% and a median PFS of 9 months. These results suggest that these 2 agents may be given safely in combination and produce efficacy improvements that are additive but not synergistic.[39] Sorafenib and IFN have been combined in 2 separate single-arm phase II trials.[40,41] These trials showed objective response rates of 18% and 35%. Toxicity observed was typical of that observed with each single agent with a notable reduction in hand-foot syndrome compared with sorafenib monotherapy data. The benefit/toxicity ratio of this combination regimen awaits further investigation in randomized trials.

INVESTIGATIONAL IMMUNOTHERAPY IN RCC TUMOR VACCINES

Metastatic RCC is a setting in which there has been great interest in testing novel immunotherapies. Several such approaches, including vaccination and allogeneic bone marrow transplantation, have been tested over the past 2 decades. The initial reports evaluating allogeneic bone marrow transplantation were encouraging; however, further clinical trials have highlighted the potential toxicity and limited applicability of this approach.[6,42,43]

The use of tumor vaccines has been explored in RCC, in an effort to limit treatment-related toxicity and enhance tumor-specific immune responses. A variety of antigens associated with RCC have been identified, including MAGE-A6, MAGE 9, PRAME, and MUC1.[44–51] Therefore, early clinical trials evaluated irradiated tumor cells or tumor lysate as a means of inducing antitumor responses.[5,52–57] In the first published clinical trial reporting results of 120 patients, no improvement in PFS or overall survival was observed with treatment with irradiated autologous tumor cells given BCG.[53] In contrast, results of a large multicenter randomized controlled trial evaluating an autologous tumor lysate-based vaccine in patients with high-risk nonmetastatic kidney cancer showed an improvement in PFS in vaccinated patients (5-year PFS 77.4% in vaccinated patients vs 67.8% in controls, $P = .02$).[54] In a recent study, May and colleagues[58] published results of 495 patients treated with an autologous tumor lysate-based vaccine in the adjuvant setting after undergoing radical nephrectomy for high-risk disease. Results were compared with a control group of 495 matched patients treated with nephrectomy alone. Overall survival at 5 and 10 years was 80.6% and 68.9%, respectively, in vaccinated patients, and 79.2% and 62.1%, respectively, in the control group ($P = .066$). A statistically significant increase in overall survival was observed in the subset of patients with pT3 tumors (5-year overall survival 71.3% in vaccinated patients vs 65.4% in controls, $P = .022$). These data have yet to be confirmed in a randomized, controlled phase III trial.

Despite the presence of tumor-specific antigens, tumor cells lack appropriate costimulatory molecules and stimulatory cytokines to elicit an effective immune response. Therefore, in an attempt to augment effective immune response to vaccination, the use of renal carcinoma cells that have been genetically engineered to encode stimulatory cytokines and/or costimulatory molecules have been evaluated in phase I and II studies.[59–65] Vaccination was well tolerated, and both complete and partial responses were observed, although in a minority of patients. Recently, tumor antigens have been engineered into vaccinia virus vectors. Trovax, a modified vaccinia Ankara (MVA) encoding the human oncofetal antigen 5T4, has been studied in phase I and II trials, which revealed suggestions of clinical efficacy.[66–68] In a recent phase III clinical trial, 733 patients with metastatic RCC were randomized to receive Trovax versus placebo in combination with either sunitinib, IL-2, or IFN-γ. However, no difference in overall survival was observed in the Trovax-treated cohort. The magnitude of immune response to vaccination was associated with improved survival.[69]

An alternative means of augmenting tumor antigen presentation and reversing tumor-induced anergy lies in the use of dendritic cell-based vaccines. Dendritic cells are potent antigen-presenting cells, uniquely capable of eliciting primary immune responses.[70] Dendritic cell vaccines present tumor antigens in the context of dendritic cell-derived costimulatory molecules, resulting in effective antitumor immune responses. Several clinical studies have evaluated the ability of dendritic cell-based vaccines to elicit immunologic and clinical responses in patients with metastatic RCC.[52,71–90] In a recent study, 18 patients with metastatic RCC were treated with autologous ex vivo generated dendritic cells loaded with autologous tumor lysate.

Patients were treated with 5 cycles of intranodal injection with vaccine, in conjunction with a day continuous infusion of IL-2 (18 MiU/m^2) and 3 injections of IFN-α 2a every other day. Three patients showed a complete response, 6 patients showed a partial response, and 6 patients showed stable disease.[91] Avigan[46] has conducted studies evaluating a dendritic cell/tumor fusion vaccine, in which ex vivo generated dendritic cells are fused to patient-derived tumor cells. In 1 study, 23 patients were treated (10 patients with breast cancer, 13 renal patients with renal cancer) with escalating doses of dendritic cell /tumor fusion cells, ranging from 1 × 10^6 – 4 × 10^6 fusion cells. No significant treatment-related toxicity was observed. Tumor-specific immunity was assessed by measuring IFN-γ secretion by T cells after ex vivo exposure to autologous tumor lysate. Immunologic responses, defined as a 2-fold or greater increase in IFN-γ secretion by CD4 and or CD8 T-cell populations, was observed in more than half of patients. Five patients with renal cancer showed disease stabilization. In a subsequent study, patients with metastatic RCC underwent vaccination with allogeneic dendritic cell/tumor fusions. Of 24 patients who underwent vaccination, 2 patients showed a partial response, and 8 patients showed stable disease. A correlation between clinical and immunologic response was observed.[92]

Although dendritic cell-based vaccines show promise, clinical responses are observed in a minority of patients. This finding may be in part because of the paradoxic increase in regulatory T cells that is observed in response to vaccination. In a recent study, peripheral blood mononuclear cells were isolated from 25 patients enrolled in a clinical trial in which patients with metastatic RCC were treated with autologous dendritic cells pulsed with tumor antigens given in conjunction with low-dose IL-2. The proportion of regulatory T cells increased more than 7-fold after vaccination compared with pretreatment levels.[93] Strategies to deplete regulatory T cells and inhibit the effect of inhibitory pathways may be required to augment clinical response to vaccination strategies.

OVERCOMING OBSTACLES TO EFFECTIVE IMMUNOTHERAPY IN RCC

An improved understanding of the molecular mechanisms that govern the interaction between a tumor and host immune response has provided insight into why immunotherapies too often fail to achieve satisfactory results. In RCC, obstacles to effective immunotherapy likely include the physiologic downmodulation of the immune response through the increased expression of molecules such as cytotoxic T-lymphocyte antigen 4 (CTLA-4) on the surface of activated T cells, the proliferation of regulatory (CD4+CD25+) T cells (T-regs) in response to nonspecific cytokine administration, and the immunosuppressive effects of increased circulating VEGF levels and myeloid-derived suppressor cells (MDSC).[94–102] These insights have encouraged investigators to pursue agents that block T-cell regulation (eg, programmed death 1 [PD-1] and CTLA-4 antibodies), inhibit tumor-induced immunosuppression (eg, transforming growth factor beta [TGF-β] antibody, PD ligand 1 [PD-L1] antibody) and more specifically activate T cells (eg, CD137 antibody, IL-21), and dendritic cells (eg, toll-like receptor agonists) (**Table 2**).[103–109] Several of these approaches have shown encouraging efficacy in early trials both as single agents and in combination with standard therapies.

INVESTIGATIONAL TARGETED IMMUNOTHERAPY

In a single-institution phase II trial, the CTLA-4 antibody ipilimumab produced major tumor regressions but also significant toxicities in patients with metastatic RCC who had failed previous immunotherapy.[104] Toxicities associated with CTLA-4 antibodies,

Table 2
Investigational immunotherapeutic approaches to the treatment of metastatic RCC

Target	Drug	Class	Development Phase
Blockade of T-cell regulation			
PD-1 antibody[103]	BMS-936558	Fully human mAb	Phase I
CTLA-4 antibody[104]	Ipilimumab	Fully human IgG1 mAb	Phase III (melanoma)
Inhibition of tumor-induced T-cell function			
TGF-β[105]	GC1008	Fully human mAb	Phase I
TGF-β2	AP12009	Fully human mAb	Phase I
T-cell activation			
CD137[106]	BMS-663,513	mAb	Phase I
Cytokines[107]	IL-21	Recombinant molecule	Phase II (melanoma)
Dendritic cell activation			
Toll-like receptor[108]	HYB2055	TLR9 agonist	Phase II
Dendritic cell-tumor fusions[109]	AGS-003	Dendritic cell based immunotherapy	Phase III

Abbreviations: IgG1, immunoglobulin 1; mAb, monoclonal antibodies; TLR9, toll-like receptor 9.

including enteritis, skin rash, and hypophysitis, have occasionally been life threatening and have also been associated with tumor response. Combination of cytokines and agents that block immune downregulation may prove particularly effective in select patients. A recent report of high-dose IL-2 and ipilimumab (CTLA-4 antibody) in patients with metastatic melanoma revealed manageable toxicity with a complete response rate of 17%, suggesting a potential role for this combination in patients with RCC.[110] However, the combination of another CTLA-4 antibody (tremelimumab) and a VEGF tyrosine kinase inhibitor (TKI; sunitinib) proved more toxic than expected, in large part because of acute renal toxicity.[111] Investigators at the Dana-Farber Harvard Cancer Center have recently launched a phase I trial of the combination of ipilimumab and bevacizumab in patients with metastatic melanoma. Should this combination prove tolerable, it should represent a rational combination for investigation in patients with RCC.

One of the most critical and promising pathways responsible for tumor-induced immune suppression in RCC is the interaction between B7-1, otherwise known as PD-1, and its ligand B7-H1 (PD-L1) interaction, which serves to restrict the cytolytic function of tumor-infiltrating T lymphocytes. Renal tumors that express B7-H1 have been shown to behave more aggressively, which leads to a shorter survival (**Fig. 1**).[112] Blocking the receptor (PD-1)/ligand (PD-L1) interaction with monoclonal antibodies (eg, PD-1 antibody BMS-936558, PD-L1 antibody MDX–1105), may facilitate immunotherapy and represents one of the most promising therapeutic strategies being studied in patients with RCC. These agents have recently completed phase I testing.[103]

PD-1/PD-L1 BIOLOGY

The PD-1/PD-L1 pathway is an important inhibitory pathway that regulates T-cell activation and mediates T-cell tolerance (**Fig. 2**).[113] The PD-1 receptor is expressed on

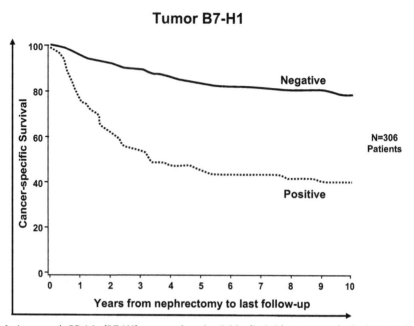

Fig.1. Increased PD-L1 (B7-H1) expression in RCC diminishes survival. (*Adapted from* Thompson RH, Gillett MD, Cheville JC, et al. Costimulatory B7-H1 in renal cell carcinoma patients: indicator of tumor aggressiveness and potential therapeutic target. Proc Natl Acad Sci U S A 2004;101:17174–9; with permission.)

T cells, B cells, monocytes, and natural killer T cells after activation. PD-L1 (B7-H1) and PD-L2 (B7-dendritic cell), the 2 ligands for PD-1, are expressed on antigen-presenting cells, including dendritic cells and macrophages. In addition, PD-L1 is expressed on nonhematopoietic cells, including pancreatic islet cells, endothelial cells, and epithelial cells, and they play a role in protecting tissue from immune-mediated injury.[114]

The critical role that PD-1 plays in blunting activated T-cell responses was first shown by the autoimmune phenotypes that develop in PD-1 knockout mice, including cardiomyopathy, diabetes, glomerulonephritis, and arthritis.[113,115–118] PD-L1 expression on nonhematopoietic cells, including renal tubular epithelial cells, inhibits immune-mediated tissue damage, which indicates that the PD-1/PD-L1 pathway is a critical mediator of tissue tolerance.[114,119–121] The PD-1/PD-L1 pathway plays an important role in modulating immune response to infection. T-cell expression of PD-1 is upregulated during chronic viral infection, which results in an exhausted T-cell phenotype. The lymphocytic choriomeningitis virus model was the first to show the impact of the PD-1/PD-L1 pathway in limiting clearance of virally infected cells.[114,122]

PD-1 AND TUMOR IMMUNITY

There has been increasing interest in exploring the contribution of the PD-1/PD-L1 pathway to tumor evasion of host immunity. Tumor cells secrete inhibitory cytokines, including TGF-β and IL-10, which creates an immunosuppressive milieu and limits effective antitumor immunity.

Recent studies suggest that tumor expression of PD-L1 may play an important role in contributing to tumor-mediated immunosuppression. A variety of tumors have been shown to express PD-L1, including renal, melanoma, stomach, breast, and lung

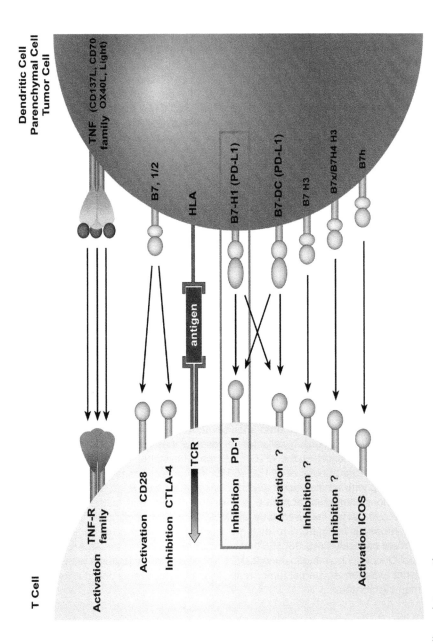

Fig. 2. T-cell regulatory pathways.

carcinoma.[112,123–133] In addition, PD-LI expression on tumor cells has been shown to correlate with a poor prognosis not only in RCC but also in breast, pancreatic, stomach, and ovarian cancer.[112,127,129–133]

Ahmadzadeh and colleagues[134] showed in a melanoma model that PD-1 expression on tumor-infiltrating lymphocytes (TIL) is significantly higher than on a T cell isolated from the peripheral blood or normal tissue of the same individuals. In this study, PD-1+ TIL were shown to have impaired effector function, as measured by IFN-γ secretion, which suggests that PD-1 expression on TIL limits their capacity to mount an effective immune response. Blank and colleagues[118] also showed higher levels of PD-1 expression on TIL than on peripheral blood lymphocytes isolated from patients with melanoma. In addition, PD-1 blockade increased IFN-γ secretion by T-cell populations in response to stimulation by antigen-loaded dendritic cells. In a murine model of chronic myelogenous leukemia (CML), leukemia-specific cytotoxic T lymphocytes were shown to express high levels of PD-1, and were functionally exhausted. PD-L1 blockade was shown to restore the function of CML-specific cytotoxic T lymphocytes, and prolong survival.[135] The effect of PD-1 blockade on enhancing activated antitumor T-cell responses makes it an ideal therapeutic target to study in the setting of malignancy.

PD-L1 expression on RCC may play a significant role in promoting T-cell tolerance by binding PD-1 on activated T cells and suppressing their capacity to secrete stimulatory cytokines. Inhibition of this pathway may significantly augment the capacity of tumor-reactive T cells to eliminate tumor cells. Monoclonal antibodies that target the PD-1/PD-L1 interaction are being evaluated in clinical studies, and hold promise as an important immunotherapeutic approach in RCC.

BMS-936558 IN PHASE I TRIALS

Brahmer and colleagues[103] reported the first human phase I/II trial of BMS-936558 (MDX-1106, ONO-4538), a fully human IgG4 anti-PD-1 blocking antibody, in patients with selected refractory or relapsed malignancies. This single-dose trial established the maximum tolerated dose (MTD) of BMS-936558 at 10 mg/kg without evidence of serious toxicity (arthritic symptoms: 2 patients; thyroid-stimulating hormone increase: 1 patient). Flow cytometric analysis showed sustained occupancy of most PD-1 molecules on patient T cells for at least 3 months after a single dose. In a dose expansion cohort at the MTD, patients with stable disease or better were able to receive repeat doses of BMS-936558. Tumor responses were seen in melanoma and RCC without increased toxicity. One patient with RCC, who had received several previous therapies, achieved a partial remission that lasted more than 18 months despite having received only 3 BMS-936558 infusions. This small efficacy signal prompted investigators to include a larger cohort of patients with RCC in a subsequent biweekly BMS-936558 trial that reported results at the American Society of Clinical Oncology meeting in June 2010.[136] In the cohort of patients with RCC, 5 of 16 patients experienced partial tumor responses that have remained durable for 8 to more than 17 months.

VACCINATION PLUS IMMUNE CHECKPOINT BLOCKADE

To realize the full potential of a vaccine approach in RCC, combinations with immune stimulants (eg, granulocyte macrophage colony-stimulating factor) and inhibitors of natural T-cell regulation pathways (eg, CTLA4 blockade, T-reg depletion) may be necessary.

The PD-1/PD-L1 pathway may play an important role in blunting immune response to tumor vaccines. PD-1 is upregulated on T-cell populations in response to antigenic and nonantigenic stimulation. Study findings suggest that stimulation with dendritic cell/tumor fusion cells results in increased T-cell expression of PD-1, which potentially blunts response to vaccination.[137] In preclinical studies, stimulation of T cells with a dendritic cell/tumor fusion vaccine in the presence of PD-1 blockade results in an increase in Th1 cytokines, a decrease in regulatory T cells, and enhanced tumor killing.[137] As such, combining dendritic cell-based tumor vaccines with PD-1 blockade may be an effective means of enhancing immunologic and clinical response to vaccination. A clinical trial is planned in which patients with metastatic RCC will be treated with dendritic cell/tumor fusion vaccination in conjunction with PD-1 blockade after debulking nephrectomy.

COMBINATION OF INVESTIGATIONAL IMMUNOTHERAPY AND TARGETED/ANTIANGIOGENIC THERAPY

Although VEGF pathway targeted therapies (eg, sunitinib, bevacizumab) have significantly improved outcomes for patients with RCC, disease progression is inevitable. Although the mechanisms of treatment resistance are poorly understood, the immunosuppressive effects of increased VEGF levels and MDSC may play an important role in the process.[99–101] Recent preclinical and correlative investigations have provided new insights into the potentially favorable effect that VEGF receptor TKIs (eg, sunitinib) may have on reversing tumor-induced immunosuppression by reducing the numbers of MDSC and limiting the negative impact of circulating VEGF.[102,138] Building on this work, several investigational immunotherapeutic agents are being studied in combination with sunitinib in hopes of enhancing their therapeutic benefit. AGS-003, an immunotherapy created by fusing patient-derived dendritic cells with autologous tumor, was recently combined with sunitinib in a single-arm phase II trial.[109] In a preliminary report, the investigators reported that the combination was well tolerated and associated with encouraging clinical outcomes (median PFS 12.5 months) in this small group of patients with RCC. In a recent study, the in vivo effect of sorafenib on circulating immune effector cells was assessed in a cohort of 35 patients with metastatic RCC. In 1 study, sorafenib treatment was shown to result in a decrease in circulating regulatory T-cell populations in vivo, suggesting that this drug may enhance the efficacy of tumor vaccines.[139] However, when sorafenib was compared with sunitinib in 1 mouse (C57BL/6) study, sorafenib reduced induction of antigen-specific T cells and inhibited dendritic cell function, whereas sunitinib reduced the number of regulatory T cells. Therefore, the investigators concluded that sunitinib was more suitable for combination with immunotherapy than sorafenib.[140] Confirmation of the potential benefit of this VEGF TKI-based combination regimen requires testing in larger randomized trials.

SUMMARY

RCC has long been considered an immunologically influenced malignancy and thus served as a platform for the clinical testing of anticancer immunotherapy. The nonspecific cytokines, IL-2 and IFN-α, have undergone the most testing and produced only modest benefits for unselected patients. High-dose IL-2 remains the only approach to produce durable responses in patients with metastatic RCC and can thus be considered in appropriately selected patients. For patients unlikely to benefit from, unable to receive, or who progress after IL-2, the emergence of molecularly targeted therapies offers hope for improved clinical outcome.[15–18] Additional opportunities for molecular and pathologic selection exist for cytokines, but considerable validation work is needed before these selection features can be used clinically. Optimally, cytokine therapy should be given in the context of a clinical trial investigating combination therapy and/or patient selection to maximize the benefit of this approach. Targeted immunotherapeutic strategies have been tested in metastatic RCC, but definitive evidence of clinical benefit is only emerging.

In recent years, the list of effective therapies (eg, angiogenesis inhibition; signal transduction inhibition, and immunotherapy) for metastatic RCC has increased substantially. The advent of targeted therapy in RCC does not eliminate the potential usefulness of immunotherapy in RCC but rather requires a rational refinement of this therapy through patient selection, combination regimens, and novel agents that together may extend overall survival and increase the remission rate for patients with this disease.

REFERENCES

1. Gleave ME, Elhilali M, Fradet Y, et al. Interferon gamma-1b compared with placebo in metastatic renal-cell carcinoma. Canadian Urologic Oncology Group. N Engl J Med 1998;338:1265–71.
2. Vogelzang NJ, Priest ER, Borden L. Spontaneous regression of histologically proved pulmonary metastases from renal cell carcinoma: a case with 5-year followup. J Urol 1992;148:1247–8.
3. Chang AE, Li Q, Jiang G, et al. Phase II trial of autologous tumor vaccination, anti-CD3-activated vaccine-primed lymphocytes, and interleukin-2 in stage IV renal cell cancer. J Clin Oncol 2003;21:884–90.
4. Lesimple T, Moisan A, Guille F, et al. Treatment of metastatic renal cell carcinoma with activated autologous macrophages and granulocyte–macrophage colony-stimulating factor. J Immunother 2000;23:675–9.
5. Schwaab T, Heaney JA, Schned AR, et al. A randomized phase II trial comparing two different sequence combinations of autologous vaccine and human recombinant interferon gamma and human recombinant interferon alpha2B therapy in patients with metastatic renal cell carcinoma: clinical outcome and analysis of immunological parameters. J Urol 2000;163:1322–7.
6. Childs R, Chernoff A, Contentin N, et al. Regression of metastatic renal-cell carcinoma after nonmyeloablative allogeneic peripheral-blood stem-cell transplantation. N Engl J Med 2000;343:750–8.
7. Rosenberg SA, Mule JJ, Spiess PJ, et al. Regression of established pulmonary metastases and subcutaneous tumor mediated by the systemic administration of high-dose recombinant interleukin 2. J Exp Med 1985;161:1169–88.
8. Fisher RI, Rosenberg SA, Fyfe G. Long-term survival update for high-dose recombinant interleukin-2 in patients with renal cell carcinoma. Cancer J Sci Am 2000;6(Suppl 1):S55–7.
9. Margolin KA, Rayner AA, Hawkins MJ, et al. Interleukin-2 and lymphokine-activated killer cell therapy of solid tumors: analysis of toxicity and management guidelines. J Clin Oncol 1989;7:486–98.
10. Escudier B, Eisen T, Stadler WM, et al. Sorafenib in advanced clear-cell renal-cell carcinoma. N Engl J Med 2007;356:125–34.
11. Motzer RJ, Hutson TE, Tomczak P, et al. Sunitinib versus interferon alfa in metastatic renal-cell carcinoma. N Engl J Med 2007;356:115–24.
12. Hudes G, Carducci M, Tomczak P, et al. Temsirolimus, interferon alfa, or both for advanced renal-cell carcinoma. N Engl J Med 2007;356:2271–81.

13. Escudier B, Pluzanska A, Koralewski P, et al. Bevacizumab plus interferon alfa-2a for treatment of metastatic renal cell carcinoma: a randomised, double-blind phase III trial. Lancet 2007;370:2103–11.
14. Fyfe G, Fisher RI, Rosenberg SA, et al. Results of treatment of 255 patients with metastatic renal cell carcinoma who received high-dose recombinant interleukin-2 therapy. J Clin Oncol 1995;13:688–96.
15. Rosenberg SA, Yang JC, White DE, et al. Durability of complete responses in patients with metastatic cancer treated with high-dose interleukin-2: identification of the antigens mediating response. Ann Surg 1998;228:307–19.
16. Belldegrun A, Webb DE, Austin HA 3rd, et al. Renal toxicity of interleukin-2 administration in patients with metastatic renal cell cancer: effect of pre-therapy nephrectomy. J Urol 1989;141:499–503.
17. Neidhart JA. Interferon therapy for the treatment of renal cancer. Cancer 1986; 57:1696–9.
18. Muss HB. Interferon therapy for renal cell carcinoma. Semin Oncol 1987;14: 36–42.
19. Muss HB, Costanzi JJ, Leavitt R, et al. Recombinant alfa interferon in renal cell carcinoma: a randomized trial of two routes of administration. J Clin Oncol 1987; 5:286–91.
20. Negrier S, Caty A, Lesimple T, et al. Treatment of patients with metastatic renal carcinoma with a combination of subcutaneous interleukin-2 and interferon alfa with or without fluorouracil. Groupe Francais d'Immunotherapie, Federation Nationale des Centres de Lutte Contre le Cancer. J Clin Oncol 2000;18: 4009–15.
21. Interferon-alpha and survival in metastatic renal carcinoma: early results of a randomised controlled trial. Medical Research Council Renal Cancer Collaborators. Lancet 1999;353:14–7.
22. Pyrhonen S, Salminen E, Ruutu M, et al. Prospective randomized trial of interferon alfa-2a plus vinblastine versus vinblastine alone in patients with advanced renal cell cancer. J Clin Oncol 1999;17:2859–67.
23. Coppin C, Porzsolt F, Awa A, et al. Immunotherapy for advanced renal cell cancer. Cochrane Database Syst Rev 2005;1:CD001425.
24. Negrier S, Escudier B, Lasset C, et al. Recombinant human interleukin-2, recombinant human interferon alfa-2a, or both in metastatic renal-cell carcinoma. Groupe Francais d'Immunotherapie. N Engl J Med 1998;338:1272–8.
25. Yang JC, Sherry RM, Steinberg SM, et al. Randomized study of high-dose and low-dose interleukin-2 in patients with metastatic renal cancer. J Clin Oncol 2003;21:3127–32.
26. McDermott DF, Regan MM, Clark JI, et al. Randomized phase III trial of high-dose interleukin-2 versus subcutaneous interleukin-2 and interferon in patients with metastatic renal cell carcinoma. J Clin Oncol 2005;23:133–41.
27. Negrier S, Perol D, Ravaud A, et al. Medroxyprogesterone, interferon alfa-2a, interleukin 2, or combination of both cytokines in patients with metastatic renal carcinoma of intermediate prognosis: results of a randomized controlled trial. Cancer 2007;110:2468–77.
28. Cangiano T, Liao J, Naitoh J, et al. Sarcomatoid renal cell carcinoma: biologic behavior, prognosis, and response to combined surgical resection and immunotherapy. J Clin Oncol 1999;17:523–8.
29. Motzer RJ, Bacik J, Mariani T, et al. Treatment outcome and survival associated with metastatic renal cell carcinoma of non-clear-cell histology. J Clin Oncol 2002;20:2376–81.

30. Upton MP, Parker RA, Youmans A, et al. Histologic predictors of renal cell carcinoma response to interleukin-2-based therapy. J Immunother 2005;28:488–95.
31. Bui MH, Seligson D, Han KR, et al. Carbonic anhydrase IX is an independent predictor of survival in advanced renal clear cell carcinoma: implications for prognosis and therapy. Clin Cancer Res 2003;9:802–11.
32. Atkins M, Regan M, McDermott D, et al. Carbonic anhydrase IX expression predicts outcome of interleukin 2 therapy for renal cancer. Clin Cancer Res 2005;11:3714–21.
33. Pantuck AJ, Fang Z, Liu X, et al. Gene expression and tissue microarray analysis of interleukin-2 complete responders in patients with metastatic renal cell carcinoma. Proc Am Soc Clin Oncol 2005;4:535.
34. Jones J, Otu HH, Grall F, et al. Proteomic identification of interleukin-2 therapy response in metastatic renal cell cancer. J Urol 2008;179:730–6.
35. McDermott. The high-dose Aldesleukin (HD IL-2) "SELECT" trial in patients with metastatic renal cell carcinoma (mRCC). J Clin Oncol 2010;28:15s [abstract: 4514].
36. Yang JC, Haworth L, Sherry RM, et al. A randomized trial of bevacizumab, an anti-vascular endothelial growth factor antibody, for metastatic renal cancer. N Engl J Med 2003;349:427–34.
37. Rini BI, Halabi S, Rosenberg JE, et al. Phase III trial of bevacizumab plus interferon alfa versus interferon alfa monotherapy in patients with metastatic renal cell carcinoma: final results of CALGB 90206. J Clin Oncol 2010;28:2137–43.
38. Escudier B, Bellmunt J, Negrier S, et al. Phase III trial of bevacizumab plus interferon alfa-2a in patients with metastatic renal cell carcinoma (AVOREN): final analysis of overall survival. J Clin Oncol 2010;28:2144–50.
39. Dandamudi A. Phase II study of bevacizumab and high dose bolus aldesleukin (IL-2) in metastatic renal cell carcinoma patients: a Cytokine Working Group Study. J Clin Oncol 2010;28:15s [abstract: 5044].
40. Gollob JA, Rathmell WK, Richmond TM, et al. Phase II trial of sorafenib plus interferon alfa-2b as first- or second-line therapy in patients with metastatic renal cell cancer. J Clin Oncol 2007;25:3288–95.
41. Ryan CW, Goldman BH, Lara PN Jr, et al. Sorafenib with interferon alfa-2b as first-line treatment of advanced renal carcinoma: a phase II study of the Southwest Oncology Group. J Clin Oncol 2007;25:3296–301.
42. Childs R, Srinivasan R. Advances in allogeneic stem cell transplantation: directing graft-versus-leukemia at solid tumors. Cancer J 2002;8:2–11.
43. Rini BI, Zimmerman T, Stadler WM, et al. Allogeneic stem-cell transplantation of renal cell cancer after nonmyeloablative chemotherapy: feasibility, engraftment, and clinical results. J Clin Oncol 2002;20:2017–24.
44. Asemissen AM, Brossart P. Vaccination strategies in patients with renal cell carcinoma. Cancer Immunol Immunother 2009;58:1169–74.
45. Gouttefangeas C, Stenzl A, Stevanovic S, et al. Immunotherapy of renal cell carcinoma. Cancer Immunol Immunother 2007;56:117–28.
46. Avigan D. Dendritic cell-tumor fusion vaccines for renal cell carcinoma. Clin Cancer Res 2004;10:6347S–52S.
47. Brossart P, Stuhler G, Flad T, et al. Her-2/neu-derived peptides are tumor-associated antigens expressed by human renal cell and colon carcinoma lines and are recognized by in vitro induced specific cytotoxic T lymphocytes. Cancer Res 1998;58:732–6.
48. Flad T, Spengler B, Kalbacher H, et al. Direct identification of major histocompatibility complex class I-bound tumor-associated peptide antigens of a renal

carcinoma cell line by a novel mass spectrometric method. Cancer Res 1998; 58:5803–11.

49. Neumann E, Engelsberg A, Decker J, et al. Heterogeneous expression of the tumor-associated antigens RAGE-1, PRAME, and glycoprotein 75 in human renal cell carcinoma: candidates for T-cell-based immunotherapies? Cancer Res 1998;58:4090–5.

50. Vissers JL, De Vries IJ, Schreurs MW, et al. The renal cell carcinoma-associated antigen G250 encodes a human leukocyte antigen (HLA)-A2.1-restricted epitope recognized by cytotoxic T lymphocytes. Cancer Res 1999;59:5554–9.

51. Tso CL, Zisman A, Pantuck A, et al. Induction of G250-targeted and T-cell-mediated antitumor activity against renal cell carcinoma using a chimeric fusion protein consisting of G250 and granulocyte/monocyte-colony stimulating factor. Cancer Res 2001;61:7925–33.

52. Itsumi M, Tatsugami K. Immunotherapy for renal cell carcinoma. Clin Dev Immunol 2010;2010:284581.

53. Galligioni E, Quaia M, Merlo A, et al. Adjuvant immunotherapy treatment of renal carcinoma patients with autologous tumor cells and bacillus Calmette-Guerin: five-year results of a prospective randomized study. Cancer 1996;77:2560–6.

54. Jocham D, Richter A, Hoffmann L, et al. Adjuvant autologous renal tumour cell vaccine and risk of tumour progression in patients with renal-cell carcinoma after radical nephrectomy: phase III, randomised controlled trial. Lancet 2004; 363:594–9.

55. Dudek AZ, Mescher MF, Okazaki I, et al. Autologous large multivalent immunogen vaccine in patients with metastatic melanoma and renal cell carcinoma. Am J Clin Oncol 2008;31:173–81.

56. Dillman R, Barth N, Vandermolen L, et al. Autologous tumor cell line-derived vaccine for patient-specific treatment of advanced renal cell carcinoma. Cancer Biother Radiopharm 2004;19:570–80.

57. Van Poppel H, Joniau S, Van Gool SW. Vaccine therapy in patients with renal cell carcinoma. Eur Urol 2009;55:1333–42.

58. May M, Brookman-May S, Hoschke B, et al. Ten-year survival analysis for renal carcinoma patients treated with an autologous tumour lysate vaccine in an adjuvant setting. Cancer Immunol Immunother 2010;59:687–95.

59. Simons JW, Jaffee EM, Weber CE, et al. Bioactivity of autologous irradiated renal cell carcinoma vaccines generated by ex vivo granulocyte-macrophage colony-stimulating factor gene transfer. Cancer Res 1997;57:1537–46.

60. Wittig B, Marten A, Dorbic T, et al. Therapeutic vaccination against metastatic carcinoma by expression-modulated and immunomodified autologous tumor cells: a first clinical phase I/II trial. Hum Gene Ther 2001;12:267–78.

61. Antonia SJ, Seigne J, Diaz J, et al. Phase I trial of a B7-1 (CD80) gene modified autologous tumor cell vaccine in combination with systemic interleukin-2 in patients with metastatic renal cell carcinoma. J Urol 2002;167:1995–2000.

62. Tani K, Azuma M, Nakazaki Y, et al. Phase I study of autologous tumor vaccines transduced with the GM-CSF gene in four patients with stage IV renal cell cancer in Japan: clinical and immunological findings. Mol Ther 2004;10: 799–816.

63. Pizza G, De Vinci C, Lo Conte G, et al. Allogeneic gene-modified tumour cells in metastatic kidney cancer. Report II. Folia Biol (Praha) 2004;50:175–83.

64. Moiseyenko VM, Danilov AO, Baldueva IA, et al. Phase I/II trial of gene therapy with autologous tumor cells modified with tag7/PGRP-S gene in patients with disseminated solid tumors: miscellaneous tumors. Ann Oncol 2005;16:162–8.

65. Fishman M, Hunter TB, Soliman H, et al. Phase II trial of B7-1 (CD-86) trans-duced, cultured autologous tumor cell vaccine plus subcutaneous interleukin-2 for treatment of stage IV renal cell carcinoma. J Immunother 2008;31:72–80.
66. Hawkins RE, Macdermott C, Shablak A, et al. Vaccination of patients with meta-static renal cancer with modified vaccinia Ankara encoding the tumor antigen 5T4 (TroVax) given alongside interferon-alpha. J Immunother 2009;32:424–9.
67. Amato RJ, Shingler W, Goonewardena M, et al. Vaccination of renal cell cancer patients with modified vaccinia Ankara delivering the tumor antigen 5T4 (TroVax) alone or administered in combination with interferon-alpha (IFN-alpha): a phase 2 trial. J Immunother 2009;32:765–72.
68. Kaufman HL, Taback B, Sherman W, et al. Phase II trial of Modified Vaccinia An-kara (MVA) virus expressing 5T4 and high dose Interleukin-2 (IL-2) in patients with metastatic renal cell carcinoma. J Transl Med 2009;7:2.
69. Amato RJ, Hawkins RE, Kaufman HL, et al. Vaccination of metastatic renal cancer patients with MVA-5T4: a randomized, double-blind, placebo-controlled phase III study. Clin Cancer Res 2010;16:5539–47.
70. Avigan D. Dendritic cells: development, function and potential use for cancer immunotherapy. Blood Rev 1999;13:51–64.
71. Oosterwijk-Wakka JC, Tiemessen DM, Bleumer I, et al. Vaccination of patients with metastatic renal cell carcinoma with autologous dendritic cells pulsed with autologous tumor antigens in combination with interleukin-2: a phase 1 study. J Immunother 2002;25:500–8.
72. Marten A, Flieger D, Renoth S, et al. Therapeutic vaccination against metastatic renal cell carcinoma by autologous dendritic cells: preclinical results and outcome of a first clinical phase I/II trial. Cancer Immunol Immunother 2002; 51:637–44.
73. Holtl L, Zelle-Rieser C, Gander H, et al. Immunotherapy of metastatic renal cell carcinoma with tumor lysate-pulsed autologous dendritic cells. Clin Cancer Res 2002;8:3369–76.
74. Azuma T, Horie S, Tomita K, et al. Dendritic cell immunotherapy for patients with metastatic renal cell carcinoma: University of Tokyo experience. Int J Urol 2002; 9:340–6.
75. Marten A, Renoth S, Heinicke T, et al. Allogeneic dendritic cells fused with tumor cells: preclinical results and outcome of a clinical phase I/II trial in patients with metastatic renal cell carcinoma. Hum Gene Ther 2003;14:483–94.
76. Su Z, Dannull J, Heiser A, et al. Immunological and clinical responses in meta-static renal cancer patients vaccinated with tumor RNA-transfected dendritic cells. Cancer Res 2003;63:2127–33.
77. Gitlitz BJ, Belldegrun AS, Zisman A, et al. A pilot trial of tumor lysate-loaded dendritic cells for the treatment of metastatic renal cell carcinoma. J Immunother 2003;26:412–9.
78. Barbuto JA, Ensina LF, Neves AR, et al. Dendritic cell-tumor cell hybrid vaccina-tion for metastatic cancer. Cancer Immunol Immunother 2004;53:1111–8.
79. Avigan D, Vasir B, Gong J, et al. Fusion cell vaccination of patients with meta-static breast and renal cancer induces immunological and clinical responses. Clin Cancer Res 2004;10:4699–708.
80. Pandha HS, John RJ, Hutchinson J, et al. Dendritic cell immunotherapy for urological cancers using cryopreserved allogeneic tumour lysate-pulsed cells: a phase I/II study. BJU Int 2004;94:412–8.
81. Arroyo JC, Gabilondo F, Llorente L, et al. Immune response induced in vitro by CD16- and CD16+ monocyte-derived dendritic cells in patients with metastatic

renal cell carcinoma treated with dendritic cell vaccines. J Clin Immunol 2004; 24:86–96.

82. Holtl L, Ramoner R, Zelle-Rieser C, et al. Allogeneic dendritic cell vaccination against metastatic renal cell carcinoma with or without cyclophosphamide. Cancer Immunol Immunother 2005;54:663–70.

83. Wierecky J, Muller MR, Wirths S, et al. Immunologic and clinical responses after vaccinations with peptide-pulsed dendritic cells in metastatic renal cancer patients. Cancer Res 2006;66:5910–8.

84. Bleumer I, Tiemessen DM, Oosterwijk-Wakka JC, et al. Preliminary analysis of patients with progressive renal cell carcinoma vaccinated with CA9-peptide-pulsed mature dendritic cells. J Immunother 2007;30:116–22.

85. Wei YC, Sticca RP, Li J, et al. Combined treatment of dendritoma vaccine and low-dose interleukin-2 in stage IV renal cell carcinoma patients induced clinical response: a pilot study. Oncol Rep 2007;18:665–71.

86. Matsumoto A, Haraguchi K, Takahashi T, et al. Immunotherapy against metastatic renal cell carcinoma with mature dendritic cells. Int J Urol 2007;14:277–83.

87. Kim JH, Lee Y, Bae YS, et al. Phase I/II study of immunotherapy using autologous tumor lysate-pulsed dendritic cells in patients with metastatic renal cell carcinoma. Clin Immunol 2007;125:257–67.

88. Berntsen A, Trepiakas R, Wenandy L, et al. Therapeutic dendritic cell vaccination of patients with metastatic renal cell carcinoma: a clinical phase 1/2 trial. J Immunother 2008;31:771–80.

89. Tatsugami K, Eto M, Harano M, et al. Dendritic-cell therapy after non-myeloablative stem-cell transplantation for renal-cell carcinoma. Lancet Oncol 2004;5:750–2.

90. Zhou J, Weng D, Zhou F, et al. Patient-derived renal cell carcinoma cells fused with allogeneic dendritic cells elicit anti-tumor activity: in vitro results and clinical responses. Cancer Immunol Immunother 2009;58:1587–97.

91. Schwaab T, Schwarzer A, Wolf B, et al. Clinical and immunologic effects of intranodal autologous tumor lysate-dendritic cell vaccine with Aldesleukin (Interleukin 2) and IFN-{alpha}2a therapy in metastatic renal cell carcinoma patients. Clin Cancer Res 2009;15:4986–92.

92. Avigan DE, Vasir B, George DJ, et al. Phase I/II study of vaccination with electrofused allogeneic dendritic cells/autologous tumor-derived cells in patients with stage IV renal cell carcinoma. J Immunother 2007;30:749–61.

93. Berntsen A, Brimnes MK, thor Straten P, et al. Increase of circulating CD4+CD25highFoxp3+ regulatory T cells in patients with metastatic renal cell carcinoma during treatment with dendritic cell vaccination and low-dose interleukin-2. J Immunother 2010;33:425–34.

94. Thompson CB, Allison JP. The emerging role of CTLA-4 as an immune attenuator. Immunity 1997;7:445–50.

95. Walunas TL, Lenschow DJ, Bakker CY, et al. CTLA-4 can function as a negative regulator of T cell activation. Immunity 1994;1:405–13.

96. Krummel MF, Allison JP. CD28 and CTLA-4 have opposing effects on the response of T cells to stimulation. J Exp Med 1995;182:459–65.

97. Chambers CA, Sullivan TJ, Allison JP. Lymphoproliferation in CTLA-4-deficient mice is mediated by costimulation-dependent activation of CD4+ T cells. Immunity 1997;7:885–95.

98. Cesana GC, DeRaffele G, Cohen S, et al. Characterization of CD4+CD25+ regulatory T cells in patients treated with high-dose interleukin-2 for metastatic melanoma or renal cell carcinoma. J Clin Oncol 2006;24:1169–77.

99. Gabrilovich DI, Ishida T, Nadaf S, et al. Antibodies to vascular endothelial growth factor enhance the efficacy of cancer immunotherapy by improving endogenous dendritic cell function. Clin Cancer Res 1999;5:2963–70.

100. Gabrilovich D. Mechanisms and functional significance of tumour-induced dendritic-cell defects. Nat Rev Immunol 2004;4:941–52.

101. Zea AH, Rodriguez PC, Atkins MB, et al. Arginase-producing myeloid suppressor cells in renal cell carcinoma patients: a mechanism of tumor evasion. Cancer Res 2005;65:3044–8.

102. Ko JS, Zea AH, Rini BI, et al. Sunitinib mediates reversal of myeloid-derived suppressor cell accumulation in renal cell carcinoma patients. Clin Cancer Res 2009;15:2148–57.

103. Brahmer JR, Topalian S, Wollner I, et al. Safety and activity of MDX-1106 (ONO-4538), an anti-PD-1 monoclonal antibody, in patients with selected refractory or relapsed malignancies. J Clin Oncol 2008;26(May 20 Suppl) [abstract: 3006].

104. Yang JC, Hughes M, Kammula U, et al. Ipilimumab (anti-CTLA4 antibody) causes regression of metastatic renal cell cancer associated with enteritis and hypophysitis. J Immunother 2007;30:825–30.

105. Morris J, Shapiro G, Tan A, et al. Phase I/II study of GC1008: a human anti-transforming growth factor-beta (TGFβ) monoclonal antibody (MAb) in patients with advanced malignant melanoma (MM) or renal cell carcinoma (RCC). J Clin Oncol 2008;26(May 20 Suppl) [abstract: 9028].

106. Sznol M, Hodi F, Margolin K, et al. Phase I study of BMS-663513, a fully human anti-CD137 agonist monoclonal antibody, in patients (pts) with advanced cancer (CA). J Clin Oncol 2008;26(May 20 Suppl) [abstract: 3007].

107. Schmidt H, Selby P, Mouritzen U, et al. Subcutaneous (SC) dosing of recombinant human interleukin-21 (rIL-21) is safe and has clinical activity: results from a dose-escalation study in stage 4 melanoma (MM) or renal cell cancer (RCC). J Clin Oncol 2008;26(May 20 Suppl) [abstract: 3041].

108. Moore DJ, Hwang J, McGreivy J, et al. Phase I trial of escalating doses of the TLR9 agonist HYB2055 in patients with advanced solid tumors. J Clin Oncol 2005;23(Suppl):2503 ASCO Annual Meeting Proceedings.

109. Amin A, Dudek T, Logan RS, et al. A phase II study testing the safety and activity of AGS-003 as an immunotherapeutic in subjects with newly diagnosed advanced stage renal cell carcinoma in combination with sunitinib. J Clin Oncol 2010;28:4588.

110. Prieto PA, Yang JC, Sherry RM, et al. Cytotoxic T lymphocyte-associated antigen 4 blockade with ipilimumab: long-term follow-up of 179 patients with metastatic melanoma. J Clin Oncol 2010;28:15s [abstract: 8544].

111. Rini BI, Stein M, Shannon P, et al. Phase 1 dose-escalation trial of tremelimumab plus sunitinib in patients with metastatic renal cell carcinoma. Cancer 2011;117:758–67.

112. Thompson RH, Gillett MD, Cheville JC, et al. Costimulatory B7-H1 in renal cell carcinoma patients: indicator of tumor aggressiveness and potential therapeutic target. Proc Natl Acad Sci U S A 2004;101:17174–9.

113. Keir ME, Francisco LM, Sharpe AH. PD-1 and its ligands in T-cell immunity. Curr Opin Immunol 2007;19:309–14.

114. Keir ME, Butte MJ, Freeman GJ, et al. PD-1 and its ligands in tolerance and immunity. Annu Rev Immunol 2008;26:677–704.

115. Okazaki T, Honjo T. The PD-1-PD-L pathway in immunological tolerance. Trends Immunol 2006;27:195–201.

116. Nishimura H, Nose M, Hiai H, et al. Development of lupus-like autoimmune diseases by disruption of the PD-1 gene encoding an ITIM motif-carrying immunoreceptor. Immunity 1999;11:141–51.
117. Nishimura H, Okazaki T, Tanaka Y, et al. Autoimmune dilated cardiomyopathy in PD-1 receptor-deficient mice. Science 2001;291:319–22.
118. Blank C, Kuball J, Voelkl S, et al. Blockade of PD-L1 (B7-H1) augments human tumor-specific T cell responses in vitro. Int J Cancer 2006;119:317–27.
119. Grabie N, Gotsman I, DaCosta R, et al. Endothelial programmed death-1 ligand 1 (PD-L1) regulates CD8+ T-cell mediated injury in the heart. Circulation 2007; 116:2062–71.
120. Keir ME, Freeman GJ, Sharpe AH. PD-1 regulates self-reactive CD8+ T cell responses to antigen in lymph nodes and tissues. J Immunol 2007;179:5064–70.
121. Keir ME, Liang SC, Guleria I, et al. Tissue expression of PD-L1 mediates peripheral T cell tolerance. J Exp Med 2006;203:883–95.
122. Barber DL, Wherry EJ, Masopust D, et al. Restoring function in exhausted CD8 T cells during chronic viral infection. Nature 2006;439:682–7.
123. Brown JA, Dorfman DM, Ma FR, et al. Blockade of programmed death-1 ligands on dendritic cells enhances T cell activation and cytokine production. J Immunol 2003;170:1257–66.
124. Oflazoglu E, Swart DA, Anders-Bartholo P, et al. Paradoxical role of programmed death-1 ligand 2 in Th2 immune responses in vitro and in a mouse asthma model in vivo. Eur J Immunol 2004;34:3326–36.
125. Fukushima A, Yamaguchi T, Azuma M, et al. Involvement of programmed death-ligand 2 (PD-L2) in the development of experimental allergic conjunctivitis in mice. Br J Ophthalmol 2006;90:1040–5.
126. Dong H, Strome SE, Salomao DR, et al. Tumor-associated B7-H1 promotes T-cell apoptosis: a potential mechanism of immune evasion. Nat Med 2002;8:793–800.
127. Hamanishi J, Mandai M, Iwasaki M, et al. Programmed cell death 1 ligand 1 and tumor-infiltrating CD8+ T lymphocytes are prognostic factors of human ovarian cancer. Proc Natl Acad Sci U S A 2007;104:3360–5.
128. Strome SE, Dong H, Tamura H, et al. B7-H1 blockade augments adoptive T-cell immunotherapy for squamous cell carcinoma. Cancer Res 2003;63:6501–5.
129. Inman BA, Sebo TJ, Frigola X, et al. PD-L1 (B7-H1) expression by urothelial carcinoma of the bladder and BCG-induced granulomata: associations with localized stage progression. Cancer 2007;109:1499–505.
130. Konishi J, Yamazaki K, Azuma M, et al. B7-H1 expression on non-small cell lung cancer cells and its relationship with tumor-infiltrating lymphocytes and their PD-1 expression. Clin Cancer Res 2004;10:5094–100.
131. Nakanishi J, Wada Y, Matsumoto K, et al. Overexpression of B7-H1 (PD-L1) significantly associates with tumor grade and postoperative prognosis in human urothelial cancers. Cancer Immunol Immunother 2007;56:1173–82.
132. Nomi T, Sho M, Akahori T, et al. Clinical significance and therapeutic potential of the programmed death-1 ligand/programmed death-1 pathway in human pancreatic cancer. Clin Cancer Res 2007;13:2151–7.
133. Wu C, Zhu Y, Jiang J, et al. Immunohistochemical localization of programmed death-1 ligand-1 (PD-L1) in gastric carcinoma and its clinical significance. Acta Histochem 2006;108:19–24.
134. Ahmadzadeh M, Johnson LA, Heemskerk B, et al. Tumor antigen-specific CD8 T cells infiltrating the tumor express high levels of PD-1 and are functionally impaired. Blood 2009;114:1537–44.

135. Mumprecht S, Schurch C, Schwaller J, et al. Programmed death 1 signaling on chronic myeloid leukemia-specific T cells results in T-cell exhaustion and disease progression. Blood 2009;114:1528–36.

136. Sznol. Safety and antitumor activity of bi-weekly MDX1106 in patients with advanced or refractory malignancies. J Clin Oncol 2010;28(Suppl):15s [abstract 2506].

137. Rosenblatt J, Glotzbecker B, Mills H, et al. CT-011, anti-PD-1 antibody, enhances ex-vivo T cell responses to autologous dendritic/myeloma fusion vaccine developed for the treatment of multiple myeloma. Blood 2009;114: 781 (ASH Annual Meeting Abstracts).

138. Ko JS, Rayman P, Ireland J, et al. Direct and differential suppression of myeloid-derived suppressor cell subsets by sunitinib is compartmentally constrained. Cancer Res 2010;70:3526–36.

139. Busse A, Asemissen AM, Nonnenmacher A, et al. Immunomodulatory effects of sorafenib on peripheral immune effector cells in metastatic renal cell carcinoma. Eur J Cancer 2011;47:690–6.

140. Hipp MM, Hilf N, Walter S, et al. Sorafenib, but not sunitinib, affects function of dendritic cells and induction of primary immune responses. Blood 2008;111: 5610–20.

Vascular Endothelial Growth Factor–Targeted Therapies in Advanced Renal Cell Carcinoma

Laurence Albiges, MD[a,1], Mohamed Salem, MD[b,1], Brian Rini, MD[b], Bernard Escudier, MD[a,*]

KEYWORDS

- Renal cell carcinoma • Clear cell carcinoma
- Vascular endothelial growth factor • HIF • Bevacizumab
- Sunitinib • Sorafenib • Pazopanib

Improved understanding of the biology and pathogenesis of renal cell carcinoma (RCC) has confirmed the role of vascular endothelial growth factor (VEGF) and its related pathway elements in the angiogenesis that promotes RCC pathogenesis. RCC tumor proliferation and survival have been shown to be largely mediated through this pathway. Therefore, inhibition of the VEGF signaling pathway is a therapeutic target for patients with RCC.

Targeted agents directed toward VEGF/VEGF receptor (VEGFR) pathways have become the mainstay of systemic treatment for metastatic RCC (mRCC), having largely replaced cytokine therapy because of improvements in both efficacy and tolerability. VEGF pathway inhibition relies either on VEGF ligand-binding blockade or on inhibition of its receptor, VEGFR.

Several questions are currently being assessed in this setting: which VEGF/VEGFR inhibitor is more potent and well tolerated? can this combination be sustained? what are the future promising agents for VEGF-targeting strategies to combat RCC? and lastly what is the best sequence of VEGF inhibitors to use?

This article focuses on the development, underlying rationale, and clinical data for the FDA-approved VEGF ligand-binding antibody (bevacizumab), small-molecule tyrosine kinase inhibitors (sunitinib, sorafenib, and pazopanib), and other drugs under

[a] Medical Oncology Department, Institut Gustave Roussy, 114 Rue Edouard Vaillant, Villejuif 94805, France
[b] Department of Solid Tumor Oncology, Cleveland Clinic Taussig Cancer Institute, 9500 Euclid Avenue, Cleveland, OH 44195, USA
[1] These two authors are co–first authors and have contributed equally to the work.
* Corresponding author.
E-mail address: Bernard.escudier@igr.fr

development (axitinib and tivozanib) that block the intracellular domain of the VEGFR in the management of patients with RCC.

VEGF BIOLOGY
Von Hippel-Lindau and VEGF

First isolated in the hereditary syndrome Von Hippel-Lindau (VHL) disease, the importance of the VHL tumor-suppressor gene emerged in sporadic clear cell RCC.[1–3] VHL gene inactivation has been observed in 84% to 98% of sporadic RCCs.[4–6] These observations are specific to clear cell RCC histology; VHL mutations have not been observed in other subtypes of RCC. Biallellic VHL gene inactivation has, therefore, been considered a key event in clear cell RCC oncogenesis according to the two-hits carcinogenesis Knudson model. The VHL protein regulates normal cellular responses to hypoxia via hypoxia-inducible factor α (HIF-α).[7–9] When oxygen levels are normal, oxygen content in the blood regulates the formation of VHL protein complexes, which target HIF-α for degradation by proteasomes. Therefore, proangiogenic factors are not released. However, mutation or inactivation of the VHL protein disrupts the ability to degrade HIF-α in the presence of normal oxygen levels, leading to excess accumulation of HIF-α, and resulting in the overproduction of proangiogenic factors, such as VEGF. Therefore, inactivation of VHL function activates the hypoxia-response pathway.[9–11] This pathway corresponds to transcriptional activation of a variety of genes involved in tumor proliferation, including VEGF (**Fig. 1**). VEGF is a key player in promoting tumor-associated angiogenesis.[12]

VEGF Function

VEGF is a growth factor that exerts its biologic effects primarily on vascular endothelial cells.[13] It is part of the VEGF family of ligands, including VEGF-B, VEGF-C, and VEGF-D, which bind to one or more of the various VEGFRs (see **Fig. 1**). On ligation to its receptor, VEGFR-2 can induce growth, proliferation, and migration of endothelial cells, and promote the survival of immature endothelial cells via inhibition of apoptosis. It also increases vascular permeability. As a key proangiogenic molecule, VEGF plays an important role in several physiologic processes, such as embryogenesis, skeletal growth, and wound healing, and is the key mediator of angiogenesis in cancer.

Taken together, these scientific findings have led to the development of therapeutic inhibitors of VEGF in RCC.[14–16] VEGF inhibition strategies rely either on VEGF blockade or on inhibition either of the VEGFR or of signaling of the downstream VEGFR. These approaches and their therapeutic results are described (see **Fig. 1**).

VEGF BINDING AGENTS
Bevacizumab

Bevacizumab (Avastin, Genentech, South San Francisco, CA, USA) is a recombinant monoclonal antibody (mAb) IgG1 antibody that has been developed for humans from murine anti-VEGF mAb A4.6.1. The murine mAb A4.6.1 is specific for human VEGF, binding to all of the known isoforms of the ligand (eg, VEGF121, VEGF165, VEGF181, VEGF206). It is formed through alternative gene splicing, preventing it from binding to VEGFRs on vascular endothelial cells. In 1997, murine anti-VEGF mAb A4.6.1 was adapted for human use by site-directed mutagenesis, resulting in the production of bevacizumab.[17] Bevacizumab is 93% human and 7% murine, and recognizes all of the major isoforms of human VEGF with a binding affinity of $Kd = 8 \times 10^{-10}$ M (a similar affinity to the murine antibody). The binding ability of bevacizumab for VEGF is restricted to human, nonhuman primate, and rabbit VEGF. Sustained

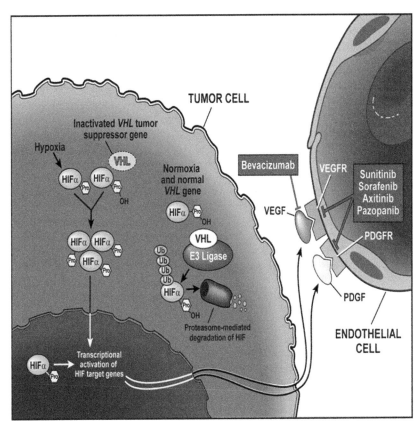

Fig. 1. VEGF pathway and the targeted agents. (*From* Rini B, Campbell S, Escudier B. Renal cell carcinoma. Lancet 2009;373:1119–32; with permission.)

inhibition of VEGF with bevacizumab results in the regression of existing tumor microvasculature and normalization of surviving tumor vasculature, and inhibits the formation of new vasculature. It may also revert tumor-associated immune suppression and improve concomitant drug delivery into the tumor.

Bevacizumab has a terminal half-life of 17 to 21 days, with no dose-limiting toxicity when used as a single agent. The low interpatient variability and the modest effects of covariates on the clearance and volume distribution of bevacizumab support the current strategy of dosing bevacizumab based on body weight (mg/kg).

Phase II trials
Two key phase II trials have been conducted on bevacizumab use in treating RCC: AVF0890s and the RACE trial. The first trial,[18] AVF0890s, was a randomized, placebo-controlled, double-blind trial of bevacizumab monotherapy conducted in patients with metastatic, predominantly clear cell RCC who were not optimal candidates for an interleukin (IL)-2 therapy or had not previously experienced response to this therapy. Between October 1998 and September 2001, 116 patients were randomized to one of three treatment arms: placebo (n = 40) or bevacizumab at either 3 mg/kg (n = 37) or 10 mg/kg (n = 39). This trial showed that the median time to progression was significantly longer for the 10-mg/kg bevacizumab arm than for the placebo

arm (4.8 vs 2.5 months; hazard ratio [HR], 2.55; P<.001). The median time to progression for the 3-mg/kg bevacizumab arm was 3 months, and was not significantly greater than the placebo arm (HR, 1.26; P = .053). Four (10%) patients in the 10-mg/kg bevacizumab arm experienced partial responses of variable duration (6, 9, 15, and >39 months, respectively). This trial provided the rationale for the using 10 mg/kg of bevacizumab in treating RCC.

The phase II RACE trial evaluated bevacizumab in combination with erlotinib in patients with mRCC[19] based on the rationale that VEGF has been implicated to have anti-epidermal growth factor receptor resistance. A randomized, double-blind, placebo-controlled trial was conducted at 21 sites in the United States. Eligible patients were enrolled from March 2004 through October 2004 to receive bevacizumab, 10 mg/kg, every 2 weeks, plus either erlotinib, 150 mg orally daily, or a placebo daily. The median progression-free survival (PFS) was not significantly improved by the addition of erlotinib to bevacizumab (8.5 months with bevacizumab plus placebo vs 9.9 months with bevacizumab plus erlotinib; HR, 0.86; 95% CI, 0.50–1.49). Furthermore, the addition of erlotinib to bevacizumab resulted in a similar overall response rate, which was 13% with bevacizumab plus placebo versus 14% with bevacizumab plus erlotinib. The addition of erlotinib to bevacizumab did not result in an improved duration of objective response (6.7 vs 9.1 months) or time to symptom progression (HR, 1.172; P = .5076). This efficacy has been the basis for testing bevacizumab in phase III trials.

Phase III trials
AVOREN trial AVOREN was the pivotal phase III trial to evaluate the efficacy and safety of adding bevacizumab to interferon for treating mRCC.[20,21] Bevacizumab was tested in combination with interferon to determine whether it would add efficacy to one of the standard treatments at the time of the trial's design. Between June 2004 and October 2005, the trial enrolled 649 patients from 18 countries. Eligible patients had mRCC with a predominantly clear cell histology (>50% clear cells if mixed), underwent prior nephrectomy for primary RCC, a measurable or nonmeasurable disease according to Response Evaluation Criteria in Solid Tumors (RECIST), a Karnofsky performance status of at least 70%, and no proteinuria at baseline (<0.5 g of protein in a 24-hour urine collection). Patients were randomized on a 1:1 basis to receive interferon (9 million international units) three times weekly plus a placebo, or bevacizumab at 10 mg/kg every 2 weeks plus interferon. The final analysis of PFS, which was performed at the scheduled time point for overall survival, showed that it was significantly improved by the addition of bevacizumab to interferon, for 5.4 to 10.2 months (HR, 0.63; P = .0001). This finding represents an 89% improvement in median PFS with bevacizumab plus interferon. The addition of bevacizumab to interferon also improves the overall response rate compared with interferon plus a placebo (31% vs 13%). Analyses of patient subgroups suggested that the addition of bevacizumab to interferon improves PFS in all subgroups analyzed. Improvements in PFS were observed in both favorable (n = 180) and intermediate (n = 363) Memorial Sloan-Kettering Cancer Center (MSKCC) risk categories (median PFS, 12.9 vs 7.6 months; HR, 0.60; P = .0039, and median PFS, 10.2 vs 4.5 months; HR, 0.55; P<.0001, respectively). A significant improvement was not seen in patients in the poor MSKCC risk category (n = 54; median PFS, 2.2 months with bevacizumab plus interferon vs 2.1 months with interferon plus placebo; HR, 0.81; P = .457). An improvement in PFS was observed in patients receiving bevacizumab plus interferon who either had a clear cell RCC histology (n = 564; median PFS, 10.2 vs 5.5 months; HR, 0.64; 95% CI, 0.53–0.77) or a mixed RCC histology (n = 85; median PFS, 5.7 vs 2.9 months; HR,

0.60; 95% CI, 0.33–0.85). Patients aged 65 years or older (n = 239; HR, 0.77; 95% CI, 0.58–1.03) and those younger than 65 years (n = 410; HR, 0.54; 95% CI, 0.43–0.68) had significant improvement in PFS, indicating that age did not affect the response to PFS. In addition, PFS did not seem to be affected by reduced kidney function, as assessed through creatinine clearance (CCr) or VEGF levels. Patients with both high/normal CCr (n = 131) or low CCr (n = 191) benefited from bevacizumab plus interferon (HR, 0.60; 95% CI, 0.46–0.79 and HR, 0.65; 95% CI, 0.51–0.82, respectively). Baseline VEGF levels were established based on recruitment, and improvements in PFS were observed in patients with VEGF levels below the median baseline level (HR, 0.44; 95% CI, 0.32–0.64) and above the median level (HR, 0.66; 95% CI, 0.49–0.93).

The tolerability profile for bevacizumab plus interferon in the AVOREN trial was consistent with the side effects previously reported for both agents. The dose intensity (percentage of planned total dose) of bevacizumab/placebo and interferon was similar in the two arms (92% bevacizumab plus interferon vs 96% interferon plus placebo for the bevacizumab/placebo arms, and 91% bevacizumab plus interferon vs 96% interferon plus placebo for the interferon arms). The incidence of grade 3/4 events associated with bevacizumab therapy included hypertension (7%), proteinuria (4%), bleeding (3%), arterial and venous thromboembolic events (3%), gastrointestinal perforation (1%), and wound-healing complications (<1%). In the final report, overall survival was not significantly improved (23.3 vs 21.3 months; unstratified HR, 0.91; 95% CI, 0.76–1.10; $P = .3360$; stratified HR, 0.86; 95% CI, 0.72–1.04; $P = .1291$). However, a trend favoring the combined treatment was reported.

Cancer and Leukemia Group B 90206 Trial The Cancer and Leukemia Group B (CALGB) 90206 trial was the second major randomized open-label phase III trial to compare the efficacy and safety of bevacizumab plus interferon against interferon alone in patients with mRCC (n = 732).[22,23] This study differed from the AVOREN study in that it was not placebo-controlled or blinded. The results from this trial confirmed the PFS data observed in the AVOREN trial, whereby the addition of bevacizumab to interferon improves PFS (median PFS for bevacizumab plus interferon was 8.5 months compared with 5.2 months for interferon alone; HR, 0.71; 95% CI, 0.61–0.83). The PFS data for subgroups, including those based on MSKCC risk, were also confirmed. The phase III CALGB 90206 trial showed no new safety signals with the bevacizumab plus interferon regimen (**Table 1**). Similar to the AVOREN trial, no

Table 1
Pivotal phase III trials with bevacizumab and interferon

Treatment	Line	No. of Patients	Response Rate	PFS (mo)	OS (mo)
Anti-VEGF					
AVOREN[20,21] Bevacizumab + interferon versus interferon + placebo	First	649	PR: 31% versus 13% CR: 1%	10.2 versus 5.4 HR: 0.63	23.3
CALGB 90206[22,23] Bevacizumab + interferon versus interferon	First	732	PR: 25.5% versus 13% CR: <1%	8.5 versus 5.2 HR: 0.71	18.3

Abbreviations: CR, complete response; HR, hazard ratio; OS, overall survival (median); PFS, progression-free survival; PR, partial response.

differences in overall survival were seen between the combined arm and the interferon-alone arm.

Bevacizumab combined with interferon received an approval as a first-line treatment for patients with advanced or metastatic RCC by the European Medicines Agency in December 2007 and the U.S. Food and Drug Administration (FDA) in July 2009.

Bevacizumab-based combination regimen

Bevacizumab, combined with a second targeted agent, has been evaluated with either tyrosine kinase inhibitors or mammalian target of rapamycin (mTOR) inhibitors (Table 2).

From the rationale of dual inhibition of the VEGF and mTOR pathways in RCC, phase I studies have been performed that have shown the feasibility of combining bevacizumab with one of the mTOR inhibitors, temsirolimus or everolimus. Based on preliminary encouraging data, several randomized trials have been designed.

The TORAVA phase II trial was a three-armed combination trial of bevacizumab plus interferon (n = 40) versus bevacizumab plus temsirolimus (n = 80) versus sunitinib (n = 40). The primary objective was nonprogression of RCC at 48 weeks. However, this trial reported a high frequency of grade 1 to 3 adverse events, especially anal fistulization. These combinations were discontinued in 41% of patients in the investigational arm because of toxicity. In terms of efficacy, the results were negative, with a median PFS of 8.2 months in the experimental arm compared with 16.8 and 8.2 months in the bevacizumab plus interferon and sunitinib arms, respectively. A phase III trial (INTORACT) comparing this combination with a combination of bevacizumab plus interferon was completed and should be reported shortly.

The combination of bevacizumab plus everolimus either as first-line treatment or after treatment with sunitinib or sorafenib in patients with advanced clear cell RCC was evaluated in a phase II trial.[2] A total of 80 patients were enrolled in the trial. All patients received bevacizumab, 10 mg/kg intravenously every 2 weeks, and everolimus 10 mg, orally daily; patients with an objective response or stable disease continued treatment until disease progression or unacceptable toxicity occurred. Median PFS in patients who were treatment-naïve (n = 50) was 9.1 months versus 7.1 months in those previously treated (n = 30). Overall response rates were similar in both groups. Generally the combination regimen was well tolerated and, except

Table 2			
Combination trials with bevacizumab			
	Second Agent	**Reference, Phase I Trial**	**Ongoing Phase II–III Combination Trials**
Bevacizumab + tyrosine kinase inhibitor			
Bevacizumab	Sunitinib	Feldman et al,[54] 2009	–
Bevacizumab 5 mg	Sorafenib (200 mg)	Sosman et al,[55] 2008	BeST (NCT00378703)
Bevacizumab + mTOR inhibitor			
Bevacizumab, 10 mg	Temsirolimus, 25 mg	Merchan et al,[56] 2009	TORAVA (NCT00619268) INTORACT (NCT00631371)
Bevacizumab	Everolimus	Hainsworth et al,[57] 2010	RECORD-2 (NCT00719264)

for grade 3 to 4 proteinuria (25%), which led to treatment discontinuation in six patients, the toxicity profile was as expected. Despite the promising antitumor activity and good safety profile of this combination regimen, further studies are needed to compare it with sequential use of these two agents. A phase III CALGB study is investigating this combination versus everolimus alone in patients for whom prior VEGF-targeted therapy failed. The phase II trial (RECORD 2) investigating the combination of bevacizumab plus everolimus versus bevacizumab plus interferon (N = 360) has completed accrual and results are expected in 2012.

Bevacizumab in a neoadjuvant setting

Little is known about the use of bevacizumab in the neoadjuvant setting for RCC. Several retrospective analyses of perioperative complications in patients with mRCC, who had undergone cytoreductive nephrectomy after receiving various antiangiogenic agents, did not report excessive morbidity.[24] One phase II trial[25] assessed the feasibility of bevacizumab after four cycles as a neoadjuvant in 50 patients, but wound dehiscence resulted in treatment discontinuation for three patients and treatment delay for two others. Primary tumor regression of greater than 10% was observed in 10 of the 45 evaluable patients.

VEGF Trap

VEGF Trap (Regeneron Pharmaceuticals, Tarrytown, New York and sanofi-aventis, Bridgewater, New Jersey) is a fusion compound composed of the human VEGFR-1 (Flt-1) extracellular immunoglobulin domain number two and the VEGFR-2 (KDR) extracellular immunoglobulin domain number three, fused to the human IgGg1 Fc molecule. Therefore, this fusion protein acts as a soluble decoy receptor to bind VEGF and prevent subsequent VEGF binding and signaling. VEGF Trap binds to VEGF with a great affinity (Kd = 1 pmol/L) and also binds the placental growth factor, another angiogenic protein. In cultured endothelial cell assays, VEGF Trap showed inhibition of VEGF-induced VEGFR-2 phosphorylation and endothelial cell proliferation. In xenograft models, mice treated with VEGF Trap exhibited significant growth inhibition of different tumor subtypes. VEGF Trap activity has been assessed in phase I trials.[26] In two trials, patients presented with refractory solid tumors. In the first report, 38 patients, including 9 with mRCC, received one or two subcutaneous doses of VEGF Trap, followed 4 weeks later with 6 weekly injections (escalating dose levels of 0.025, 0.05, 0.1, 0.2, 0.4, and 0.8 mg/kg) or six twice-weekly (0.8 mg/kg) injections. Drug-related grade 3 adverse events included hypertension and proteinuria, although a maximum tolerated dose was not determined. No anti–VEGF Trap antibodies were detected. No objective responses were observed in this trial. Of the 24 assessable patients, 14, including 5 of 6 at the highest dose level, maintained stable disease for 10 weeks. In the second trial, 30 patients were treated with intravenous VEGF Trap every 2 weeks at one of five different dose levels (0.3, 1.0, 2.0, 3.0, and 4.0 mg/kg). Drug-related grade 3 adverse events included arthralgia and fatigue. One patient with mRCC maintained a stable disease for more than 11 months (at the 1.0 mg/kg dose level). Dynamic contrast-enhanced magnetic resonance vascular imaging performed at baseline and after 24 hours indicated effective inhibition of tumor perfusion at the higher dose levels (2.0 mg/kg). Complete binding of circulating VEGF was documented at higher dose levels (2.0 mg/kg), with more free than bound VEGF Trap observed in the plasma. Further investigation is ongoing through an Eastern Cooperative Oncology Group (ECOG) phase II trial (ECOG-E4805, NCT00357760) that randomized 120 patients with mRCC to two different doses of VEGF Trap, with a primary end point of PFS at 8 weeks.

Ramucirumab (IMC-1121B; ImClone Systems Corporation, Branchburg, New Jersey) is a human mAb that specifically inhibits VEGFR-2; which is a critical receptor involved in malignant angiogenesis. Multiple clinical trials have been conducted to investigate the antitumor activity of ramucirumab in a variety of tumor types, such as RCC, colon cancer, non–small cell lung cancer, and hepatocellular carcinoma. A phase II study was recently presented of treatment with ramucirumab after tyrosine kinase inhibitors failed in patients with mRCC.[3] Among 40 patients enrolled in the trial, 54% had received prior sunitinib, 10% received prior sorafenib, and 36% received both sunitinib and sorafenib. Patients received ramucirumab, 8 mg/kg, intravenously every 2 weeks. Overall response rate was 5%, and 38% of patients had stable disease. The preliminary median was 8.3 months, with a median follow-up of more than 1 year.

Common toxicities were headache, fatigue, epistaxis, peripheral edema, nausea, and dyspnea. Serious adverse events included grade 2 proteinuria and grade 2 hemoptysis in a patient with endobronchial metastases. Grade 3 or 4 adverse events occurred in 23% of patients and included grade 4 myocardial infarction and grade 3 syncope, hypertension, fatigue, dyspnea, sensory neuropathy, headache, back pain, polyneuropathy, decreased hemoglobin, and anorexia. Grade 4 cardiopulmonary arrest followed by death 13 months after the initiation of study therapy was reported in two patients with underlying cardiovascular disease. These results suggested that ramucirumab could have clinical activity as second- or third-line treatment in patients with mRCC refractory to tyrosine kinase inhibitors.

VEGFR TYROSINE KINASE INHIBITORS

Better understanding of the biology of VEGF and its related pathway in the pathogenesis of RCC led to the era of small molecule tyrosine kinase inhibitors (sunitinib, sorafenib, and pazopanib, and axitinib and tivozanib, which are currently being evaluated), which block the intracellular domain of the VEGFR, in the management of RCC.

Sunitinib

Sunitinib is a highly potent, oral, multitargeted, selective tyrosine kinase inhibitor of the VEGFR (types 1–3), the platelet-derived growth-factor receptors (PDGFRs) α and β, and other tyrosine kinases.[27]

The activity and safety of sunitinib in patients with mRCC in the post–cytokine therapy setting was evaluated in two multi-institutional phase II studies.[28,29] These studies enrolled 63 patients with mRCC who experienced progression on first-line cytokine therapy, with the primary end point of overall response rate.[28] Per RECIST criteria, 25 (40%) of the 63 patients showed partial response; 8 of whom remained progression-free for 21 to 24 months. The median time to tumor progression was 8.7 months, and the median survival duration for the entire group was 16.4 months.

The most common grade 3 or greater toxicities observed were fatigue (11%), diarrhea (3%), hypertension (2%), stomatitis (2%), lymphopenia without infection (32%), and elevated serum lipase (21%), without clinical signs or symptoms of pancreatitis. Notably, 4 patients had a decline in cardiac ejection fraction; 3 of them were asymptomatic, and 1 patient had dyspnea. A dose reduction from 50 to 37.5 mg/d was required in 22 patients (35%) because of hyperlipasemia or hyperamylasemia (11 patients) and fatigue (5 patients), and the dose for 2 of these patients was further reduced to 25 mg/d. No patient developed adrenal insufficiency. A second trial conducted to evaluate the efficacy of sunitinib in 106 patients with mRCC[29] showed similar results, with an overall response rate of 34% and a median time to progression of 8.3 months.

Subsequently, a randomized phase III trial was conducted to compare sunitinib with interferon α as a first-line therapy for patients with mRCC.[30] A total of 750 patients with treatment-naïve mRCC were enrolled into the international multicenter trial. Patients were randomly assigned to a 1:1 ratio to receive either a 6-week cycle of sunitinib (50 mg daily for 4 weeks, followed by 2 weeks off), or interferon α (9 million units 3 times per week). The primary end point was PFS. Secondary end points included the objective response rate, overall survival, patient-reported outcomes, and safety. Median PFS was prolonged in the sunitinib group (11 vs 5 months; 95% CI, 0.32–0.54; $P<.001$). This benefit included patients with good-risk (14.5 vs 7.9 months), intermediate-risk (10.6 vs 3.8 months), and poor-risk outcomes (3.7 vs 1.2 months), as assessed using MSKCC criteria. Furthermore, sunitinib was associated with a higher objective response rate than interferon α (31% vs 6%; $P<.001$). The final analysis showed prolonged overall survival with sunitinib (median, 26.4 vs 21.8 months; HR, 0.82; 95% CI, 0.67–1.00; $P = .051$).

Grade 3 or 4 adverse events were infrequent in both groups. Generally, except for grade 3/4 treatment-related fatigue, which was significantly higher in the interferon α group (12% vs 7%; $P<.05$), adverse events were seen more frequently in the sunitinib group. However, patients in the sunitinib group reported significantly better quality of life than those in the interferon α group ($P<.001$).

Patients in the sunitinib group had higher rates of grade 3 diarrhea (5% vs no cases), vomiting (4% vs 1%), hypertension (8% vs 1%), and hand-foot syndrome (5% vs no cases; $P<.05$ for all comparisons).

No grade 4 declines in left ventricular ejection fraction were reported, but grade 3 events were similar in the sunitinib (2%) and interferon α groups (1%). However, the decline in the sunitinib group was asymptomatic and reversible after dose modification or discontinuation of treatment.

A total of 38% of patients in the sunitinib group and 32% in the interferon α group had a dose interruption because of adverse events, whereas 32% and 21%, respectively, had a dose reduction. Based on these results, sunitinib has become a front-line standard therapy for patients with mRCC.

Sorafenib

Sorafenib (BAY 43-9006, Nexavar; Bayer Healthcare, Montville, NJ, USA; Onyx Pharmaceuticals, Emeryville, CA, USA) is a Raf kinase and VEGFR inhibitor. It was initially identified as a Raf kinase inhibitor but was subsequently found to also inhibit VEGFR-1, -2, and -3; PDGFR-β, Flt-3, c-kit protein (c-kit), and RET-receptor tyrosine kinases.

Four different phase I trials were conducted to investigate the safety of sorafenib using various dosing schedules.[31–34] The most common drug-related toxicities from phase I trials were fatigue, hand-foot syndrome, and rash, whereas the most frequently reported adverse events were gastrointestinal, dermatologic, constitutional, pain, or hepatic-related. Dose-limiting toxicities at continuous doses greater than 400 mg twice daily were diarrhea, fatigue, and skin toxicity. The recommended dose for phase II trials was 400 mg twice daily, continuously.

Preclinical studies suggested that the primary effect of sorafenib is inhibition of tumor growth rather than tumor shrinkage; therefore, the primary clinical benefit of sorafenib was believed to be disease stabilization, which was the underlying rationale for the phase II placebo-controlled randomized discontinuation trial.[35] The randomized discontinuation trial was conducted to evaluate the effects of sorafenib on tumor growth in patients with mRCC. The original trial protocol focused on patients with metastatic colorectal carcinoma. However, because of the signs of antitumor activity in patients with RCC, and low numbers of patients with colorectal carcinoma meeting the criteria for randomization after the 12-week run-in period, this shifted the study's focus toward patients with RCC (202 patients).

A total of 502 patients were enrolled into the study, 501 of whom received the study drug. Patients who had more than 25% tumor shrinkage remained on sorafenib, those with 25% tumor growth discontinued treatment, and those who had less than a 25% change in their tumor size were randomly assigned to sorafenib or a placebo for an additional 12 weeks. The primary end point of the trial was the percentage of randomly assigned patients remaining RCC progression free at 24 weeks after the initiation of sorafenib. A total of 202 patients treated during the run-in period of 12 weeks remained at the end of this period. Of these, 73 had 25% tumor shrinkage and remained on sorafenib. Of the 65 patients who had a stable disease (<25% tumor shrinkage), 32 were randomly assigned to sorafenib and 33 received a placebo. At 24 weeks, 50% of the sorafenib-treated group was progression-free versus 18% in the placebo group ($P = .007$). Median PFS after randomization to the sorafenib or placebo group was 24 versus 6 weeks, respectively ($P = .0087$). Median overall PFS was 29 weeks for the entire RCC population (n = 202). Sorafenib was administered to patients whose disease progressed while on a placebo (28 patients); these patients then continued on sorafenib until further RCC progression, for a median of 24 weeks.

The most common adverse events were fatigue, rash/desquamation, hand-foot syndrome, pain, and diarrhea. The most common grade 3/4 adverse event was hypertension (31% of patients). No patient died of toxicity.

A randomized phase III (TARGET) trial was conducted to determine the effects of sorafenib on progression-free and overall survivals in patients with advanced clear cell RCC for whom a prior standard therapy failed.[36] A total of 903 patients with advanced RCC were enrolled in the trial from November 2003 until March 2005. Of these patients, 51% had a good prognosis and 49% had intermediate-risk disease according to MSKCC criteria. Patients were randomly assigned, in a 1:1 ratio and a double-blind fashion, to receive either continuous treatment with oral sorafenib (400 mg twice daily) or a placebo. Patients who continued to receive sorafenib were followed up until either disease progression occurred or they withdrew from the study. Patients who experienced a response were eligible to continue receiving open-label treatment with the drug. In April 2005, based on the first PFS analysis, an Independent Data Monitoring Committee recommended that the study be unblinded and that patients who were assigned to receive a placebo be offered sorafenib. However, investigators and the sponsor remained unaware of the study group assignments regarding survival data.

In an interim analysis of 769 of the patients, the median PFS time was significantly longer in the sorafenib group (5.5 vs 2.8 months in the placebo group; HR for progression, 0.44; 95% CI, 0.35–0.55). However, in the final intention-to-treat analysis of all patients, overall survival with sorafenib was not significantly prolonged compared with placebo (median, 17.8 vs 15.2 months; HR, 0.88; 95% CI, 0.74–1.04).[37] Partial responses were reported as the best response in 10% of patients receiving sorafenib and in 2% of those receiving a placebo ($P<.001$). Of patients in the sorafenib group, 10% discontinued the study drug compared with 8% in the placebo group. A total of 13% of patients in the sorafenib group, compared with 3% in the placebo group ($P<.001$), had a dose reduction. Doses were interrupted because of adverse events in 21% of patients in the sorafenib group compared with 6% in the placebo group ($P<.001$).

As expected, adverse events of all grades occurred more frequently in the sorafenib group. However, the proportion of patients with grade 3 or 4 adverse events was relatively low; events were mostly grade 1 or 2. The most common events were diarrhea (43%), rash (40%), fatigue (37%), hand-foot reactions (30%), alopecia (27%), and nausea (23%). However, serious adverse events that led to hospitalization were higher among patients in the sorafenib group compared with the placebo group (34% vs 24%; P<.01). Serious adverse events associated with treatment were cardiac ischemia (or infarction), which occurred in 3% of the sorafenib group and less than 1% of the placebo group (P = .01); constitutional symptoms, which occurred in 2% of both groups; dyspnea, which occurred in 2% of both groups; and death from progressive disease, which occurred in 2% of both groups. Hypertension was the most frequent drug-related serious adverse event (17% of patients in the sorafenib group and none in the placebo group). Patients in the sorafenib group had higher rates of grade 1 bleeding than those in the placebo group (15% vs 8%). However, the incidence of serious hemorrhagic events was similar in both groups (3% and 2%, respectively). The most frequently grade 3/4 laboratory abnormalities included lymphopenia without infection (13% vs 7%) and hypophosphatemia (13% and 3%). No patient in the sorafenib group had febrile neutropenia or grade 4 thrombocytopenia. Grade 3 or 4 anemia occurred in 3% of patients in the sorafenib group and 4% in the placebo group. Elevated serum lipase level occurred in 41% of the sorafenib group and 30% of the placebo group but was rarely associated with clinical signs or symptoms of pancreatitis.

Another phase II randomized trial compared the efficacy and safety of first-line therapy with sorafenib plus interferon α in patients with untreated mRCC.[38] A total of 189 patients were randomly assigned, in a 1:1 ratio, to receive either 400 mg of sorafenib twice daily (97 patients) or 9 million units of interferon subcutaneously, three times weekly (92 patients); this was referred to as "period 1." PFS was similar in the sorafenib and interferon α groups (5.7 and 5.6 months, respectively). In period 2 (defined as patients who had progressive RCC on sorafenib, for whom the dose was escalated to 600 mg twice daily, and patients who had progressive RCC on interferon α and were switched to sorafenib at 400 mg twice daily), the median PFS was 3.6 months for patients who escalated to sorafenib at 600 mg twice daily versus 5.3 months for patients treated with interferon who crossed over to sorafenib at 400 mg twice daily. Thus, this trial failed to show a robust clinical effect of sorafenib in an unselected front-line RCC population.

Pazopanib

Pazopanib (GW786034, Votrient; GlaxoSmithKline, Middlesex, UK) is an orally potent, multitarget receptor tyrosine kinase inhibitor of VEGFR-1, -2, and -3; PDGFR-α and -β; and stem cell factor receptor (c-kit). The safety, pharmacokinetics, and clinical activity of pazopanib were evaluated in patients with advanced-stage refractory solid tumors in a phase I trial.[39] Sixty-three patients, with a variety of solid tumor types, received doses ranging from 50 mg 3 times per week, to 2000 mg daily to 400 mg twice daily.

Forty-eight (76%) patients experienced drug-related adverse events, mostly grade 1 or 2. The most frequent drug-related adverse events were hypertension (33%), diarrhea (33%), hair depigmentation (32%), and nausea (32%). Hypertension was the most frequent grade 3 adverse events. Hair depigmentation was seen in 12 patients, all of whom were treated at doses equal to 800 mg or more. Additionally, single events of gastrointestinal bleeding, pulmonary thrombosis, and deep vein thrombosis occurred. However, no patient developed hand-foot syndrome.

Clinical benefits were generally observed in patients who received doses of 800 mg (or more) once daily or 300 mg twice daily, and a plateau of steady-state exposure was observed at doses of 800 mg once daily or more. Therefore, the recommended phase II dose is 800 mg daily.

A multicenter, phase II placebo-controlled randomized discontinuation study was conducted to evaluate the efficacy and safety of pazopanib in patients with mRCC.[40] A total of 225 patients were enrolled in the study from October 2005 to September 2006, of which 155 (69%) were treatment-naïve and 70 (31%) had received one prior cytokine- or bevacizumab-containing regimen. All patients began the study with an open-label pazopanib treatment for 12 weeks as the initial run-in period. Although the study was originally designed as a randomized discontinuation study, it was changed to an open-label trial because of the results from the planned interim analysis, which indicated early activity.

The primary end point in the revised design was overall response rate. Secondary end points included duration of response and PFS. Overall response rate was 35%; median duration of response was 68 weeks. Median PFS was 52 weeks.

The PFS in the randomized comparison (n = 55) was 11.9 months for pazopanib versus 6.2 months for the placebo (P = .0128). Furthermore, the ECOG performance status of 0 and the time from diagnosis to treatment of more than 1 year were associated with prolonged PFS.

Generally, pazopanib was well tolerated; 215 patients of 225 (96%) experienced treatment-related adverse events of any grade. However, 77 patients (34%) had grade 3 adverse events and 16 (7%) had grade 4 adverse events. Two grade 5 drug-related adverse events were reported (namely large-bowel perforation and dyspnea). The most commonly reported adverse events of any grade were diarrhea in 133 patients (59%), hair color changes in 96 (43%), hypertension in 90 (40%), nausea in 83 (37%), fatigue in 83 (37%), dysgeusia in 52 (23%), anorexia in 39 (17%), vomiting in 33 (15%), rash in 28 (12%), and hand-foot syndrome in 28 (12%). The most frequent grade 3 adverse events were diarrhea in 9 patients (4%), hypertension in 19 (8%), fatigue in 9 (4%), and hand-foot syndrome in 4 (2%). Treatment was discontinued in 15% of patients because of adverse events.

Another phase II study evaluated the efficacy of pazopanib in patients with mRCC who had progressive RCC during other targeted therapies, such as sunitinib or bevacizumab.[41] Thirty-one patients who had either experienced progression on, or were intolerant of, previous treatment with sunitinib or bevacizumab were enrolled onto the trial. All patients received oral pazopanib, 800 mg daily. As of May 2010, 24 patients (77%) previously treated with sunitinib and 7 (23%) previously treated with bevacizumab were enrolled in the trial. Among 25 patients evaluated, 6 (24%) had objective responses, and the disease-control rate (objective response plus stable disease) was 72%. Overall response rate and disease-control rates after sunitinib were 21% and 68%, and were 33% and 83% after bevacizumab, respectively. The 6-month PFS probability for the entire group was 61% (95% CI, 33%–80%). The toxicity profile was similar to the above-mentioned trial.

A randomized, double-blind, global, multicenter, placebo-controlled phase III study was conducted to evaluate the efficacy and safety of pazopanib monotherapy in patients with advanced RCC who had experienced disease progression after prior cytokine-based systemic therapy, or who had undergone no prior therapy.[42] A total of 435 patients with measurable, locally advanced, or mRCC were enrolled in the trial between April 2006 and April 2007, all having clear cell or predominantly clear cell histology. A total of 233 patients were treatment-naïve (54%) and 202 were pretreated with cytokine therapy (46%). Patients were randomly assigned in a 2:1 ratio to receive either 800 mg of pazopanib once daily (n = 290) or placebo (n = 145). Patients who had progressive RCC on the placebo were allowed to receive pazopanib via an open-label study (VEG107769), which included 70 (48%) of the patients in the placebo arm.

The primary end point was PFS, from the date of randomization until the date of RCC progression or death. Secondary end points included overall survival, tumor response rate (complete response and partial response), and safety.

Median PFS for the overall study population was significantly prolonged in pazopanib compared with the placebo group (9.2 vs 4.2 months; HR, 0.46; 95% CI, 0.34–0.62; $P<.0001$) for the treatment-naïve subpopulation (11.1 vs 2.8 months; HR, 0.40; 95% CI, 0.27–0.60; $P<.0001$) and the cytokine-pretreated subpopulation (7.4 vs 4.2 months; HR, 0.54; 95% CI, 0.35–0.84; $P<.001$).The prespecified subgroup analyses showed improved PFS in patients treated with pazopanib compared with those receiving a placebo, regardless of MSKCC risk category, gender, age, or ECOG performance status (HR range, 0.40–0.52; $P<.001$). The objective response rate with pazopanib compared with placebo was 30% versus 3%, respectively ($P<.001$). The median duration of response was longer than 1 year.

The final overall survival rate, presented at the 2010 European Society for Medical Oncology meeting was a median overall survival of 22.9 versus 20.5 months in the pazopanib and placebo arms, respectively ($P = .224$).

For all patients, grade 3 or 4 adverse events were relatively low. The most common grade 3/4 adverse events in the pazopanib arm were hypertension (4%) and diarrhea (4%). The most common events reported in the pazopanib arm were diarrhea (52%), hypertension (40%), hair color change (38%), nausea (26%), anorexia (22%), and vomiting (21%). The proportion of patients who discontinued the drug because of adverse events was higher in those pretreated with cytokine therapy than in those who were treatment-naïve (19% vs 12%). However, the adverse event profile was similar in both groups; 33% of patients had grade 3 and 7% had grade 4 adverse events in the pazopanib arm (with the most common adverse events being hypertension [4%] and diarrhea [4%]) compared with 14% and 6%, respectively, in the placebo arm.

Patients in the pazopanib arm had higher rates of bleeding than those in the placebo group (13% vs 5%). Serious adverse events leading to hospitalization were higher among patients in the pazopanib group; 2% of patients had myocardial infarction (or ischemia), 1% had a cerebrovascular accident, and 1% had a transient ischemic attack compared with none in the placebo group.

Laboratory abnormalities included predominantly grade 1/2 electrolyte abnormalities, including hypophosphatemia, hypocalcaemia, hyponatremia, and hypomagnesemia. However, the most frequent laboratory abnormalities observed in the pazopanib group were elevated alanine transaminase (ALT) and aspartate transaminase levels. Of patients in the pazopanib group, 18% had ALT levels more than threefold higher than the upper limit. However, ALT was normalized in most of these patients (87%) after dose modification, interruption, or discontinuation.

Death resulting from adverse events was reported in 4% of patients in the pazopanib arm and 3% of patients in the placebo arm.

A randomized, open-label phase III study (COMPARZ; ClinicalTrials.gov, identifier NCT00720941)[43] conducted to compare pazopanib with sunitinib in approximately 876 patients with locally advanced or mRCC has completed accrual and is undergoing analysis. Another randomized, double-blind, crossover study (PISCES; ClinicalTrials.gov, identifier NCT01064310)[44] is addressing patient preferences between pazopanib and sunitinib in approximately 160 patients with mRCC who have not received any prior systemic therapy.

Axitinib

Axitinib (Pfizer Inc., New York, NY, USA) is an oral, potent, selective tyrosine kinase inhibitor of VEGFR-1, -2, and -3, PDGFRs, and c-kit. The safety, pharmacokinetics, and clinical activity of axitinib were evaluated in patients with advanced-stage refractory solid tumors in a phase I trial.[45] Thirty-six patients received doses ranging from 5 to 30 mg orally twice daily. The most frequent drug-related adverse events were hypertension, fatigue, diarrhea, stomatitis, nausea, and vomiting. The dose-limiting toxicities were hypertension and stomatitis. Two patients developed grade 3 or 4 hypertension. The maximum tolerated dose and the recommended phase II dose is 5 mg twice daily, administered in a fasted state. Three patients (two with RCC and one with adenoid cystic carcinoma) had partial responses.

A single-arm, open-label, phase II study in 52 patients, 49 of whom had previously undergone a nephrectomy, evaluated the efficacy and safety of axitinib in patients with mRCC for whom prior cytokine therapy failed.[46] All patients received axitinib at a starting dose of 5 mg twice daily. The median duration of axitinib therapy was 9.4 months and the median dose was 8.8 mg/d. The primary end point was the RECIST-defined objective response. Secondary end points were duration of response, time to progression, overall survival, safety, pharmacokinetics, and patient-reported health-related quality of life. Among patients enrolled, 23 (44.2%) had a RECIST-defined objective response (95% CI, 30.5%–58.7%), 2 had a complete response, and 21 had a partial response. The median duration of response was 23 months. Stable disease was seen in 22 patients (for at least 8 weeks). Median time to progression was 15.7 months (8.4–23.4, range 0.03–31.5) and median overall survival was 29.9 months (range 2.4–35.8).

Ten patients discontinued axitinib, and 15 had dose reductions because of adverse events, the most of common of which were fatigue, hypertension, and diarrhea. The most common treatment-related adverse events included diarrhea, hypertension, fatigue, nausea, and hoarseness. The most common grade 3/4 adverse events were hypertension (15.4%), diarrhea (9.6%), and fatigue (7.7%). Four patients had treatment-related proteinuria, and 4 patients reported hand-foot syndrome. Axitinib-related hypertension was reported in 30 patients, 8 of whom had grade 3/4 hypertension. No hematologic toxicities were reported.

Another open-label, phase II trial investigated the efficacy and safety of axitinib in patients with advanced clear cell RCC for whom a prior standard therapy with sorafenib failed.[47] The trial enrolled 62 patients between March and November 2006. All patients had undergone a nephrectomy and had received a prior sorafenib therapy, and many had received additional prior therapy regimens. Fourteen patients (22.6%) experienced a partial response to axitinib. The median duration of response was 17.5 months. Eleven patients (17.7%) had stable disease and 12 stopped axitinib before having a posttreatment scan. The median PFS was 7.4 months (95% CI, 6.7–11.0 months) and median overall survival was 13.6 months (95% CI, 8.4–18.8 months).

The most common adverse events were fatigue, diarrhea, anorexia, hypertension, and nausea. The most common grade 3/4 adverse events included hypertension (16.1%), fatigue (16.1%), hand-foot syndrome (16.1%), diarrhea (14.5%), and dyspnea (14.5%). A total of 22 patients discontinued axitinib because of adverse events. Two patients developed congestive heart failure and two had cerebral hemorrhage during the study. One patient had bowel perforation. Nine (16.4%) patients had grade 3 lymphopenia; otherwise, most hematologic toxicities were mild or of moderate (grade 1 or 2).

An open-label, randomized, phase III study (AXIS)[48] is comparing axitinib to sorafenib as a second-line therapy for mRCC after failure of a prior first-line therapy that included sunitinib, cytokines, temsirolimus, or bevacizumab/interferon α. The results were recently reported, and showed that PFS was significantly superior in patients receiving axitinib versus sorafenib (6.7 vs 4.7 months).[48]

Another phase III trial is underway to compare axitinib with sorafenib in patients with mRCC as a first- or second-line therapy after progression with either sunitinib or cytokines, or both.[49]

Preliminary data suggested that patients on axitinib who experienced a diastolic blood pressure of 90 mm Hg or greater seemed to have a higher response rate and longer overall survival than those who do not. A phase II trial investigating whether dose titration of axitinib in patients who tolerate the drug at the standard starting dose will improve the efficacy of axitinib has completed accrual, and results are expected in 2012.[50]

Tivozanib

Tivozanib (AV-951; KRN-951) is a potent, oral, small-molecule inhibitor of VEGFR-1, -2, and -3 at picomolar concentrations. In a single-center, open-label, dose-escalation, phase I clinical trial, a total of 41 patients with solid tumors[51] were consecutively enrolled into three cohorts of different dose levels. Patients received an oral dose of tivozanib once daily for 4 weeks, followed by 2 weeks of no treatment. Three dose levels were evaluated: 2.0, 1.5, and 1.0 mg. The maximum tolerated dose of tivozanib was 1.5 mg/d when given for 28 consecutive days followed by 14 days of no treatment. Hypertension was the most frequently observed toxicity, and was dose-related. No grade 4 hypertension was observed. Other dose-limiting toxicities included grade 3 dyspnea and fatigue (n = 1), grade 3 ataxia (n = 1), grade 3 transaminases (n = 2), grade 3 proteinuria (n = 1), and grade 4 intracerebral bleeding (n = 1). Clinical activity was observed in all patients with RCC (n = 9); 2 patients had a partial response, and 7 had stable disease.

A phase II, placebo-controlled, randomized discontinuation trial enrolled 272 patients, approximately 73% of whom had undergone prior nephrectomy, to evaluate the efficacy and safety of tivozanib in patients with locally advanced or mRCC.[52] All patients received tivozanib for the initial run-in period. Patients received tivozanib at 1.5 mg once daily for 3 weeks, followed by 1 week off (one cycle over 4 weeks) for the first 12 weeks. Patients who had more than 25% tumor shrinkage remained on tivozanib, those with 25% tumor growth discontinued treatment, and those who had less than a 25% change in tumor size were randomly assigned to tivozanib or

Table 3
Relative potencies of tyrosine kinase inhibitors in RCC[a]

Agent	IC$_{50}$ (nmol/L)				
	VEGFR-1	VEGFR-2	VEGFR-3	c-kit	PDGFR-β
Axitinib[58]	1.2	0.3	0.3	1.6	1.7
Sunitinib[58]	2	10	17	10	8
Pazopanib[58]	15	8	10	2.4	14
Sorafenib[58]	NA	90	20	68	80
Tivozanib[51,57,59,60]	0.2	0.2	0.2	1.6	1.7

[a] The IC$_{50}$ values for the various compound were determined with different assays and not necessarily identical conditions. Thus, the values should be viewed as approximations and comparisons are imprecise.

Abbreviation: NA, not available.

Table 4
Comparative first-line response data in RCC (independent radiology assessment)

Independent assessment of best response	Sunitinib[30]	Sorafenib[36]	Pazopanib[42]	Tivozanib[52]	Axitinib[46]
	Clear cell RCC 91% nephrectomy Phase III trial versus interferon (n = 750)	Clear cell RCC 94% nephrectomy Phase III trial versus PBO (n = 903)	Clear cell RCC 89% nephrectomy Phase III trial versus PBO (n = 435)	Clear cell RCC 100% nephrectomy Phase II RDT	Clear cell RCC 94% nephrectomy Phase II single-arm trial (n = 52)
	(n = 335)	(n = 451)	(n = 290)	(n = 176)	(n = 52)
ORR	31%	10%	30%	32%	44%
PFS (months)	11	5.5	9.2	11.8	15.7

Abbreviations: ORR, overall response rate; PBO, placebo; PFS, progression-free survival; RDT, randomized discontinuation trial.

Table 5
Comparison of reported adverse-event profiles of tyrosine kinase inhibitors

Adverse Event (≥grade 3)	Sunitinib[30] n = 375	Sorafenib[36] n = 451	Pazopanib[42] n = 290	Axitinib[46] n = 52	Tivozanib[52] n = 272
Hypertension all grades (grade >3)	30% (10%)	17% (3%)	40% (4%)	58% (15%)	50% (9%)
Mucositis/stomatitis	43% (3%)	35%[a]	10% (<1%)	17% (2%)	4% (<1%)
Hand-food syndrome	21% (5%)	30% (6%)	11% (2%)	7% (<1%)	4% (<1%)
Rash/desquamation	27% (1%)	40% (1%)	16% (<1%)	12% (0%)	6% (1%)
Fatigue	58% (9%)	37% (6%)	19% (2%)	52% (8%)	8% (2%)
Diarrhea	58% (6%)	43% (2%)	52% (4%)	60% (10%)	12% (2%)
Dose reduction	32%	13%	NA	29%	10%
Dose interruption	38%	21%	14%	NA	4%
Drug discontinuation from toxicity	8%	3%	14%	19%	Not reported

[a] Reported from phase II placebo-controlled randomized discontinuation trial of sorafenib.[35]
Abbreviation: NA, not applicable.

a placebo for an additional 12 weeks. The median PFS was 11.8 months for all patients. The subset of patients with clear cell RCC histology and a prior nephrectomy (176 patients) had a median PFS of 14.8 months. Efficacy was similar between patients who were treatment-naïve and those who were previously treated. Hypertension (50%) and dysphonia (hoarseness of voice, 21.7%) were the most common treatment-related adverse events, and were mostly grades 1 and 2. A low incidence of diarrhea (12.1%), fatigue (8.1%), stomatitis (4.4%), and hand-foot syndrome (3.7%) was seen. Few tivozanib dose reductions and interruptions occurred.

An open-label, randomized, phase III study (tivo-1 trial, NCT01030783)[53] is comparing tivozanib with sorafenib in 500 patients with advanced clear cell RCC who had undergone prior nephrectomy and had no prior VEGF treatment. The primary end point is PFS, with secondary end points including overall survival, overall response rate, and quality of life. The study has completed enrollment and results are eagerly awaited.

SUMMARY

VEGF targeted therapy is the main treatment of mRCC in 2011. Both selective VEGF blockade using bevacizumab and VEGF receptor inhibition are effective and have almost similar activities, but have different potencies (**Tables 3** and **4**) and toxicity profiles (**Table 5**). Off-target effects are important to consider for treatment decisions, and ongoing and future studies will be critical for choosing between currently available drugs (bevacizumab, sorafenib, sunitinib, pazopanib) and upcoming new drugs (axitinib, tivozanib).

REFERENCES

1. Gnarra JR, Glenn GM, Latif F, et al. Molecular genetic studies of sporadic and familial renal cell carcinoma. Urol Clin North Am 1993;20(2):207–16.
2. Linehan WM, Gnarra JR, Lerman MI, et al. Genetic basis of renal cell cancer. Important Adv Oncol 1993;47–70.

3. Gnarra JR, Lerman MI, Zbar B, et al. Genetics of renal-cell carcinoma and evidence for a critical role for von Hippel-Lindau in renal tumorigenesis. Semin Oncol 1995;22(1):3–8.

4. Shuin T, Kondo K, Torigoe S, et al. Frequent somatic mutations and loss of heterozygosity of the von Hippel-Lindau tumor suppressor gene in primary human renal cell carcinomas. Cancer Res 1994;54(11):2852–5.

5. Clifford SC, Prowse AH, Affara NA, et al. Inactivation of the von Hippel-Lindau (VHL) tumour suppressor gene and allelic losses at chromosome arm 3p in primary renal cell carcinoma: evidence for a VHL-independent pathway in clear cell renal tumourigenesis. Genes Chromosomes Cancer 1998;22(3):200–9.

6. Herman JG, Latif F, Weng Y, et al. Silencing of the VHL tumor-suppressor gene by DNA methylation in renal carcinoma. Proc Natl Acad Sci U S A 1994;91(21): 9700–4.

7. Ferrara N. Vascular endothelial growth factor: basic science and clinical progress. Endocr Rev 2004;25(4):581–611.

8. Leung DW, Cachianes G, Kuang WJ, et al. Vascular endothelial growth factor is a secreted angiogenic mitogen. Science 1989;246(4935):1306–9.

9. Kaelin WG. The von Hippel-Lindau protein, HIF hydroxylation, and oxygen sensing. Biochem Biophys Res Commun 2005;338(1):627–38.

10. George DJ, Kaelin WG. The von Hippel-Lindau protein, vascular endothelial growth factor, and kidney cancer. N Engl J Med 2003;349(5):419–21.

11. Kaelin WG. The von Hippel-Lindau tumor suppressor protein and clear cell renal carcinoma. Clin Cancer Res 2007;13(2 Pt 2):680s–4s.

12. Carmeliet P. VEGF as a key mediator of angiogenesis in cancer. Oncology 2005; 69(Suppl 3):4–10.

13. Ferrara N, Gerber H, LeCouter J. The biology of VEGF and its receptors. Nat Med 2003;9(6):669–76.

14. Kaelin WG. Treatment of kidney cancer: insights provided by the VHL tumorsuppressor protein. Cancer 2009;115(10 Suppl):2262–72.

15. Ferrara N, Kerbel RS. Angiogenesis as a therapeutic target. Nature 2005; 438(7070):967–74.

16. Iliopoulos O. Molecular biology of renal cell cancer and the identification of therapeutic targets. J Clin Oncol 2006;24(35):5593–600.

17. Presta LG, Chen H, O'Connor SJ, et al. Humanization of an anti-vascular endothelial growth factor monoclonal antibody for the therapy of solid tumors and other disorders. Cancer Res 1997;57(20):4593–9.

18. Yang JC, Haworth L, Sherry RM, et al. A randomized trial of bevacizumab, an anti-vascular endothelial growth factor antibody, for metastatic renal cancer. N Engl J Med 2003;349(5):427–34.

19. Bukowski RM, Kabbinavar FF, Figlin RA, et al. Randomized phase II study of erlotinib combined with bevacizumab compared with bevacizumab alone in metastatic renal cell cancer. J Clin Oncol 2007;25(29):4536–41.

20. Escudier B, Bellmunt J, Négrier S, et al. Phase III trial of bevacizumab plus interferon alfa-2a in patients with metastatic renal cell carcinoma (AVOREN): final analysis of overall survival. J Clin Oncol 2010;28(13):2144–50.

21. Escudier B, Pluzanska A, Koralewski P, et al. Bevacizumab plus interferon alfa-2a for treatment of metastatic renal cell carcinoma: a randomised, double-blind phase III trial. Lancet 2007;370(9605):2103–11.

22. Rini BI, Halabi S, Rosenberg JE, et al. Bevacizumab plus interferon alfa compared with interferon alfa monotherapy in patients with metastatic renal cell carcinoma: CALGB 90206. J Clin Oncol 2008;26(33):5422–8.

23. Rini BI, Halabi S, Rosenberg JE, et al. Phase III trial of bevacizumab plus interferon alfa versus interferon alfa monotherapy in patients with metastatic renal cell carcinoma: final results of CALGB 90206. J Clin Oncol 2010;28(13):2137–43.

24. Margulis V, Matin SF, Tannir N, et al. Surgical morbidity associated with administration of targeted molecular therapies before cytoreductive nephrectomy or resection of locally recurrent renal cell carcinoma. J Urol 2008;180(1):94–8.

25. Jonasch E, Wood CG, Matin SF, et al. Phase II presurgical feasibility study of bevacizumab in untreated patients with metastatic renal cell carcinoma. J Clin Oncol 2009;27(25):4076–81.

26. Lockhart AC, Rothenberg ML, Dupont J, et al. Phase I study of intravenous vascular endothelial growth factor trap, aflibercept, in patients with advanced solid tumors. J Clin Oncol 2010;28(2):207–14.

27. Faivre S, Delbaldo C, Vera K, et al. Safety, pharmacokinetic, and antitumor activity of SU11248, a novel oral multitarget tyrosine kinase inhibitor, in patients with cancer. J Clin Oncol 2006;24(1):25–35.

28. Motzer RJ, Michaelson MD, Redman BG, et al. Activity of SU11248, a multitargeted inhibitor of vascular endothelial growth factor receptor and platelet-derived growth factor receptor, in patients with metastatic renal cell carcinoma. J Clin Oncol 2006;24(1):16–24.

29. Motzer RJ, Rini BI, Bukowski RM, et al. Sunitinib in patients with metastatic renal cell carcinoma. JAMA 2006;295(21):2516–24.

30. Motzer RJ, Hutson TE, Tomczak P, et al. Sunitinib versus interferon alfa in metastatic renal-cell carcinoma. N Engl J Med 2007;356(2):115–24.

31. Awada A, Hendlisz A, Gil T, et al. Phase I safety and pharmacokinetics of BAY 43-9006 administered for 21 days on/7 days off in patients with advanced, refractory solid tumours. Br J Cancer 2005;92(10):1855–61.

32. Clark JW, Eder JP, Ryan D, et al. Safety and pharmacokinetics of the dual action Raf kinase and vascular endothelial growth factor receptor inhibitor, BAY 43-9006, in patients with advanced, refractory solid tumors. Clin Cancer Res 2005;11(15):5472–80.

33. Moore M, Hirte HW, Siu L, et al. Phase I study to determine the safety and pharmacokinetics of the novel Raf kinase and VEGFR inhibitor BAY 43-9006, administered for 28 days on/7 days off in patients with advanced, refractory solid tumors. Ann Oncol 2005;16(10):1688–94.

34. Strumberg D, Richly H, Hilger RA, et al. Phase I clinical and pharmacokinetic study of the Novel Raf kinase and vascular endothelial growth factor receptor inhibitor BAY 43-9006 in patients with advanced refractory solid tumors. J Clin Oncol 2005;23(5):965–72.

35. Ratain MJ, Eisen T, Stadler WM, et al. Phase II placebo-controlled randomized discontinuation trial of sorafenib in patients with metastatic renal cell carcinoma. J Clin Oncol 2006;24(16):2505–12.

36. Escudier B, Eisen T, Stadler WM, et al. Sorafenib in advanced clear-cell renal-cell carcinoma. N Engl J Med 2007;356(2):125–34.

37. Escudier B, Eisen T, Stadler WM, et al. Sorafenib for treatment of renal cell carcinoma: final efficacy and safety results of the phase III treatment approaches in renal cancer global evaluation trial. J Clin Oncol 2009;27(20):3312–8.

38. Escudier B, Szczylik C, Hutson TE, et al. Randomized phase II trial of first-line treatment with sorafenib versus interferon alfa-2a in patients with metastatic renal cell carcinoma. J Clin Oncol 2009;27(8):1280–9.

39. Hurwitz HI, Dowlati A, Saini S, et al. Phase I trial of pazopanib in patients with advanced cancer. Clin Cancer Res 2009;15(12):4220–7.

40. Hutson TE, Davis ID, Machiels JH, et al. Efficacy and safety of pazopanib in patients with metastatic renal cell carcinoma. J Clin Oncol 2010;28(3):475–80.
41. Hainsworth A. Phase II trial of pazopanib in patients with metastatic renal cell carcinoma previously treated with sunitinib or bevacizumab [abstract]. Available at: http://clinicaltrials.gov/show/NCT00731211.
42. Sternberg CN, Davis ID, Mardiak J, et al. Pazopanib in locally advanced or metastatic renal cell carcinoma: results of a randomized phase III trial. J Clin Oncol 2010;28(6):1061–8.
43. Pazopanib versus sunitinib in the treatment of locally advanced and/or metastatic renal cell carcinoma. Available at: http://clinicaltrials.gov/ct2/show/NCT00720941.
44. Patient preference study of pazopanib versus sunitinib in advanced or metastatic kidney cancer. Available at: http://clinicaltrials.gov/ct2/show/NCT01064310. Accessed April 23, 2011.
45. Rugo HS, Herbst RS, Liu G, et al. Phase I trial of the oral antiangiogenesis agent AG-013736 in patients with advanced solid tumors: pharmacokinetic and clinical results. J Clin Oncol 2005;23(24):5474–83.
46. Rixe O, Bukowski RM, Michaelson MD, et al. Axitinib treatment in patients with cytokine-refractory metastatic renal-cell cancer: a phase II study. Lancet Oncol 2007;8(11):975–84.
47. Rini BI, Wilding G, Hudes G, et al. Phase II study of axitinib in sorafenib-refractory metastatic renal cell carcinoma. J Clin Oncol 2009;27(27):4462–8.
48. Rini B, Escudier B, Tomczak P, et al. Axitinib vs sorafenib as second-line therapy for metastatic renal cell carcinoma (mRCC): results of phase 3 AXIS trial. ASCO 2011 [abstract: 4503].
49. Axitinib (AG-013736) for the treatment of metastatic renal cell cancer. Available at: http://clinicaltrials.gov/ct2/show/NCT00920816. Accessed April 23, 2011.
50. Axitinib (AG-013736) with or without dose titration (increase) in patients with kidney cancer. Available at: http://clinicaltrials.gov/ct2/show/NCT00835978. Accessed April 23, 2011.
51. Eskens FA. Proceedings of the 99th annual meeting of the AACR. Philadelphia: American Association of Cancer Research; 2008 [abstract: LB-201].
52. Bhargava P, Esteves B, Nosov DA, et al. Updated activity and safety results of a phase II randomized discontinuation trial (RDT) of AV-951, a potent and selective VEGFR1, 2, and 3 kinase inhibitor, in patients with renal cell carcinoma (RCC). J Clin Oncol 2008;26(Suppl 1) [abstract: 35403].
53. A study to compare tivozanib (AV-951) to sorafenib in subjects with advanced renal cell carcinoma. Available at: http://clinicaltrials.gov/ct2/show/NCT01030783. Accessed April 23, 2011.
54. Feldman DR, Baum MS, Ginsberg MS, et al. Phase I trial of bevacizumab plus escalated doses of sunitinib in patients with metastatic renal cell carcinoma. J Clin Oncol 2009;27(9):1432–9.
55. Sosman JA, Flaherty KT, Atkins MB, et al. Updated results of phase I trial of sorafenib (S) and bevacizumab (B) in patients with metastatic renal cell cancer (mRCC). J Clin Oncol 2008;26(Suppl 1) [abstract: 5011].
56. Merchan JR, Pitot HC, Qin R, et al. Phase I/II trial of CCI 779 and bevacizumab in advanced renal cell carcinoma (RCC): safety and activity in RTKI refractory RCC patients. J Clin Oncol 2009;27(Suppl 1) [abstract: 5039].
57. Hainsworth JD, Spigel DR, Burris HA, et al. Phase II trial of bevacizumab and everolimus in patients with advanced renal cell carcinoma. J Clin Oncol 2010; 28(13):2131–6.

58. Chow LQ, Eckhardt SG. Sunitinib: from rational design to clinical efficacy. J Clin Oncol 2007;25(7):884–96.
59. Data on file. AVEO Pharmaceuticals, Inc.
60. Garcia JA, Hudes GR, Choueiri TK, et al. Phase II study of IMC-1121B in patients with metastatic renal cancer (mRCC) following VEGFR-2 tyrosine kinase inhibitor (TKI) therapy (IMCL CP12–0605/NCT00515697). Presented at: 2010 Genitourinary Cancers Symposium. San Francisco (CA), March 5–7, 2010. [abstract: 326].

mTOR Inhibitors in Advanced Renal Cell Carcinoma

Martin H. Voss, MD, Ana M. Molina, MD, Robert J. Motzer, MD*

KEYWORDS

- Kidney neoplasms • mTOR • Targeted therapy
- Renal cell carcinoma • Treatment resistance

Better understanding of the genetics and molecular biology of renal cell carcinoma (RCC) has led to the development of several targeted agents, six of which have previously received US Food and Drug Administration (FDA) approval for treatment of advanced disease based on large international phase III trials.[1–6]

Four of these compounds (sunitinib, sorafenib, pazopanib, and bevacizumab) inhibit tumor angiogenesis through blockade of vascular endothelial growth factor (VEGF). A second class of agents includes the intravenously administered temsirolimus and the oral compound everolimus, which both exhibit antitumor effects through inhibition of the mammalian target of rapamycin (mTOR). The mechanisms of action, clinical data leading to approval, clinical use of mTOR inhibitors, as well as current understanding of the molecular mechanisms behind resistance to this class of drugs are reviewed here.

BIOLOGY AND MECHANISM OF ACTION

The phosphatidyl-inositol-3 kinase (PI3K)/Akt/mTOR pathway is a molecular signaling axis with key impact on various integral cellular functions, including protein synthesis, glucose metabolism, cellular migration, and cell survival. It has been implicated in promoting tumor growth.[7,8] The pathway is affected by growth factors (epidermal growth factor (EGF), insulin-like growth factor 1 (IGF-1), fibroblast growth factor [FGF]), hormones (estrogen, thyroid hormones), vitamins, integrins, intracellular calcium, and the Ras-dependent mitogen-activated protein kinase (MAPK) pathway. Binding of insulin or insulin-like growth factors to their respective receptors leads to

Financial disclosure: The authors (RJM, AM) disclose research funding from Novartis and Pfizer, In. and have no other financial disclosure to report.
Genitourinary Oncology Service, Department of Medicine, Memorial Sloan-Kettering Cancer Center, 353 East 68th Street, New York, NY 10065, USA
* Corresponding author.
E-mail address: motzerr@mskcc.org

recruitment of PI3K. Once activated, PI3K converts phosphatidylinositol-4,5-phosphate (PIP2) to phosphatidylinositol-3,4,5-phosphate (PIP3), which in turn activates Akt/PKB, a serine/threonine kinase. PI3K signaling is inhibited by action of the tumor suppressor phosphatase and tensin homolog (PTEN), which negatively affects formation of PIP3, thus limiting Akt activity.[9] Activated Akt promotes several biological processes through phosphorylation of various downstream targets and indirectly activates mTOR, a high-molecular-weight serine threonine kinase. Specifically, activated Akt phosphorylates tuberous sclerosis complex (TSC)2, leading to disassociation of the TSC1/TSC2 heterodimer complex, and inhibiting the ability of TSC2 to act as a GTPase-activating protein. This allows Rheb (Ras homologue enriched in the brain), an activator of mTOR, to remain GTP-bound and thus active.[10] In addition to and independent of upstream signaling through PI3K, mTOR integrates other stimuli including nutrients (also through TSC1/2 and Rheb), cellular energy levels, and cellular stress.[11] In normal cells, this helps to coordinate cell-cycle progression from G1 to S phase; in tumorigenesis, however, deregulation of components in this intricate system promotes growth and proliferation of malignant clones.

Once activated, mTOR exerts its action via protein synthesis and affects various cellular functions including cell growth, proliferation, angiogenesis, and metabolism.[11] The latter includes effects on glucose and lipid control,[12,13] which has implications for therapeutically targeting mTOR. mTOR has been found to act through two structurally and functionally distinct multiprotein signaling complexes, mTOR complex 1 (mTORC1, comprising mTOR and a scaffolding protein termed regulatory-associated protein of mTOR [raptor]) and mTOR complex 2 (mTORC2, comprising mTOR and a scaffolding protein termed rapamycin insensitive companion of mTOR [rictor]).[8,11]

Activation of mTORC1 takes place indirectly through inhibition of its repressor TSC2 as outlined above. The main downstream targets of mTORC1 are the ribosomal S6 kinase (p70S6K) and the eukaryotic translation initiation factor 4E-binding protein 1 (4E-BP1). Phosphorylation of 4E-BP1 through mTORC1 results in the release of 4E-BP1 from the eukaryotic translation initiation factor (eIF4E), which is then freed to interact with eIF4 G and other proteins to assemble the mammalian ribosome initiation complex eIF4F.[14] In cancer cells, 4E-BP1 phosphorylation eventually results in the initiation of translation. The activation of mTORC1 downstream targets, through its effect on protein synthesis, modulates activity of cell-cycle–regulating proteins, hypoxia-inducible factor 1 alpha (HIF1α), FGF, VEGF, signal transducer and activator of transcription 3 (STAT3), cyclin-D, and c-Myc.[15–17]

In the pathogenesis of RCC, regulation of HIF, a known oncologic driver of the disease, appears specifically relevant and possibly central to the antitumor effects of mTOR inhibitors.[18]

The details of mTORC2 functions are less well understood. Once active, mTORC2 phosphorylates the hydrophobic motif of the AGC kinase family, including Akt (S^{473}), thereby inducing Akt activation.[19] Other possible downstream targets with effect on cell survival, proliferation, and cytoskeleton include the Forkhead box, class O (FOXO) class of transcription factors,[20] protein kinase C alpha (PKCα), and the serum- and glucocorticoid–regulated kinase 1 (SGK1).[21] Translation of HIF2α depends upon the activity of mTORC2 but not mTORC1, whereas HIF1α expression depends upon both mTORC1 and mTORC2.[22] These findings are significant, as most conventional RCC possesses biallelic alterations in the VHL gene, resulting in the accumulation of both HIF1α and 2α. Despite overlapping effects on gene expression, HIF2α is more relevant to the development and progression of RCC because it preferentially activates VEGF, transforming growth factor-alpha (TGFα), the stem cell factor Oct4, and Cyclin D1.[23] In preclinical models, HIF2α suppression prevented tumor formation in von hippel lindau (VHL) defective renal carcinoma cells.[24] Importantly, mTORC2 activity is unaffected by rapamycin and its analogues, the mTOR inhibitors currently used in common practice. Consequently, HIF1α levels decrease, but HIF2α remains unaffected by rapamycin in preclinical RCC models.[25]

PI3K/AKT/mTOR IN RCC

One study examined 128 primary RCCs, 22 metastatic RCCs, and 24 nonneoplastic (normal) kidneys, and found the expression levels of p70S6K, phospho-mTOR (p-mTOR), and pAkt significantly higher in RCC than in normal kidneys, both by immunohistochemistry and protein levels.[26] Similarly, another group found increased levels of phospho-S6 and/or p-mTOR in the majority of 29 clear cell RCC tumors by immunohistochemistry.[27] A more recent report looking at 132 metastatic RCC samples, a subset with matched primary tumors, and an additional 10 sections from healthy kidney tissues found strong expression of various mTOR pathway proteins.[28] The investigators reported significantly higher immunoreactivity scores for PI3K, p-mTOR, p-AKT, and p70S6 in metastatic lesions compared to nonneoplastic proximal tubular epithelial cells. Notably, there were almost no cases of *PTEN* gene deletion in this series. There was no significant correlation between primary tumors and metastatic samples in matched pairs, suggesting that hyperactivation of the pathway may contribute to the metastatic progress. Patients with shorter disease-free intervals showed significantly higher expression of PI3K (P = .035).[28] Similarly, a separate report in primary RCC correlated mTOR pathway activation with survival and poor pathologic prognostic features.[29]

RAPAMYCIN AND ITS ANALOGUES

Rapamycin (also termed sirolimus) was originally identified as a natural antifungal antibiotic isolated from the bacteria *Streptomyces hygroscopicus* in the 1970s[30,31] and eventually led to the discovery of mTOR, the "mammalian target of rapamycin." Due to its ability to potently inhibit T-cell function, rapamycin was initially mainly used as an immunosuppressant in recipients of solid organ transplantation,[32] but subsequently was found to be an attractive candidate for application in oncology due to its antitumor activity, including preclinical models for RCC.[33–35] Several analogues of rapamycin have been developed to improve solubility and bioavailability. These include temsirolimus and everolimus, and are termed "rapalogs." They share the same mechanism of action and have been successfully applied in the treatment of various solid and hematologic malignancies.[36,37] Rapamycin and its analogues do not directly inhibit the mTOR kinase. Instead, they bind with high affinity to the FK-binding protein 12 (FKBP-12), an abundant intracellular immunophilin. The resulting complex potently inhibits the kinase activity of mTORC1, but has no suppressive effects on mTORC2.[17,38]

TEMSIROLIMUS

Temsirolimus[1] (Torisel; Pfizer, New York, NY, USA) is a water-soluble prodrug of rapamycin with an added ester at the C43 position. It is rapidly metabolized to sirolimus through de-esterification; both are potent binders of FKBP-12, and each forms an inhibitory complex with subsequent suppression of mTORC1 activity.

Phase I and II Studies

Preclinical studies demonstrating temsirolimus activity in a variety of human cancers[39–42] were fortified by promising results in phase 1 studies.[43–45] Intermittent schedules abrogated immunosuppressive effects without significant loss in antitumor activity. Responses included patients with advanced RCC. This led to a dedicated phase II trial in advanced refractory RCC.[46] With a primary endpoint of objective tumor response rate, 111 patients were randomized to 25, 75, or 250 mg of temsirolimus weekly by intravenous infusion. Patients were heavily pretreated (51% had received ≥ 2 prior immunotherapies) with extensive disease (83% had ≥ 2 sites of metastases). The objective response (OR) rate was 7% (1 complete response, 7 partial responses [PR]); 51% had stable disease (SD) for ≥ 24 weeks or an OR. Median time to progression (TTP) was 5.8 months for the entire group; 6.3, 6.7, and 5.2 for patients in the 25-, 75-, and 250-mg groups, respectively. Median overall survival (OS) was 15 months; 13.8, 11.0, and 17.5 for patients in the 25-,75-, and 250-mg groups, respectively. Maculopapular rash (76%) and mucositis (70%) were the most frequent treatment-related toxicities; the most common grade 3 or 4 adverse events (AEs) included hyperglycemia (17%), hypophosphatemia (13%), anemia (9%) and hypertriglyceridemia (6%). Importantly, overall response rates (ORR) and OS were comparable for all dose levels. Dose reductions and treatment discontinuations were more frequent at higher doses. A subgroup analysis by Memorial Sloan-Kettering Cancer Center (MSKCC) risk group, developed for patients treated with interferon (IFN)-α,[47] demonstrated greater than twofold survival differences between good or intermediate versus poor-risk patients at each dose level. Compared with historical data for IFN-α, treatment benefit was most striking for the poor-risk population.

Phase III Data

The Global Advanced Renal Cell Carcinoma (ARCC) phase III trial, conducted between 2003 and 2005, compared temsirolimus to IFN-α, or the combination, in advanced RCC.[4] Entry criteria allowed all histologic subtypes, but required participants to have at least three of six predictors of short survival (**Table 1**). Patients were randomized to one of three arms: temsirolimus 25 mg intravenously (IV) once weekly, IFN-α 3 million units subcutaneously three times per week (escalated to 18 million units three times per week, if tolerated), or a combination of temsirolimus 15 mg IV weekly and IFN 3 million units(escalated to 6 million units three times per week). Efficacy at the second planned interim analysis of the intent-to-treat population revealed superior survival for temsirolimus over IFN-α but no improved survival for the combination over IFN-α alone. Median OS was 7.3, 10.9, and 8.4 months for IFN-α, temsirolimus, and the combination group, respectively. Progression-free survival (PFS) was significantly longer in patients receiving temsirolimus, with median PFS times of 1.9, 3.8, and 3.7 months for the IFN-α, temsirolimus, and the combination group, respectively ($P<.001$). The proportion of patients with SD greater than or equal to 6 months or an OR was significantly greater for patients receiving temsirolimus alone (32.1%) or in combination (28.1%) than in the IFN-α group (15.5%; $P<.001$ and $P = .002$, respectively). In prespecified exploratory subgroup analyses, the superior survival benefit of temsirolimus was greatest for patients less than 65 years of age and for those with elevated lactate dehydrogenase.[4] The most common all-grade toxicities (**Table 2**) for the temsirolimus group were managed with supportive measures. Fewer grade 3 or 4 AEs were seen with temsirolimus alone than with IFN-α or the combination (67% vs 78% vs 87%, respectively; $P = .02$). Most dose reductions or delays were reported for the combination group. Based on this study, in May 2007, temsirolimus received FDA approval for the treatment of advanced RCC.

Table 1
Trial design and treatment efficacy of mTOR inhibitors in phase III trials in advanced RCC

	ARCC Trial[4]	RECORD 1 Trial[6,61]	
Number of Patients	626	416	—
Histologies	All	Clear cell RCC component	—
Prior Therapy	None	Sunitinib, sorafenib or both	—
Clinical Risk	All with ≥3/6 poor-risk features: LDH ≥ 1.5 × ULN decreased Hgb corrected Ca of ≥10 mg/dL time diagnosis to treatment initiation of <1 year KPS 60%–70% ≥2 metastatic sites	Favorable risk[a] 29% Intermediate risk[a] 57% Poor risk[a] 15% (well balanced between groups)	
Randomization Arms, Number of Patients	IFN: 207 Tem: 209 IFN/Tem: 210	Everolimus: 277 Placebo: 139	
Primary endpoint	OS	PFS	

Results			
Responses	**1st-Line Tem**	**1st-Line IFN**	**2nd-Line Everolimus**	**2nd-Line Placebo**
---	---	---	---	---
mPFS (mo)	3.8 (CI 3.6–5.2)[b]	1.9 (CI 1.9–2.2)[b]	4.9 (CI 4.0–5.5)[c]	1.9 (CI 1.8–1.9)[c]
mOS (mo)	10.9 (CI 8.6–12.7)[d]	7.3 (CI 6.1–8.8)[d]	14.8[e]	14.4[f]
Response	ORR: 9% (CI 4.8–12.4) Benefit[g]: 32% (CI 25.7–38.4)	ORR: 5% (CI 1.9–7.8) Benefit[g]: 16% (CI 10.5–20.4)	Best response: PR: 2% SD: 67% (CI not reported)	Best response: PR: 0% SD: 32% (CI not reported)

Abbreviations: ARRC, Global Advanced Renal Cell Carcinoma; Ca, serum calcium; Hgb, hemoglobin; HR, hazard ratio; KPS, Karnofsky performance status; LDH, lactate dehydrogenase; mOS, median overall survival; mPFS, median progression-free survival; RECORD, REnal Cell Cancer Treatment with Oral Rad001 given Daily; Tem, temsirolimus; ULN, upper limit of normal.
[a] Risk stratification per MSKCC clinical risk score.[47]
[b] HR not reported.
[c] HR: 0.33; CI 0.25–0.43; $P<.001$.
[d] HR: 0.73; CI 0.58–0.92; $P = .008$.
[e] HR: 0.87; CI 0.65–1.15; $P = .16$.
[f] Rank preserving structural failure time approach estimated true mOS for placebo group to be 10.0 months.
[g] Clinical benefit defined as ORR or SD × ≥24 weeks.

This study included patients with both conventional and non-clear cell histologies. Patients with histologies other than clear cell RCC accounted for 17% and 18% in the temsirolimus and interferon group, respectively. An unplanned secondary analysis for this patient subset was undertaken and suggested superior median OS and PFS for temsirolimus versus IFN-α with a hazard ratio (HR) of 0.49 (95% CI, 0.29–0.85) and 0.38 (95% CI, 0.23–0.62), respectively.[48] Whereas median OS was shorter in non-clear cell histologies compared with conventional RCC, the benefit of temsirolimus appeared more pronounced with non-clear cell or indeterminate primary cell types.[48] This may be because IFN has fewer efficacies in this group.[49]

Table 2
Adverse events in phase III trials of mTOR inhibitors in advanced RCC

Adverse Events	1st-Line Temsirolimus in Poor-risk Patients[4]		2nd-Line Everolimus after Prior VEGF TKI[61]	
	All Grades (%)	Grade 3 or 4 (%)	All Grades (%)	Grade 3 or 4 (%)
Asthenia	51	11	33	3–4
Fatigue	NR		31	5
Rash	47	4	29	1
Nausea	37	2	26	1
Anorexia	32	3	25	1
Pain	28	5	NR	
Dyspnea	28	9	24	7
Infection	27	5	37	7
Diarrhea	27	1	30	1
Constipation	20	0	NR	
Peripheral edema	27	2	24	<1
Cough	26	1	30	<1
Dyspnea	NR		24	7
Pneumonitis[a]	NR		14[a]	4[a]
Fever	24	1	20	<1
Abdominal Pain	21	4	NR	
Stomatitis	20	1	44	4–5
Vomiting	19	2	20	2
Headache	15	1	19	0–2
Epistaxis	NR		18	0
Pruritus	NR		14	<1
Dysgeusia	NR		10	0
Laboratory Abnormalities				
Anemia	45	20	92	13
Thrombocytopenia	14	1	23	1
Lymphopenia	NR		51	16
Neutropenia	7	3	14	<1
Increased Creatinine	14	3	50	1
Hyperlipidemia	27	3	73	<1
Hypercholesterolemia	24	1	77	4
Hyperglycemia	26	11	57	15–16
Increased AST	8	1	25	0–2
Hypophosphatemia	NR		37	6

Abbreviations: AST, aspartate amino-transaminase; NR, not reported.
[a] Includes interstitial lung disease, lung infiltration, pneumonitis, pulmonary alveolar hemorrhage, alveolitis, and pulmonary toxicity.

Temsirolimus in Second-line Setting

A randomized phase III trial has completed accrual (clinicaltrials.gov; NCT00474786), comparing temsirolimus with sorafenib in advanced RCC of any histology after progression on sunitinib, but no prospective second-line data have been reported thus far. The largest retrospective series reported outcome for 87 patients treated at North American centers through the Torisel Compassionate Use Program.[50] The majority of patients had been pretreated with sunitinib (85%) or sorafenib (51%), 63% had pure clear cell histology. The study population overall had unfavorable clinical features, mostly with either intermediate (53%) or poor (36%) MSKCC risk status[51]; 13% of patients had an Eastern Cooperative Oncology Group (ECOG) performance status of three. The reported ORR was 5% (all PR); best response of SD was 65%. The median TTP was 3.9; median OS was 11.2 months. Benefit was seen for both clear cell and non-clear cell histologies.

EVEROLIMUS
Phase I and II Studies

Everolimus[1] (Afinitor; Novartis, Basel, Switzerland) is a derivate of rapamycin and, unlike temsirolimus, is not converted to sirolimus in vivo. It has been studied as an immunosuppressant for solid organ transplantation.[52–54] Based on preclinical data with weekly treatment schedules,[55] a phase I trial determined safety for weekly dosing up to 70 mg and daily dosing up to 10 mg.[56] Clinical efficacy was seen for several RCC patients, including one confirmed PR, one unconfirmed PR, and 5 of 10 RCC patients progression-free at 6 months.[56] Whereas pharmacodynamic profiling in this trial confirmed target inhibition for both dosing schedules, additional studies incorporating a direct-link pharmacokinetic-pharmacodynamic model using tumor-bearing rats demonstrated more sustained S6K1 inhibition with daily rather than weekly everolimus.[57] Subsequently, a single-arm phase II trial enrolled 41 RCC patients with one or no prior regimen to be treated on everolimus 10 mg daily.[58] The trial reported a median PFS and OS of 11.2 and 22.1 months, respectively; ORR was 14%, and 70% of patients had either response or SD for greater than or equal to 6 months.[58] Treatment was well tolerated with low-grade toxicities primarily managed with supportive care. The most common AEs included anorexia, nausea, diarrhea, stomatitis, and rash. Grade 3 pneumonitis (19%) was managed with dose delays and reductions. Four of the patients were successfully re-escalated to 10 mg.

Phase III Data

A multicenter, international, placebo-controlled phase III trial was conducted to investigate everolimus in patients who progressed on sunitinib, sorafenib, or both tyrosine kinase inhibitors (TKIs) ("refractory").[6] The RECORD-1 trial (REnal Cell Cancer Treatment with Oral Rad001 given Daily) assigned 410 patients with advanced RCC to either everolimus 10 mg daily or placebo by 2:1 randomization, both in conjunction with best supportive care (see **Table 1**). All subjects had clear cell RCC that had progressed on or within 6 months of therapy with VEGF receptor (VEGFR) TKIs (sunitinib, sorafenib, or both). The primary endpoint was PFS, and the trial was terminated after second interim analysis suggested that the study goal was met. The median duration of treatment was 95 days in the everolimus group versus 57 days in the placebo group, and PFS was significantly longer for patients receiving study drug with HR of 0.3 (95% CI, 0.22–0.40; $P<.0001$). Median PFS was 4.0 and 1.9 months for everolimus and placebo, respectively. PFS benefit was maintained through various predefined subgroups, including MSKCC-risk status, prior type of therapy (sunitinib vs sorafenib vs both), and demographic differences. Partial responses were seen in 1% of patients receiving everolimus, none with placebo. There was no significant difference in OS, likely because 81% of all patients who progressed on placebo went on to receive everolimus.[6] The trial assessed health-related quality-of-life,[59,60] and failed to demonstrate significant time differences to outcome deterioration between the treatment and placebo groups. More toxicity was seen with everolimus, including higher rates of grade 3 or 4 AEs. Treatment discontinuation due to AEs was reported in 10% of patients receiving everolimus and 4% of patients in the placebo group.

Recently, updated efficacy and safety results of RECORD-1 were reported for 416 patients with mature OS data 13 months after interim analysis cutoff.[61] Median PFS for everolimus and placebo were 4.9 months and 1.9 months, respectively (HR, 0.33; 95% CI, 0.25–0.43; P<.001), with a 25% probability of remaining progression free after 10 months with everolimus. Again, benefit was seen in all MSKCC-risk groups regardless of prior therapy. PR rates were 1.8% and 0%, respectively. A post hoc exploratory OS analysis used rank-preserving structural failure time analysis estimates to correct for bias introduced by crossover from placebo to everolimus after progression and thus provided an estimate of treatment effect per the original randomization. By this assessment, survival time with everolimus was estimated as 1.9-fold longer than for placebo if no crossover occurred. The corrected OS for the placebo group was 10.0 months versus 14.8 months in the everolimus group.[61] Safety analysis was consistent with the original findings of the second interim analysis (see **Table 2**). Seven percent of the everolimus patients required dose modifications. Noninfectious pneumonitis was diagnosed in 14% (grade 3 in 4%) with a median time to onset of pneumonitis of 108 days (range 24–257 days). Clinical and demographic factors were investigated as prognostics for both PFS and OS. Poor prognostic factors included prior treatment with sunitinib, MSKCC intermediate-risk or poor-risk status, elevated neutrophil or alkaline phosphatase levels, and metastases to liver or bone.[61]

Everolimus for Other Indications

The utility of using single-agent everolimus in the first-line setting is being investigated in the RECORD-3 trial, an international multicenter phase II trial randomizing treatment-naïve patients with advanced RCC to receive either the current standard of care, that is, first-line treatment with sunitinib followed by second-line therapy with everolimus when disease progression is seen, versus the opposite (ie, everolimus followed by sunitinib), with a primary endpoint of PFS after first-line therapy.[62] The drug is also being studied in the neoadjuvant setting (clinicaltrials.gov: NCT01107509). Finally, an adjuvant intergroup trial for locally advanced disease is in preparation.

COMBINATION THERAPY WITH OTHER TARGETED AGENTS

Concurrent treatment of RCC with mTOR inhibitors and other targeted agents has been studied in hopes of enhancing antitumor effects by parallel inhibition of multiple oncogenic signaling pathways. Unfortunately, this has been limited by treatment-associated toxicity. Several trials have evaluated the safety of combining an mTOR inhibitor with a VEGF TKI, which has typically required attenuated dosing schedules. In a phase I trial of sunitinib plus temsirolimus,[63] dose-limiting toxicities (DLTs) were seen in two out of three patients at the starting dose of temsirolimus 15 mg weekly and sunitinib 25 mg daily (one grade 3 acneiform rash, one grade 3 cellulitis). Other AEs included hemorrhage, thrombocytopenia, gastrointestinal toxicity, and severe infection. Because of efficacy concerns at lower doses, the study was terminated early.[63] The combination of sunitinib and everolimus proved toxic in a separate phase I trial,[64] and investigators switched to a weekly schedule of everolimus, as two out of two patients suffered DLT even at attenuated doses of sunitinib 37.5 mg and everolimus 5 mg. Even so, chronic treatment was only tolerable at the lowest weekly dosing schedule of everolimus 20 mg weekly, with sunitinib 37.5 mg daily (4 weeks on,

2 weeks off). DLTs included mucositis, vomiting, and leukopenia. Five patients (25%) achieved PR, three of these had non-clear cell RCC.[64]

In a phase I trial of sorafenib plus temsirolimus in advanced solid tumors, investigators reported nine DLTs in 23 patients treated up to a level of temsirolimus 25 mg weekly and sorafenib 400 mg twice daily. Toxicities were predominantly mucocutaneous, but also included thrombocytopenia and loss in renal function.[65] Sorafenib was better tolerated when combined with everolimus, as per preliminary reports of another dose-finding study.[66] Still, two out of four patients in the second cohort suffered DLTs (grade 4 uricemia and grade 3 elevation in lipase with concurrent pancreatitis, respectively) with everolimus 5 mg daily plus sorafenib 400 mg twice daily. Three of 10 evaluable patients achieved PR, two had SD, and five showed evidence of progression.

The combination of temsirolimus and tivozanib, a novel VEGFR TKI, appears to be better tolerated per recent reports of an ongoing phase I study in pretreated RCC patients.[67] Better tolerance was also seen for combinations with bevacizumab. A phase I/II trial of temsirolimus and bevacizumab[68] established safety at standard doses (temsirolimus 25 mg IV weekly, bevacizumab 10 mg/kg IV every 2 weeks) with one DLT in six patients (grade 3 mucositis). The tolerability at full doses[68] prompted ongoing randomized studies. In the phase III INTORACT (Investigation of Torisel and Avastin Combination Therapy) trial, targeting accrual of approximately 800 subjects, treatment-naïve patients are randomized to receive bevacizumab plus temsirolimus versus bevacizumab plus IFN-α (clinicaltrials.gov; NCT00631371). Similarly, the TORAVA (TORisel and AVAstin) phase II trial is comparing bevacizumab plus temsirolimus versus single-agent sunitinib versus bevacizumab plus IFN-α in the first-line setting. Preliminary findings have been presented[69] and revealed higher drop-out rates but no improvement in efficacy for the combination over the two control arms. The ECOG BeST (Bevacizumab Sorafenib Temsirolimus) is an ongoing 4-arm phase II trial of bevacizumab-temsirolimus versus bevacizumab-sorafenib versus sorafenib-temsirolimus versus sorafenib alone (clinicaltrials.gov; NCT00378703).

The combination of everolimus and bevacizumab is tolerated at full doses as demonstrated in a phase I trial with no reported DLT and mostly grade 1 or 2 toxicities.[70] A subsequent phase II study in pretreated advanced RCC[71] yielded an ORR of 30% and 23% with median PFS of 9.1 months and 7.1 month in the untreated and pretreated groups, respectively. The study aim of raising the PFS rate from 50% (phase II data for single-agent bevacizumab in pretreated patients) to 70% was met at 5 months. Median PFS and OS were reported at 9.1 and 21.3 months for untreated patients, 7.1 and 14.5 months for the pretreated group, respectively.[72] The most common grade 3 or 4 toxicities included proteinuria (26%), mucositis (15%), fatigue (12%), and diarrhea (9%). The final PFS findings for this trial are not superior to that reported in the first-line setting for phase III studies of bevacizumab plus IFN-α.[5,73] The latter is currently being addressed in the phase II RECORD-2 trial comparing bevacizumab plus everolimus to bevacizumab plus IFN-α in untreated clear cell RCC.[74] Similarly, the Cancer and Leukemia Group B (CALGB) is conducting a phase III trial randomizing patients to receive everolimus plus bevacizumab versus placebo after progression on VEGF TKI (clinicaltrials.gov; NCT01198158).

INCIDENCE AND MANAGEMENT OF AEs SPECIFIC TO mTORC1 INHIBITORS

Several class-specific effects, primarily metabolic and pulmonary toxicities, have occurred with rapamycin and its analogues, and require close attention while treating patients with these agents.[75]

The attenuating effects of the PI3K/Akt/mTOR cascade on insulin signaling has been established,[76,77] and mTOR has been implicated in insulin resistance.[78] As expected, clinical trials of temsirolimus and everolimus have noted AEs on glucose metabolism. The ARCC trial reported hyperglycemia in 26% of patients.[4] Investigators attributed hyperglycemia to the study drug in 18% (all grades) and 9% (grades 3 or 4) of subjects.[79] RECORD-1[61] reported hyperglycemia in 57% of patients receiving everolimus, grade 3 or 4 glucose intolerance in 15%. There are no official recommendations guiding management of treatment-associated hyperglycemia. Instead, physicians should adhere to good clinical practice, which includes adequate glucose control before initiation of mTOR-directed treatment, education of patients on the symptoms of hyperglycemia, and intermittent monitoring of fasting glucose levels. Laboratory testing, interpretation of levels, and management should mirror that of type 2 diabetes mellitus.[75,80,81]

Effects of lipid metabolism can be explained through the roles of mTOR in cell metabolism.[11] In the phase III trial leading to its registration, temsirolimus caused hypercholesterolemia and hypertriglyceridemia in 21% and 25% of patients, respectively; primarily in grades 1 to 2.[79] The reported incidence was higher for everolimus; cholesterol and triglycerides were elevated in 77%, and 73% of patients treated with the drug on the pivotal trial, respectively (the majority grades 1–2). As for the management of hyperglycemia, no standardized guidance has been issued for rapalogs-induced hyperlipidemia. Most investigators have adapted target levels and management of abnormally high levels from general medical practice.[82] Prescribing physicians should ascertain adequate levels prior to starting treatments and monitor patients for development of hyperlipidemia.

Mild hypophosphatemia has been reported in 6% of patients using temsirolimus and 37% for patients using everolimus in phase III trials.[6,79] Severely low levels can impair neurologic and myocardial function and should be replenished.

Much attention has been given to nonspecific interstitial pneumonitis, which has been associated with the use of mTOR inhibitors. Although this is often asymptomatic or only presents with mild dyspnea and/or cough, it can be life-threatening in extent. In severe cases, systemic corticosteroids have been found to be beneficial. The original design of the ARCC trial paid limited attention to nonspecific interstitial pneumonitis[4]; however, a subsequent independent, blinded review of 178 patients in the temsirolimus group revealed drug-induced pneumonitis in 29% (vs 6% of 138 in the IFN-α group; $P<.0001$).[83] Most (60%) occurred within the first 8 weeks of treatment; only 31% were symptomatic. The incidence of noninfectious pneumonitis on RECORD-1 was 13.5% (3.6% grade 3, none grade 4) with a median time to occurrence of 108 days.[61] Forty-three percent of symptomatic patients received corticosteroids, 54% underwent dose-modification of study drug, and 27% discontinued treatment permanently. Clinical pneumonitis was fully reversible in 54% of cases. This trial contained a prospective, independent monitoring of patients for pneumonitis that was reported separately.[84] On blinded review of serial images obtained with the study, baseline radiographic abnormalities were present in 17% of all patients, in 24% of those who went on to develop clinical pneumonitis, and in 50% of those with subsequent grade 3 pneumonitis. New or worsening radiographic changes suggestive of pneumonitis were detected in 53.9% of patients on everolimus, which included 38.9% of patients without clinical suspicion for pneumonitis. All patients had undergone pulmonary function tests at baseline, which did not help predict likelihood of developing clinical pneumonitis. Chest radiographs were found to be less sensitive than CT scans in detecting abnormalities in asymptomatic patients or confirming clinical pneumonitis by radiographic changes. Based on their observations, the investigators issued specific management guidelines (**Table 3**).[84]

Table 3
Management of everolimus-associated noninfectious pneumonitis

Severity	Definition	Intervention	Imaging or Further Diagnostic Workup
Grade 1	Radiographic Changes with Few or No Symptoms	• Continue without dose adjustment, maintain close clinical follow-up[a]	• Obtain chest CT scan, PFT • Repeat CT scan or CXR every 2 cycles until back to baseline
Grade 2	Moderate Symptoms	• Reduce dose to 5 mg/d until ≤ grade 1 • Consider interruption if symptoms troublesome to patient • Discontinue treatment if no improvement in ≥3 weeks • Consider corticosteroid, if above is ineffective[b]	• Obtain chest CT scan, PFT • Repeat every cycle until return to baseline • In appropriate clinical setting, rule out causes, such as infection (bronchoscopy), PE, or cardiac cause

Grade 3	Severe Symptoms	• Interrupt everolimus until ≤ grade 1
		• Initiate corticosteroids[c]
		  ○ High-dose IV methylprednisolone for respiratory distress
		  ○ Lower dose in less severe cases
		• Upon resolution of toxicity, consider reinitiating everolimus at attenuated dose
			• Obtain CT chest, PFT
			• Repeat every cycle until return to baseline
			• Bronchoscopy
			• Consider workup for other causes (eg, PE, cardiac)

Grade 4	Life-threatening	• Discontinue everolimus permanently • Initiate corticosteroids[c] • Do not restart	• Obtain chest CT scan, PFT • Repeat every cycle until return to baseline • Bronchoscopy • Consider workup for other causes (eg, PE, cardiac)

Abbreviations: CXR, chest radiograph; PE, pulmonary embolism; PFT, pulmonary function test.
[a] Except if findings extensive or baseline pneumonitis worsening. In either case, consider interruption or dose modification.
[b] Prior to initiation of corticosteroids, exclude infectious process, cardiac cause, or pulmonary embolism, if appropriate.
[c] Infectious cause or pulmonary embolism should be excluded if either suggested by clinical presentation; however, this should not delay initiation of steroids.
Data from White DA, Camus P, Endo M, et al. Noninfectious pneumonitis after everolimus therapy for advanced renal cell carcinoma. Am J Respir Crit Care Med 2010;182(3):396–403.

Other potentially class-related toxicities were recognized but not reported with the registration trials. These include increased risk of angioedema with angiotensin-converting enzyme (ACE) inhibitors[85] and rapalogs-associated enteritis.[86]

MECHANISMS OF RESISTANCE

Although clinical studies have proven efficacy for rapalogs in advanced RCC, patients eventually acquire resistance to therapy. Preclinical models and experiments using patient tumor samples have suggested that mTORC1 inhibitors activate Akt and its downstream substrates through a feedback loop involving the insulin-like growth factor I receptor (IGF-IR).[87–90] Active mTOR signaling promotes receptor dissociation and protein degradation of IRS-1, an effect mitigated by inhibition of mTORC1. Such inhibition leads to enhanced IGF-1 signaling.[88] This is mediated through the mTORC1 downstream effector S6K and requires PI3K function, but was found to be independent of TSC-2.[87,90,91] These findings propose the following mechanism: inhibition of mTORC1, through decreased activity of S6K, stabilizes insulin receptor substrate 1 (IRS-1) association with its receptor, leading to activation of PI3K and subsequent phosphorylation of Akt (T^{308}).

A different mechanism of resistance to mTORC1 inhibition relates to the equilibrium between mTORC1 and mTORC2 signaling,[92,93] which shifts toward mTORC2 in treatment with rapalogs, subsequently leading to Akt (S^{473}) phosphorylation and activation.[94] Preclinical studies in non-Hodgkin lymphoma have confirmed such rapamycin-induced, mTORC2-mediated activation of Akt and demonstrated this effect to be independent of PI3K signaling.[95]

A third proposed mechanism of resistance involves a negative feedback loop with a separate signaling pathway. Data from a small number of patients receiving everolimus for breast cancer, melanoma, and colorectal cancer suggested that such treatment can activate the MAPK-signaling cascade, a separate well established oncogenic pathway.[96] MAPK feedback activation was found to be PI3K-dependent.[96]

Current drug development incorporates an understanding of these mechanisms, and ongoing efforts include strategies for combined inhibition of mTORC1 and PI3K, mTORC1 and 2, as well as PI3K-mTOR and MAPK.

FUTURE DIRECTIONS

Study of temsirolimus and everolimus continues. Both drugs are being tested in combination with other targeted agents and outside of their currently approved indication for advanced RCC. Considering the potential mechanisms of resistance to rapalogs, several novel agents targeting PI3K/Akt/mTOR are being developed for anticancer therapy in early phase clinical trials.[97,98] These include PI3K inhibitors (eg, CAL-101, BKM-120, XL-147), Akt inhibitors (eg, MK-2206, perifosine), mTORC1 inhibitors (eg, ridaforolimus), ATP-competitive inhibitors of the mTOR kinase domain that target both mTORC1 and mTORC2 (eg, PP242, Torin-1), as well as combined PI3K/mTORC1/mTORC2 inhibitors (eg, BEZ235, XL765, GDC-0980).

Several biomarkers have been tested for prognostic value, particularly their potential to predict response to RCC treatment with mTOR inhibitors. Hyperactivation of the PI3K/Akt/mTOR pathway assessed by immunohistochemistry on 375 RCC nephrectomy specimens adversely affected outcome, independent of stage.[29] Tumor tissue from greater than 50% of patients in the ARCC trial[4] was tested for baseline PTEN and HIF1α levels, but no correlation with treatment benefit for temsirolimus was seen.[99] A smaller study investigated PI3K/Akt/mTOR pathway in 20 RCC patients treated with temsirolimus, and suggested that pS6K levels and possibly pAkt can help predict response to temsirolimus.[100] Mutation analysis in preclinical models and a small series of patients with various solid tumors have shown that deregulation of phosphoinositide-3-kinase catalytic α peptide (PIK3CA) and KRAS can attenuate response to everolimus.[101] Importantly, this report did not include RCC patients, and mutations in PIK3CA or KRAS are uncommon in RCC.[102–105]

Identification of new, more effective agents is one of the major goals for the coming years. The other will be to apply our growing understanding of the molecular changes behind pathogenesis and treatment resistance successfully to optimize drug selection for individual patients.

REFERENCES

1. Escudier B, Eisen T, Stadler WM, et al. Sorafenib in advanced clear-cell renal-cell carcinoma. N Engl J Med 2007;356(2):125–34.
2. Motzer RJ, Hutson TE, Tomczak P, et al. Sunitinib versus interferon alfa in meta-static renal-cell carcinoma. N Engl J Med 2007;356(2):115–24.
3. Sternberg CN, Davis ID, Mardiak J, et al. Pazopanib in locally advanced or metastatic renal cell carcinoma: results of a randomized phase III trial. J Clin Oncol 2010;28(6):1061–8.
4. Hudes G, Carducci M, Tomczak P, et al. Temsirolimus, interferon alfa, or both for advanced renal-cell carcinoma. N Engl J Med 2007;356(22):2271–81.
5. Escudier B, Pluzanska A, Koralewski P, et al. Bevacizumab plus interferon alfa-2a for treatment of metastatic renal cell carcinoma: a randomised, double-blind phase III trial. Lancet 2007;370(9605):2103–11.
6. Motzer RJ, Escudier B, Oudard S, et al. Efficacy of everolimus in advanced renal cell carcinoma: a double-blind, randomised, placebo-controlled phase III trial. Lancet 2008;372(9637):449–56.
7. Katso R, Okkenhaug K, Ahmadi K, et al. Cellular function of phosphoinositide 3-kinases: implications for development, homeostasis, and cancer. Annu Rev Cell Dev Biol 2001;17:615–75.
8. Gibbons JJ, Abraham RT, Yu K. Mammalian target of rapamycin: discovery of rapamycin reveals a signaling pathway important for normal and cancer cell growth. Semin Oncol 2009;36(Suppl 3):S3–17.
9. Sansal I, Sellers WR. The biology and clinical relevance of the PTEN tumor suppressor pathway. J Clin Oncol 2004;22(14):2954–63.
10. Manning BD, Cantley LC. AKT/PKB signaling: navigating downstream. Cell 2007;129(7):1261–74.
11. Wullschleger S, Loewith R, Hall MN. TOR signaling in growth and metabolism. Cell 2006;124(3):471–84.
12. Peng T, Golub TR, Sabatini DM. The immunosuppressant rapamycin mimics a starvation-like signal distinct from amino acid and glucose deprivation. Mol Cell Biol 2002;22(15):5575–84.
13. Kim JE, Chen J. Regulation of peroxisome proliferator-activated receptor-gamma activity by mammalian target of rapamycin and amino acids in adipo-genesis. Diabetes 2004;53(11):2748–56.
14. Hay N, Sonenberg N. Upstream and downstream of mTOR. Genes Dev 2004; 18(16):1926–45.
15. Hudes GR. Targeting mTOR in renal cell carcinoma. Cancer 2009;115(Suppl 10): 2313–20.
16. Azim H, Azim HA Jr, Escudier B. Targeting mTOR in cancer: renal cell is just a beginning. Target Oncol 2010;5:269–80.
17. Guertin DA, Sabatini DM. Defining the role of mTOR in cancer. Cancer Cell 2007; 12(1):9–22.
18. Thomas GV, Tran C, Mellinghoff IK, et al. Hypoxia-inducible factor deter-mines sensitivity to inhibitors of mTOR in kidney cancer. Nat Med 2006; 12(1):122–7.
19. Sarbassov DD, Guertin DA, Ali SM, et al. Phosphorylation and regulation of Akt/PKB by the rictor-mTOR complex. Science 2005;307(5712):1098–101.

20. Birkenkamp KU, Coffer PJ. Regulation of cell survival and proliferation by the FOXO (Forkhead box, class O) subfamily of Forkhead transcription factors. Biochem Soc Trans 2003;31(Pt 1):292–7.
21. Sarbassov DD, Ali SM, Kim DH, et al. Rictor, a novel binding partner of mTOR, defines a rapamycin-insensitive and raptor-independent pathway that regulates the cytoskeleton. Curr Biol 2004;14(14):1296–302.
22. Toschi A, Lee E, Gadir N, et al. Differential dependence of hypoxia-inducible factors 1 alpha and 2 alpha on mTORC1 and mTORC2. J Biol Chem 2008; 283(50):34495–9.
23. Gordan JD, Simon MC. Hypoxia-inducible factors: central regulators of the tumor phenotype. Curr Opin Genet Dev 2007;17(1):71–7.
24. Kondo K, Kim WY, Lechpammer M, et al. Inhibition of HIF2alpha is sufficient to suppress pVHL-defective tumor growth. PLoS Biol 2003;1(3):E83.
25. Bhatt RS, Landis DM, Zimmer M, et al. Hypoxia-inducible factor-2alpha: effect on radiation sensitivity and differential regulation by an mTOR inhibitor. BJU Int 2008;102(3):358–63.
26. Lin F, Zhang PL, Yang XJ, et al. Morphoproteomic and molecular concomitants of an overexpressed and activated mTOR pathway in renal cell carcinomas. Ann Clin Lab Sci 2006;36(3):283–93.
27. Robb VA, Karbowniczek M, Klein-Szanto AJ, et al. Activation of the mTOR signaling pathway in renal clear cell carcinoma. J Urol 2007;177(1):346–52.
28. Abou Youssif T, Fahmy MA, Koumakpayi IH, et al. The mammalian target of rapamycin pathway is widely activated without PTEN deletion in renal cell carcinoma metastases. Cancer 2011;117(2):290–300.
29. Pantuck AJ, Seligson DB, Klatte T, et al. Prognostic relevance of the mTOR pathway in renal cell carcinoma: implications for molecular patient selection for targeted therapy. Cancer 2007;109(11):2257–67.
30. Sehgal SN, Baker H, Vezina C. Rapamycin (AY-22,989), a new antifungal antibiotic. II. Fermentation, isolation and characterization. J Antibiot (Tokyo) 1975; 28(10):727–32.
31. Vezina C, Kudelski A, Sehgal SN. Rapamycin (AY-22,989), a new antifungal antibiotic. I. Taxonomy of the producing streptomycete and isolation of the active principle. J Antibiot (Tokyo) 1975;28(10):721–6.
32. Sehgal SN, Molnar-Kimber K, Ocain TD, et al. Rapamycin: a novel immunosuppressive macrolide. Med Res Rev 1994;14(1):1–22.
33. Bjornsti MA, Houghton PJ. The TOR pathway: a target for cancer therapy. Nat Rev Cancer 2004;4(5):335–48.
34. Eng CP, Sehgal SN, Vezina C. Activity of rapamycin (AY-22,989) against transplanted tumors. J Antibiot (Tokyo) 1984;37(10):1231–7.
35. Luan FL, Ding R, Sharma VK, et al. Rapamycin is an effective inhibitor of human renal cancer metastasis. Kidney Int 2003;63(3):917–26.
36. Meric-Bernstam F, Gonzalez-Angulo AM. Targeting the mTOR signaling network for cancer therapy. J Clin Oncol 2009;27(13):2278–87.
37. Panwalkar A, Verstovsek S, Giles FJ. Mammalian target of rapamycin inhibition as therapy for hematologic malignancies. Cancer 2004;100(4):657–66.
38. Abraham RT, Gibbons JJ. The mammalian target of rapamycin signaling pathway: twists and turns in the road to cancer therapy. Clin Cancer Res 2007;13(11):3109–14.
39. Dudkin L, Dilling MB, Cheshire PJ, et al. Biochemical correlates of mTOR inhibition by the rapamycin ester CCI-779 and tumor growth inhibition. Clin Cancer Res 2001;7(6):1758–64.

40. Geoerger B, Kerr K, Tang CB, et al. Antitumor activity of the rapamycin analog CCI-779 in human primitive neuroectodermal tumor/medulloblastoma models as single agent and in combination chemotherapy. Cancer Res 2001;61(4): 1527–32.

41. Shi Y, Gera J, Hu L, et al. Enhanced sensitivity of multiple myeloma cells containing PTEN mutations to CCI-779. Cancer Res 2002;62(17):5027–34.

42. Yu K, Toral-Barza L, Discafani C, et al. mTOR, a novel target in breast cancer: the effect of CCI-779, an mTOR inhibitor, in preclinical models of breast cancer. Endocr Relat Cancer 2001;8(3):249–58.

43. Buckner JC, Forouzesh B, Erlichman C, et al. Phase I, pharmacokinetic study of temsirolimus administered orally to patients with advanced cancer. Invest New Drugs 2010;28(3):334–42.

44. Raymond E, Alexandre J, Faivre S, et al. Safety and pharmacokinetics of escalated doses of weekly intravenous infusion of CCI-779, a novel mTOR inhibitor, in patients with cancer. J Clin Oncol 2004;22(12):2336–47.

45. Hidalgo M, Buckner JC, Erlichman C, et al. A phase I and pharmacokinetic study of temsirolimus (CCI-779) administered intravenously daily for 5 days every 2 weeks to patients with advanced cancer. Clin Cancer Res 2006; 12(19):5755–63.

46. Atkins MB, Hidalgo M, Stadler WM, et al. Randomized phase II study of multiple dose levels of CCI-779, a novel mammalian target of rapamycin kinase inhibitor, in patients with advanced refractory renal cell carcinoma. J Clin Oncol 2004; 22(5):909–18.

47. Motzer RJ, Bacik J, Murphy BA, et al. Interferon-alfa as a comparative treatment for clinical trials of new therapies against advanced renal cell carcinoma. J Clin Oncol 2002;20:289–96.

48. Dutcher JP, de Souza P, McDermott D, et al. Effect of temsirolimus versus interferon-alpha on outcome of patients with advanced renal cell carcinoma of different tumor histologies. Med Oncol 2009;26(2):202–9.

49. Motzer RJ, Bacik J, Mariani T, et al. Treatment outcome and survival associated with metastatic renal cell carcinoma of non-clear-cell histology. J Clin Oncol 2002;20(9):2376–81.

50. Mackenzie MJ, Rini BI, Elson P, et al. Temsirolimus in VEGF-refractory metastatic renal cell carcinoma. Ann Oncol 2011;22(1):145–8.

51. Motzer RJ, Bacik J, Schwartz LH, et al. Prognostic factors for survival in previously treated patients with metastatic renal cell carcinoma. J Clin Oncol 2004; 22(3):454–63.

52. Eisen HJ, Tuzcu EM, Dorent R, et al. Everolimus for the prevention of allograft rejection and vasculopathy in cardiac-transplant recipients. N Engl J Med 2003;349(9):847–58.

53. Neuhaus P, Klupp J, Langrehr JM. mTOR inhibitors: an overview. Liver Transpl 2001;7(6):473–84.

54. Pascual J. Everolimus in clinical practice—renal transplantation. Nephrol Dial Transplant 2006;21(Suppl 3):iii18–23.

55. Boulay A, Zumstein-Mecker S, Stephan C, et al. Antitumor efficacy of intermittent treatment schedules with the rapamycin derivative RAD001 correlates with prolonged inactivation of ribosomal protein S6 kinase 1 in peripheral blood mononuclear cells. Cancer Res 2004;64(1):252–61.

56. O'Donnell A, Faivre S, Burris HA 3rd, et al. Phase I pharmacokinetic and pharmacodynamic study of the oral mammalian target of rapamycin inhibitor everolimus in patients with advanced solid tumors. J Clin Oncol 2008;26(10):1588–95.

57. Tanaka C, O'Reilly T, Kovarik JM, et al. Identifying optimal biologic doses of everolimus (RAD001) in patients with cancer based on the modeling of preclinical and clinical pharmacokinetic and pharmacodynamic data. J Clin Oncol 2008;26(10):1596–602.

58. Amato RJ, Jac J, Giessinger S, et al. A phase 2 study with a daily regimen of the oral mTOR inhibitor RAD001 (everolimus) in patients with metastatic clear cell renal cell cancer. Cancer 2009;115(11):2438–46.

59. Cella D, Yount S, Brucker PS, et al. Development and validation of a scale to measure disease-related symptoms of kidney cancer. Value Health 2007;10(4):285–93.

60. Aaronson NK, Ahmedzai S, Bergman B, et al. The European Organization for Research and Treatment of Cancer QLQ-C30: a quality-of-life instrument for use in international clinical trials in oncology. J Natl Cancer Inst 1993; 85(5):365–76.

61. Motzer RJ, Escudier B, Oudard S, et al. Phase 3 trial of everolimus for metastatic renal cell carcinoma: final results and analysis of prognostic factors. Cancer 2010;116:4256–65.

62. Knox JJ, Kay AC, Schiff E, et al. First-line everolimus followed by second-line sunitinib versus the opposite treatment sequence in patients with metastatic renal cell carcinoma (mRCC). Proc Am Soc Clinical Oncol 2010;28(Suppl 15) [abstract: TPS232].

63. Patel PH, Senico PL, Curiel RE, et al. Phase I study combining treatment with temsirolimus and sunitinib malate in patients with advanced renal cell carcinoma. Clin Genitourin Cancer 2009;7(1):24–7.

64. Molina AM, Feldman DR, Ginsberg MS, et al. Phase I trial sunitinib plus everolimus in patients with metastatic renal cell carcinoma (mRCC). J Clin Oncol 2011;29(Suppl) [abstract: 311].

65. Patnaik A, Ricart A, Cooper JS, et al. A phase I, pharmacokinetic and pharmacodynamic study of sorafenib (S), a multi-targeted kinase inhibitor in combination with temsirolimus (T), an mTOR inhibitor in patients with advanced solid malignancies. Annual Meeting Proceedings Part I. J Clin Oncol 2007;25(Suppl 18) [abstract: 3512].

66. Rosenberg JE, Weinberg VK, Claros C, et al. Phase I study of sorafenib and RAD001 for metastatic clear cell renal cell carcinoma. J Clin Oncol 2008; 26(Suppl) [abstract: 5109].

67. Kabbinavar FF, Srinivas S, Hauke RJ, et al. A phase I trial of combined tivozanib (AV-951) and temsirolimus therapy in patients (pts) with renal cell carcinoma (RCC). J Clin Oncol 2011;29(Suppl 7) [abstract: 330].

68. Merchan JR, Liu G, Fitch T, et al. Phase I/II trial of CCI-779 and bevacizumab in stage IV renal cell carcinoma: phase I safety and activity results. Annual Meeting Proceedings Part I. J Clin Oncol 2007;25(Suppl 18) [abstract: 5034].

69. Escudier B, Negrier S, Gravis G, et al. Can the combination of temsirolimus and bevacizumab improve the treatment of metastatic renal cell carcinoma (mRCC)? Result of the randomized TORAVA phase II trial. J Clin Oncol 2010;28(Suppl 15) [abstract: 4516].

70. Zafar Y, Bendell J, Lager J, et al. Preliminary results of a phase I study of bevacizumab (BV) in combination with everolimus (E) in patients with advanced solid tumors. J Clin Oncol 2006;24(Suppl 18) [abstract: 3097].

71. Hainsworth JD, Spigel DR, Burris HA 3rd, et al. Phase II trial of bevacizumab and everolimus in patients with advanced renal cell carcinoma. J Clin Oncol 2010;28(13):2131–6.

72. Yang JC, Haworth L, Sherry RM, et al. A randomized trial of bevacizumab, an anti-vascular endothelial growth factor antibody, for metastatic renal cancer. N Engl J Med 2003;349(5):427–34.

73. Rini BI, Halabi S, Rosenberg JE, et al. Bevacizumab plus interferon alfa compared with interferon alfa monotherapy in patients with metastatic renal cell carcinoma: CALGB 90206. J Clin Oncol 2008;26:5422–8.

74. Ravaud A, Bajetta E, Kay AC, et al. Everolimus with bevacizumab versus interferon alfa-2a plus bevacizumab as first-line therapy in patients with metastatic clear cell renal cell carcinoma. J Clin Oncol 2010;28(Suppl 15) [abstract: TPS238].

75. Rodriguez-Pascual J, Cheng E, Maroto P, et al. Emergent toxicities associated with the use of mTOR inhibitors in patients with advanced renal carcinoma. Anti-cancer Drugs 2010;21(5):478–86.

76. Li J, DeFea K, Roth RA. Modulation of insulin receptor substrate-1 tyrosine phosphorylation by an Akt/phosphatidylinositol 3-kinase pathway. J Biol Chem 1999; 274(14):9351–6.

77. Ozes ON, Akca H, Mayo LD, et al. A phosphatidylinositol 3-kinase/Akt/mTOR pathway mediates and PTEN antagonizes tumor necrosis factor inhibition of insulin signaling through insulin receptor substrate-1. Proc Natl Acad Sci U S A 2001;98(8):4640–5.

78. Manning BD. Balancing Akt with S6K: implications for both metabolic diseases and tumorigenesis. J Cell Biol 2004;167(3):399–403.

79. Bellmunt J, Szczylik C, Feingold J, et al. Temsirolimus safety profile and management of toxic effects in patients with advanced renal cell carcinoma and poor prognostic features. Ann Oncol 2008;19(8):1387–92.

80. American Diabetes Association. Standards of medical care in diabetes—2010. Diabetes Care 2010;33(Suppl 1):S11–61.

81. Nathan DM, Buse JB, Davidson MB, et al. Medical management of hyperglycemia in type 2 diabetes: a consensus algorithm for the initiation and adjustment of therapy: a consensus statement of the American Diabetes Association and the European Association for the Study of Diabetes. Diabetes Care 2009; 32(1):193–203.

82. Grundy SM, Cleeman JI, Merz CN, et al. Implications of recent clinical trials for the National Cholesterol Education Program Adult Treatment Panel III guidelines. Circulation 2004;110(2):227–39.

83. Pablo M, Hudes G, Dutcher J, et al. Radiographic findings of drug-induced pneumonitis and clinical correlation in patients with advanced renal cell carcinoma treated with temsirolimus. Eur J Cancer 2009;7(Suppl 2):426–7.

84. White DA, Camus P, Endo M, et al. Noninfectious pneumonitis after everolimus therapy for advanced renal cell carcinoma. Am J Respir Crit Care Med 2010; 182(3):396–403.

85. Duerr M, Glander P, Diekmann F, et al. Increased incidence of angioedema with ACE inhibitors in combination with mTOR inhibitors in kidney transplant recipients. Clin J Am Soc Nephrol 2010;5(4):703–8.

86. Parithivel K, Ramaiya N, Jagannathan JP, et al. Everolimus- and temsirolimus-associated enteritis: report of three cases. J Clin Oncol 2011;29(14):e404–6.

87. Wan X, Harkavy B, Shen N, et al. Rapamycin induces feedback activation of Akt signaling through an IGF-1R-dependent mechanism. Oncogene 2007;26(13): 1932–40.

88. Shi Y, Yan H, Frost P, et al. Mammalian target of rapamycin inhibitors activate the AKT kinase in multiple myeloma cells by up-regulating the insulin-like growth

factor receptor/insulin receptor substrate-1/phosphatidylinositol 3-kinase cascade. Mol Cancer Ther 2005;4(10):1533–40.

89. Tamburini J, Chapuis N, Bardet V, et al. Mammalian target of rapamycin (mTOR) inhibition activates phosphatidylinositol 3-kinase/Akt by up-regulating insulin-like growth factor-1 receptor signaling in acute myeloid leukemia: rationale for therapeutic inhibition of both pathways. Blood 2008;111(1):379–82.

90. O'Reilly KE, Rojo F, She QB, et al. mTOR inhibition induces upstream receptor tyrosine kinase signaling and activates Akt. Cancer Res 2006;66(3):1500–8.

91. Sun SY, Rosenberg LM, Wang X, et al. Activation of Akt and eIF4E survival pathways by rapamycin-mediated mammalian target of rapamycin inhibition. Cancer Res 2005;65(16):7052–8.

92. Hay N. The Akt-mTOR tango and its relevance to cancer. Cancer Cell 2005;8(3):179–83.

93. Huang J, Manning BD. A complex interplay between Akt, TSC2 and the two mTOR complexes. Biochem Soc Trans 2009;37(Pt 1):217–22.

94. Breuleux M, Klopfenstein M, Stephan C, et al. Increased AKT S473 phosphorylation after mTORC1 inhibition is rictor dependent and does not predict tumor cell response to PI3K/mTOR inhibition. Mol Cancer Ther 2009;8(4):742–53.

95. Gupta M, Ansell SM, Novak AJ, et al. Inhibition of histone deacetylase overcomes rapamycin-mediated resistance in diffuse large B-cell lymphoma by inhibiting Akt signaling through mTORC2. Blood 2009;114(14):2926–35.

96. Carracedo A, Ma L, Teruya-Feldstein J, et al. Inhibition of mTORC1 leads to MAPK pathway activation through a PI3K-dependent feedback loop in human cancer. J Clin Invest 2008;118(9):3065–74.

97. Albert S, Serova M, Dreyer C, et al. New inhibitors of the mammalian target of rapamycin signaling pathway for cancer. Expert Opin Investig Drugs 2010;19(8):919–30.

98. Courtney KD, Corcoran RB, Engelman JA. The PI3K pathway as drug target in human cancer. J Clin Oncol 2010;28(6):1075–83.

99. Figlin RA, de Souza P, McDermott D, et al. Analysis of PTEN and HIF-1alpha and correlation with efficacy in patients with advanced renal cell carcinoma treated with temsirolimus versus interferon-alpha. Cancer 2009;115(16):3651–60.

100. Cho D, Signoretti S, Dabora S, et al. Potential histologic and molecular predictors of response to temsirolimus in patients with advanced renal cell carcinoma. Clin Genitourin Cancer 2007;5(6):379–85.

101. Di Nicolantonio F, Arena S, Tabernero J, et al. Deregulation of the PI3K and KRAS signaling pathways in human cancer cells determines their response to everolimus. J Clin Invest 2010;120(8):2858–66.

102. MacConaill LE, Campbell CD, Kehoe SM, et al. Profiling critical cancer gene mutations in clinical tumor samples. PLoS One 2009;4(11):e7887.

103. Thomas RK, Baker AC, Debiasi RM, et al. High-throughput oncogene mutation profiling in human cancer. Nat Genet 2007;39(3):347–51.

104. Gattenlohner S, Etschmann B, Riedmiller H, et al. Lack of KRAS and BRAF mutation in renal cell carcinoma. Eur Urol 2009;55(6):1490–1.

105. Rochlitz CF, Peter S, Willroth G, et al. Mutations in the ras protooncogenes are rare events in renal cell cancer. Eur J Cancer 1992;28(2–3):333–6.

Systemic Therapy for Metastatic Non–Clear-Cell Renal Cell Carcinoma: Recent Progress and Future Directions

Simon Chowdhury, MA, MRCP, PhD[a], Marc R. Matrana, MD, MS[b],
Christopher Tsang, BA[a], Bradley Atkinson, PharmD[b],
Toni K. Choueiri, MD[c], Nizar M. Tannir, MD[b],*

KEYWORDS

- Non–clear-cell renal cell carcinoma • Targeted therapy
- Papillary • Chromophobe • Unclassified
- Renal medullary carcinoma • Collecting duct carcinoma
- Sarcomatoid dedifferentiation

Renal cell carcinoma (RCC) affects more than 40,000 patients in the United States each year.[1] Localized disease is curable with surgery, but a significant proportion of patients relapse or present with metastatic disease that is largely incurable.[2–4] Until relatively recently all adult renal epithelial tumors were labeled as "renal cell carcinomas" or "kidney cancers." Over the last 15 years RCC has increasingly been recognized as a heterogeneous disease with several distinct subtypes that have differing clinical, pathologic, and molecular characteristics.

RCCs can be divided into clear-cell (CCRCC, 70%–80%), and non–clear-cell (NCCRCC) histologies. The latter mainly include papillary (PRCC, 10%–15%), chromophobe (ChRCC, 5%), unclassified (5%), collecting duct, and medullary (CDRCC, MRCC, <5%).[5] In the era of immunotherapy, metastatic CCRCC was perceived to have a better outcome than PRCC,[6,7] but this has been contradicted by a large study of 1001 patients with metastatic RCC (82 of which had PRCC), showing similar 5-year

[a] Department of Medical Oncology, Guy's Hospital, London SE1 9RT, UK
[b] Department of Genitourinary Medical Oncology, The University of Texas MD Anderson Cancer Center, 1515 Holcombe Boulevard - Unit 1374, Houston, TX, USA
[c] Dana-Farber Cancer Institute, Harvard Medical School, Boston, MA, USA
* Corresponding author.
E-mail address: ntannir@mdanderson.org

Hematol Oncol Clin N Am 25 (2011) 853–869
doi:10.1016/j.hoc.2011.05.003   **hemonc.theclinics.com**
0889-8588/11/$ – see front matter © 2011 Elsevier Inc. All rights reserved.

survival rates of around 10% irrespective of clear-cell or papillary histology.[4] ChRCC is acknowledged to have the best overall prognosis compared with other subtypes, in both local and metastatic disease, and the same study confirmed this, indicating 5-year survival rates of 87.9% in ChRCC compared with 73.2% in CCRCC.

In the past decade, various targeted therapies such as tyrosine kinase inhibitors (TKIs), mammalian target of rapamycin (mTOR) inhibitors, and vascular endothelial growth factor (VEGF) monoclonal antibodies have changed the paradigm of CCRCC management. However, a key unresolved issue is whether these therapies can replicate their efficacy in NCCRCC. Indeed, most clinical trials to date have focused on patients with clear-cell histology. Retrospective analysis of these trials has indicated potential activity of targeted agents in NCCRCC and, as such, prospective trials have been initiated. This review outlines the different subtypes of NCCRCC, as well as the latest therapeutic developments in NCCRCC.

DEVELOPMENT OF TARGETED AGENTS

Improved understanding of the molecular biology underlying RCC has led to the development of several drugs that specifically target distinct pathways, and there is now convincing evidence that they are of benefit in patients with clear-cell histology.[8,9] This evidence raises the question of whether VEGF is a valid target in NCCRCC. Despite the fact that VHL inactivation and the subsequent overexpression of hypoxia-inducible genes such as VEGF are hallmarks of CCRCC, patients with papillary, chromophobe, and medullary histology can still demonstrate high expression of VEGF, VEGF receptor 1 (VEGFR1), and VEGFR2 (especially in more advanced stages) that is correlated with worse survival, making VEGF-targeted therapy an attractive therapeutic option.[10–13] There are currently two major classes of targeted agents of particular interest for treatment of NCCRCC.

Tyrosine Kinase Inhibitors

Kinase inhibitors are drugs that generally inhibit tyrosine kinase (TK) enzymes, which catalyze the transfer of phosphate groups from adenosine triphosphate (ATP) to tyrosine residues on proteins.[14] This process can be an activating event for proteins involved in signaling, and leads to increased cellular proliferation and the promotion of angiogenesis and metastasis. Receptor tyrosine kinases (RTKs) such as the epidermal growth factor receptor (EGFR) are located in the cell membrane and transduce signals from the extracellular environment to the cell interior.[14] Numerous downstream signaling pathways such as RAS/RAF/MEK/ERK and PI3K (phosphoinositol 3'-kinase)/Akt may be activated by ligand binding to a RTK.[15] Nonreceptor tyrosine kinases such as c-ABL are located intracellularly and can be activated by mechanisms such as phosphorylation. TKIs disrupt TK signaling by preventing the binding of either protein substrates or ATP,[14] and examples of TKIs with activity in NCCRCC include sunitinib, sorafenib, erlotinib, and pazopanib.

mTOR Inhibitors

mTOR is a nonreceptor serine/threonine kinase in the PI3K/Akt pathway that controls the translation of specific messenger RNA; mTOR activation has multiple downstream effects including increasing HIF-1α gene expression.[16] Furthermore, reduced PTEN expression has been demonstrated in some renal cell carcinomas,[17,18] and loss of PTEN function results in Akt phosphorylation with downstream effects on cell growth and proliferation that may be blocked using rapamycin derivatives.[19] There is therefore a strong rationale for using mTOR inhibitors in RCC.

SPORADIC PAPILLARY RCC
Pathology and Molecular Biology

Sporadic PRCC is itself a heterogeneous entity with at least 2 and possibly 3 distinct subtypes, both at the morphologic and genetic levels, which appear to have different clinical characteristics.[5,20,21] As might be expected, most of these tumors have a papillary, tubular, or tubulopapillary growth pattern.

From a histologic standpoint, two different subtypes of PRCC are identified, type 1 with small cells and pale cytoplasm and type 2 with large cells and eosinophilic cytoplasm.[20,22] Similarly, these two subtypes have distinct cytogenetic and molecular profiles that distinguish them from other renal epithelial tumors. Although only about 10% of sporadic type I PRCC have been reported to show somatic mutations in the c-MET gene, a genetic abnormality commonly seen as a germline mutation in hereditary cases,[23] the c-*Met* pathway can be activated in many sporadic PRCC in the absence of c-*Met* mutation.[24] The group from the National Institutes of Health described the genetic abnormality associated with the hereditary form of the type 2 papillary RCC, consisting of mutations in the fumarate hydratase (*FH*) gene.[25] The contribution of this mutation to the pathogenesis of sporadic papillary type 2 RCC remains unknown.

More recently, Yang and colleagues[21] proposed a refinement of the former (type I/type II) classification and introduced a molecular classification. Using gene expression profiling, they identified two highly distinct molecular PRCC subclasses with morphologic correlation. The first class, with excellent survival, corresponded to 3 histologic subtypes: type 1, low-grade type 2, and mixed type 1/low-grade type 2 tumors. The second class, with poor survival, corresponded to high-grade type 2 tumors. Dysregulation of G1-S and G2-M checkpoint genes were found in class 1 and 2 tumors, respectively. c-Met was differentially expressed, with higher expression in class 1 tumors. This refined classification of PRCC based on morphologic and molecular characteristics may be more relevant and is likely to aid diagnosis, prognosis, treatment, and analysis of clinical trials for advanced PRCC.

Treatment

Sunitinib inhibits the RTKs VEGFR2, platelet-derived growth factor receptor (PDGFR), FLT-3, and c-KIT (**Table 1**).[26,27] A dose of 50 mg orally once a day for 4 weeks followed by a 2-week break was the recommended phase 2 dose based on two phase 1 studies.[28,29] It has subsequently been shown to significantly increase progression-free

Table 1	
Selected targeted agents demonstrating activity in papillary renal cell carcinoma	
Agent	**Target**
Sorafenib	VEGFR2, VEGFR3, PDGFR, FLT-3, c-KIT, CRAF, wtBRAF, V600E BRAF
Sunitinib	VEGFR2, PDGFR, FLT-3, c-KIT
Temsirolimus	mTOR
Erlotinib	EGFR
Foretinib (GSK1363089) (previously XL880)	MET, VEGFR2

Abbreviations: EGFR, epidermal growth factor receptor; MET, mesenchymal epithelial transition factor; mTOR, mammalian target of rapamycin; PDGFR, platelet-derived growth factor receptor; VEGFR, vascular endothelial growth factor receptor; VEGF, vascular endothelial growth factor.

survival (PFS) in patients with metastatic CCRCC and has become a first-line standard of care for these patients.[9]

A worldwide expanded access trial of sunitinib has been undertaken, with a primary purpose to make the drug available to patients before regulatory approval. More than 4000 patients have been enrolled into this study, giving an important database especially for subgroup analysis. In May 2007, Gore and colleagues[30] presented data on 2341 patients, the majority of whom (78%) had received prior cytokine therapy. A subgroup analysis of patients with non–clear-cell histology was performed and 276 patients (11.8%) with non–clear-cell histology were identified, although distinction between different subtypes was not made. A response rate of 5.4%, clinical benefit (defined as response and stable disease >3 months) of 47% and median PFS of 6.7 months was seen in this subgroup. This result compared with an overall response rate for the entire patient group of 9.3%, clinical benefit of 52.3%, and median PFS of 8.9 months. The investigators concluded that sunitinib was active in the non–clear-cell subgroup; however, these data need to be interpreted with caution because of the nonrandomization of patients in the expanded access trial and the lack of pathology verification.

In light of the results of the retrospective subgroup analysis, further trials have been initiated to provide additional data on sunitinib activity in NCCRCC. In 2008, Plimack and colleagues[31] reported preliminary results from a phase 2 study of sunitinib in patients with NCCRCC. In a cohort of 26 patients of whom 13 had PRCC there were no objective responses, although 8 patients did experience stable disease. Moreover, the response rate and median PFS (48 days) were disappointing. Recently, updated results from this trial have been reported.[32] The trial has been expanded to include 48 patients, with analysis focused on the patients with PRCC (23). Unfortunately, the results remained disappointing; among the PRCC patients the median PFS was 1.6 months (95% confidence interval [CI] 1.3–12), the median overall survival (OS) was 10.8 months (95% CI, 6.2 to not evaluable), and no major responses were observed, with the best response being stable disease (seen in 8 patients).

The SUPAP study is another phase 2 trial investigating sunitinib activity in type 1 and 2 PRCC.[33] Twenty-eight patients were enrolled, and of the 23 patients with type 2 PRCC, 1 had a partial response and 13 had stable disease (lasting for ≥12 weeks in 4 patients). Five patients had type 1 PRCC, and although none experienced a partial response, 3 had stable disease. Based on these results, the investigators concluded that sunitinib did have some activity in PRCC, albeit inferior compared with CCRCC.

These conclusions have been supported by the results of another phase 2 study conducted in a cohort of 23 NCCRCC patients by Molina and colleagues.[34] There were 8 patients with PRCC, and in this subgroup no partial responses were seen, with a median PFS of 5.6 months (95% CI 1.4–7.1). The data from recent phase 2 studies has therefore tempered the initial optimism raised by the retrospective subgroup analysis, and it appears that sunitinib at best has modest activity in PRCC. Nevertheless, there are still several ongoing phase 2 trials investigating sunitinib therapy for PRCC, and their results will be useful in clarifying the role of sunitinib in NCCRCC (Clinicaltrials.gov identifier NCT00465179, NCT01034878, and NCT01219751). One study of 9 patients from Korea was preliminarily presented at the 2011 Genitourinary Cancers Symposium, and showed a response rate of 38% and a time to progression of 6.4 months. The investigators considered the primary end point has been met, and suggested that sunitinib has promising activity in patients with NCCRCC.[35]

Sorafenib inhibits the RTKs VEGFR2, VEGFR3, FLT-3, c-KIT, and PDGFR, and the nonreceptor serine threonine kinases BRAF and CRAF (see **Table 1**).[36] The BRAF and CRAF kinases are members of the RAF/MEK/ERK signaling cascade, which is involved in the survival and proliferation of tumor cells and is a therapeutic target in cancer,[37] although it is not known to be of major importance in RCC. Sorafenib has subsequently been shown to significantly increase PFS in patients with metastatic CCRCC who had progressed on cytokine therapy, and is licensed for the treatment of metastatic RCC.[8]

Ratain and colleagues[38] were among the first to administer sorafenib for metastatic PRCC. In a phase 2 randomized discontinuation study; they treated 15 PRCC patients out of a total of 202 patients. From this subgroup, 2 patients achieved a partial response and 3 had tumor shrinkage of 25% to 49%; this was comparable to the entire population and indicated sorafenib activity in PRCC.

In one of the largest detailed series to date, Choueiri and colleagues[39] reported on the efficacy of sunitinib and sorafenib in metastatic papillary and chromophobe RCC. This retrospective analysis identified 53 patients who had been treated with either sunitinib or sorafenib at 5 different cancer centers in the United States and France. In contrast to the expanded access studies, expert genitourinary pathologists from each institution reviewed the cases to confirm the histopathological diagnosis of NCCRCC. Forty-one patients had PRCC; 13 were treated with sunitinib and of these, 2 patients achieved a partial response (15% response rate), with durations of 12 months and more than 8 months. No responses were seen in the 28 patients treated with sorafenib. In total, 27 patients (68%) achieved stable disease for more than 3 months after 2 cycles of treatment with sunitinib or sorafenib. Minor responses ranging from −4% to −25% were seen in 9 patients. PRCC patients had a PFS of 7.6 months, and it was observed that treatment with sunitinib resulted in a superior PFS compared with sorafenib (PFS 11.9 vs 5.1 months, respectively; $P<.001$), and this remained statistically significant even after adjusting for other important prognostic factors in metastatic RCC such as hemoglobin and the number of metastatic sites.

A worldwide expanded access trial of sorafenib has also been undertaken. Response data on the Advanced Renal Cell Carcinoma Sorafenib (ARCCS) expanded access trial in North America has recently been reported on 1891 patients out of a total of 2504 patients enrolled.[40] This study contained a subgroup of 107 PRCC patients with valid data. Within this subgroup, 3 patients (3%) exhibited partial responses, with 87 patients (81%) experiencing stable disease lasting for at least 8 weeks. This study also included an extension protocol for which NCCRCC patients and patients who had not received prior therapy were eligible, although specific distinctions between NCCRCC subtypes were not made. Data were available for 248 patients in this extension protocol; NCCRCC patients (n = 26) had a PFS of 46 weeks (95% CI 30–59; censorship rate 39%) compared with first-line patients who had a PFS of 36 weeks (95% CI 33–45; censorship rate 56%). Overall in the whole trial, toxicities for NCCRCC patients did not differ from those seen in patients with CCRCC, and sorafenib was well tolerated in both groups. Moreover, it was concluded that sorafenib appeared to have activity against PRCC.

A similar European expanded access study of sorafenib was undertaken (the European ARCCS).[41] This study included 118 patients with PRCC of whom 104 were evaluable for response. The disease control rate was 66.4% and the median PFS was 5.8 months for PRCC compared with 75.7% and 7.5 months for patients with CCRCC, respectively.

Overall, currently available data from retrospective and expanded access studies suggest that sorafenib may possess activity against PRCC. Smaller-scale studies have also supported this impression. Unnithan and colleagues[42] investigated cell lines established from primary and metastatic tumors from a patient with type II PRCC, and reported that sorafenib inhibited cell growth and expression of angiogenic genes such as VEGF and PDGF. Given its apparent promising activity, further trials may be necessary to confirm whether sorafenib is suitable for NCCRCC therapy.

Temsirolimus, a derivative of sirolimus (rapamycin), inhibits mTOR (see **Table 1**). Temsirolimus has been studied in a 3-arm phase 3 study comparing temsirolimus, interferon-α (IFN-α), and the combination of the two agents as first-line therapy for poor-risk patients with metastatic RCC.[43] Response rates were similar in all 3 arms and ranged between 7% and 11%, but median OS was longer in the temsirolimus single-agent arm in comparison with the other 2 arms (10.9 months for temsirolimus, 7.3 months for IFN-α, and 8.4 months for the combination; hazard ratio [HR] 0.73, $P = .0069$ for single-agent temsirolimus). The investigators concluded that temsirolimus as a single agent significantly improves OS of patients with metastatic RCC and poor-risk features as compared with IFN-α, but the combination of the two drugs does not improve OS.

In this study, approximately 20% of all patients had non–clear-cell histology. Of these patients, 75% had PRCC. A subset analysis has been performed to determine the effect of temsirolimus versus IFN-α on OS and PFS in patients with clear-cell or other histologies.[44] For NCCRCC patients (n = 73), those in the temsirolimus group had a longer OS and PFS than those in the IFN-α group (median OS 11.6 vs 4.3 months, respectively; HR 0.49; median PFS 7.0 vs 1.8 months, respectively; HR 0.38). Thus, it seems that temsirolimus may benefit patients irrespective of histology and warrants further study in patients with non–clear-cell histologies. Unfortunately, this study had no central review of the histology and therefore there was no detailed differentiation between different non–clear-cell subtypes.

More recently, Yang and colleagues[45] performed further retrospective analysis, focusing on quality of life data gathered using the EuroQoL-5D utility score (EQ-5D index) and EQ-5D visual analog scale (EQ-VAS). It was observed that the mean EQ-5D score was higher in the temsirolimus arm compared with the IFN-α arm in NCCRCC patients.

The possibility that mTOR inhibitors have clinical activity regardless of RCC histology has led to the development of studies aimed at patients with non–clear-cell histology, and a phase 2 trial comparing temsirolimus against sunitinib as first-line therapies is currently recruiting (NCT00979966). Everolimus is another mTOR inhibitor that is being investigated by several trials. Most notably, the RAPTOR study aims to evaluate everolimus as a first-line therapy for PRCC (NCT00688753). Other ongoing trials are also investigating the use of everolimus alone, or in comparison with sunitinib, for treatment of NCCRCC (NCT00830895, NCT01185366, NCT01108445). The randomized phase 2 studies comparing mTOR inhibitors with sunitinib may help to clarify the relative role of each agent in NCCRCC.

The rationale for the use of erlotinib, an oral EGFR TKI, in PRCC stems from a study by Perera and colleagues.[46] These investigators demonstrated that blockade of the EGFR by an anti-EGFR monoclonal antibody resulted in significant growth inhibition in NCCRCC-derived cell lines, suggesting that EGFR blockade may provide a potential therapeutic approach. In a study led by the Southwest Oncology Group (SWOG), Gordon and colleagues[47] treated 45 patients with PRCC with erlotinib (150 mg/d). Five patients achieved a partial response for an overall response rate of 11% (95% CI 3–24) with a disease control rate (DCR) of 64% (5 partial response + 24 stable). Median OS time was 27 months (95% CI 13–36). There was no correlation between EGFR expression and disease outcome, and the drug was generally well tolerated. Although the RECIST response rate of 11% did not exceed prespecified estimates (≥20% response rate) for further study, single-agent erlotinib yielded encouraging DCR and OS results. As a result of its promising activity, two phase 2 trials are now under way to investigate erlotinib alone and in combination with bevacizumab in patients with PRCC (NCT01130519, NCT00060307).

Foretinib (GSK1363089) is a novel inhibitor of RTKs targeting MET and VEGFR. In a phase 1 study partial responses were noted in 2 out of 4 patients with PRCC, lasting for longer than 48 and 12 months.[48] This finding has led to the initiation of a multicenter phase 2 study of foretinib (240 mg/d orally for 5 days on/9 days off) in patients with histologically confirmed PRCC.[49] After enrollment, patients were stratified into two strata based on the presence or absence of a genetic aberration in c-MET (A: evidence of c-MET pathway activation; B: without evidence of activation). Thirty-one patients were enrolled (15 strata A and 16 strata B), and of 25 evaluable patients, 24 had at least stable disease and 20 had decreases in tumor size (range 4%–35%). Two patients had confirmed partial response and 2 had unconfirmed partial response pending independent confirmation. The same trial has expanded to investigate the efficacy and safety of two dosing regimens (240 mg 5 days on/9 days off vs 80 mg daily) of foretinib for PRCC.[50] Of 37 enrolled patients in the 5-day-on/9-day-off cohort, 35 were evaluable; 4 patients experienced confirmed partial responses and 27 had stable disease. Enrollment is incomplete in cohort 2; however, among 9 evaluable patients, 2 had partial responses and 7 had stable disease. The investigators concluded that foretinib was well tolerated and displayed promising antitumor activity. Therefore, it appears that foretinib may be an effective therapy for PRCC. The final results from this study are eagerly awaited.

CHROMOPHOBE RCC
Pathology and Molecular Biology

ChRCC is a subtype of RCC distinguished from CCRCC and other forms of NCCRCC by a distinct set of clinicopathological and molecular features. ChRCC arises from renal intercalated cells and can be divided into 3 subtypes: classic, eosinophilic, and mixed. All subtypes are characterized by a sheet-like histologic appearance, and vary depending on whether they possess a pale or eosinophilic cytoplasm. ChRCC was first identified by Bannasch and colleagues[51] in experimental renal tumor models in rats. These tumors arose in the rat model after exposure to nitrosomorpholine, and had a characteristic cloudy cytoplasm. Similar neoplasms were later found in humans by Thoenes and colleagues.[52] The World Health Organization classification recognized ChRCC as a distinct subset of RCC in 2004.

Epidemiologically, ChRCC makes up about 4% of RCC. It is most often diagnosed in the sixth decade of life, but may occur more frequently than other forms of RCC in younger patients. Unlike other forms of RCC, male-to-female ratio is approximately equal. ChRCC, like other forms of RCC, is most often found incidentally on imaging. Radiographically, ChRCC are typically hypovascular tumors that compress the renal vasculature, and usually have a homogeneous appearance. Pathologically, ChRCC tumors tend to be beige uniform masses lacking necrosis and hemorrhage.[53]

Genetically, ChRCC cells tend to be hypodyploid, and often feature loss of heterozygosity involving chromosomes 1, 3p, 6, 10, 13, 17, and 21.[54] In addition, ChRCC is a feature of Birt-Hogg-Dubé (BHD) syndrome. This autosomal dominant condition involves mutations in the *BHD* gene, resulting in benign cutaneous tumors, RCCs (especially with chromophobe histology), and spontaneous pneumothoraces. *BHD* encodes folliculin, a tumor suppressor, and it has been reported that *BHD* is also mutated in sporadic ChRCC.[55]

Deranged expression of the RTK KIT is also understood to be important in ChRCC. *KIT* is an oncogene involved in several cell processes including proliferation, apoptosis, and differentiation, and is known to be abnormally activated in various neoplasias. Gene expression analysis has indicated upregulated expression of KIT on ChRCC cell membranes, and therefore KIT may prove to be useful for the diagnosis and treatment of ChRCC.[56] Mutations or rearrangements of mitochondrial DNA have been frequently observed.[57] mRNA expression profiles in ChRCC are quite similar to those in oncocytomas, with ChRCC expressing more distal nephron markers. This observation suggests that ChRCC and oncocytoma may represent spectrums of differentiation from the same progenitor cells, and both are thought to be derived from intercalated cells of the collecting duct system. Both ChRCC and oncocytomas occur with increased frequency in patients with BHD syndrome, providing further evidence of the relatedness of these two tumors.

Treatment

Some of the aforementioned data described for PRCC is also applicable to ChRCC, because many trials have not distinguished between specific NCCRCC subtypes. Examples include the retrospective analysis of the sunitinib expanded access trial as well as the phase 3 temsirolimus trial. Both trials included ChRCC patients, but no definite conclusions can be drawn because the data did not differentiate between the different subtypes of NCCRCC.

In the retrospective study by Choueiri and colleagues[39] on sunitinib and sorafenib in NCCRCC, 12 of 53 patients had ChRCC. Of these, 7 were treated with sunitinib and 5 with sorafenib. Partial responses were seen in 1 patient treated with sunitinib and in 2 patients treated with sorafenib, and the remaining 9 patients all experienced stable disease for at least 3 months. The median PFS time for sorafenib-treated patients was 27.5 months, and although both agents had activity, the low number of patients precluded any firm conclusions to be drawn.

The ARCCS expanded access trial of sorafenib has also yielded valuable data on ChRCC patients. This cohort of 202 patients contained 20 ChRCC patients with available response data. No complete responses were seen, although 1 patient (5%) did have a partial response, and 17 patients (75%) had stable disease for longer than 8 weeks. Both studies therefore indicate potential activity for targeted agents in ChRCC, and as such several trials are under way (**Table 2**).

Recent data has also pointed to a possible role for chemotherapy in treatment of ChRCC. Capecitabine is a fluoropyrimidine, which is converted into 5-fluorouracil

Table 2
Targeted agents currently under evaluation in selected clinical trials

Agent	Subtype	Trial Number
Sunitinib	Metastatic NCCRCC (all types)	NCT00465179
	Metastatic NCCRCC (all types)	NCT01034878
	Metastatic PRCC, ChRCC, MRCC	NCT01219751
Temsirolimus versus sunitinib	Locally advanced and metastatic NCCRCC (all types)	NCT00979966
Everolimus	Metastatic PRCC	NCT00688753
	Metastatic NCCRCC (all types)	NCT00830895
Everolimus versus sunitinib	Metastatic PRCC, ChRCC, CDRCC	NCT01185366
	Metastatic PRCC, ChRCC	NCT01108445
Erlotinib	Local and metastatic PRCC	NCT00060307
Erlotinib and bevacizumab	Hereditary and sporadic metastatic PRCC	NCT01130519

(5-FU). 5-FU has shown activity in metastatic RCC when combined with interleukin-2 and interferon, and consequently a phase 2 study has been conducted to investigate capecitabine and docetaxel in metastatic RCC.[58] In a cohort of 25 patients, 10 (40%) experienced stable disease (90% CI 25–58). Of interest, most of the patients with prolonged stable disease had non–clear-cell histology, including one patient with ChRCC. A phase 2 trial evaluating capecitabine in metastatic NCCRCC has since completed accrual of patients, with results yet to be published (NCT01182142).

RENAL MEDULLARY CARCINOMA

Renal medullary carcinoma (RMC) is a newly recognized aggressive form of kidney cancer, which was first described in a case series by Davis and colleagues in 1995.[59] All patients in the series were younger than 40 years, black, and nearly all had sickle cell trait. This new entity was quickly designated the seventh sickle cell nephropathy (the other 6 are: gross hematuria, papillary necrosis, nephrotic syndrome, renal infarction, inability to concentrate urine, and pyelonephritis).[60]

Since the original report more than 150 additional cases have been reported, and clear clinical and epidemiologic associations noted in the original report have been confirmed. Patients diagnosed with RMC tend to be young (median age around 30 years), almost always of black race (although Hispanic/Brazilian and even a few Caucasian patients have been reported), and virtually all have sickle cell trait or sickle cell disease. A male/female ratio of 2:1 has been observed in adults, although in children the male predominance is even greater. The clinical presentation of RMC varies, but nearly all patients are symptomatic at diagnosis. Pain and hematuria are the most commonly seen symptoms. The right kidney is more often (>75%) affected than the left.[61,62]

Pathologically, the tumors are of malignant epithelial type that arise from collecting duct epithelium. The tumors tend to be solitary, gray-white masses with macroscopic necrosis and hemorrhage.[63,64]

Clinically, RMCs tend to be highly aggressive. Metastases to the lymph nodes, liver, and lungs are common at diagnosis. Treatment has proved challenging, as neither chemotherapy nor radiation therapy has been found to be particularly useful in this disease. Tannir and colleagues[65] presented a series of 22 patients with RMC from 4 major institutions at the 2011 Genitourinary Cancer Symposium. The investigators found that targeted therapy has low efficacy when given as monotherapy and noted that currently cytotoxic chemotherapy is the mainstay of treatment, but this modality provides only modest short-term palliation, with median survival of about 1 year from diagnosis. Albadine and colleagues[66] performed immunoexpression analysis of tissues and found that topoisomerase IIα was overexpressed in 11 of 13 (85%) cases, suggesting that this might be an appropriate target of therapy. Schaeffer and colleagues[67] reported results of whole-genome expression of 4 RMC tumors that showed increases of topoisomerase II in all cases. These investigators further reported a case of metastatic RMC in which a complete response was achieved for 9 months using topoisomerase II inhibitor therapy.

Genetically, the loss of INI1, a factor in the ATP-dependent chromatin-modifying complex, is seen in some RMCs as well as in renal rhabdoid tumors. The absence of INI1 expression does not appear to be predictive of rhabdoid histopathology, but is associated with aggressive behavior in RMC.[68] Rearrangement of the ALK RTK has been reported in RMC as well. Mariño-Enríquez and colleagues[69] identified a novel ALK oncoprotein in which the cytoskeletal protein vinculin (VCL) was fused to the ALK kinase domain in a case of RMC harboring a t(2;10)(p23;q22) translocation. Their report suggests a rationale for studying the treatment of RMC with targeted ALK inhibitors.

Although rare, RMC has garnered interest among oncologists, as well as physicians who treat sickle cell disease. There are currently no open clinical trials aimed solely at RMC, but a handful of trials seek to enroll patients with various forms of non–clear-cell kidney cancer. As the molecular drivers of RMC are further elucidated in the laboratory, new treatment options should emerge.

COLLECTING DUCT RCC
Pathology and Molecular Biology

CDRCC (also known as Bellini tumor) is rare and arises from the collecting ducts. By light microscopy, CDRCC is indistinguishable from RMC. Due to its rarity, few data exist, although it is known that CDRCC is genetically similar to urothelial cancers.[70]

Treatment

One of the largest trials focusing on CDRCC to date was conducted in 2007. This phase 2 study enrolled 23 patients, and investigated treatment with gemcitabine combined with either cisplatin or carboplatin. Results were encouraging, with median PFS of 7.1 months (95% CI 3–11.3) and OS of 10.5 months (95% CI 3.8–17.1). One patient experienced a complete response.

More recent data has further pointed to a potential benefit of chemotherapy in this type of cancer. Bortezomib is a proteasome inhibitor, which acts to interfere with degradation of cell cycle proteins as well as with the expression of genes involved in angiogenesis and metastasis. Phase 1 trials confirmed the safety of the drug, as well as indicating potential benefit for treatment of RCC.[71] These data prompted a phase 2 trial that enrolled 37 patients with metastatic disease, with doses of 1.5 mg/m^2 given to 25 patients and 1.3 mg/m^2 given to 12 patients.[72] Partial responses were seen in 4 patients (11%; 95% CI 3–25) and stable disease in 14 patients (38%; 95% CI 23–55). Of note, of the 4 patients with responses, 1 had RMC. Ronnen and colleagues[73] have since reported that after 7 months of treatment with bortezomib, this patient achieved a complete response and was disease-free for 27 months at the time of writing. Therefore, bortezomib may have a role in the treatment of RMC/CDRCC. Further data are required to assess its activity. One phase 2 trial of bortezomib in NCCRCC has completed accrual and results are awaited with interest (NCT00276614).

Given the rarity of both CDRCC and RMC, very few patients with either histology were treated with targeted therapy. Ansari and colleagues[74] reported a patient with metastatic CDRCC who was treated with sorafenib, resulting in PFS exceeding 13 months. Further data clearly are necessary to characterize treatments for CDRCC and RMC, and this is being addressed in ongoing trials (see **Table 2**).

UNCOMMON TYPES OF NCCRCC

Mucinous tubular and spindle-cell carcinoma (MTSCC) is a recently described type of RCC thought to arise from either the collecting duct or loop of Henle. MTSCC is characterized histologically by the presence of tubules, spindle cells, and mucinous stroma. MTSCC is associated with a 4:1 female predominance. Multiple chromosome losses have been identified in MTSCC. Some studies have shown trisomies of chromosome 7 and 17. The majority of these tumors follow an indolent course, although there are a few case reports of lymph node and visceral metastases.[75,76] MTSCC may rarely be associated with sarcomatoid dedifferentiation, and carries a poor prognosis.

Tubulocystic carcinoma is another recently described type of NCCRCC, with a strong male predominance (7:1). Tubulocystic carcinoma is histologically distinguished by the presence of tightly packed tubules and interspersed cysts. On electron microscopy, abundant microvilli with a brush border resembling proximal convoluted tubules can be seen. Other cells resembling intercalated cells of the collecting duct may also be seen. Genetic studies suggest some relationship to papillary carcinoma. Metastases have been reported in a few cases.[77] Sunitinib showed a response in a patient who failed 2 lines of cytotoxic chemotherapy.[78]

Renal translocation carcinomas are rare tumors often found in children or young adults. These tumors almost exclusively are associated with translocations involving a transcription factor, E3 located on Xp11.2, although other chromosomal transloca- tions have been described. Confirmation of the presence of a translocation, by either immunohistochemical, genetic, or molecular methods, is required for diagnosis. The tumors tend to present at advanced stages but often have a relatively indolent course,[79–81] especially in children and adolescents. There is a female preponderance, with the vast majority of patients having lymph node metastasis at presentation.[82,83] Translocation carcinoma of the kidney responds less well to targeted therapy than CCRCC, but partial responses are seen with sunitinib and other anti-VEGF agents.[82,83]

Thyroid-like or follicular renal carcinoma represents a rare and newly emerging form of kidney cancer reported in only a handful of cases. Histologically, these tumors are distinguished by the presence of a pseudocapsule, and microfollicles and macrofol- licles. Of the few cases reported, all patients remained tumor-free following surgery.[64] However, a recent case report described a patient who presented with lung and retro- peritoneal lymph node metastases at initial diagnosis.[84]

SARCOMATOID FEATURES IN RCC

"Sarcomatoid features" is likely a more appropriate nomenclature than "sarcomatoid RCC," because these features can be seen with all types of RCC. The presence of sar- comatoid dedifferentiation is now understood to reflect a final common pathway that can occur in diverse tumor types. It is associated with high-grade, aggressive tumors and short survival. The estimated median survival for patients with localized disease is 17 months, and for patients with metastatic disease only 7 months.[85]

Patients with metastatic sarcomatoid RCC do not appear to benefit from cytoreduc- tive nephrectomy. In most cases the sarcomatoid features are only identified after the nephrectomy.[86] In a single-institution series of 417 patients who underwent cytore- ductive nephrectomy at University of California Los Angeles,[87] the median OS for 62 patients with sarcomatoid RCC was 4.9 months, compared with 17.7 months for those without sarcomatoid features. Patients identified as having sarcomatoid RCC prior to cytoreductive nephrectomy might benefit from immediate systemic therapy rather than surgery.

There is currently no standard therapy for metastatic or unresectable sarcomatoid carcinoma of the kidney, and there are very few published clinical studies. In a retro- spective study, Golshayan and colleagues[88] reported the median time to progression and median OS of 43 patients with sarcomatoid RCC treated with VEGF-targeted agents. There were 8 objective responses (19%), median time to progression was 5.3 months, and median OS was 11.8 months. Patients who had CCRCC as the under- lying epithelial component and 20% or fewer sarcomatoid elements had a better outcome. In the only published phase 2 clinical trial of sarcomatoid RCC, the regimen of doxorubicin and ifosfamide produced no objective responses, with median time to progression of 2.2 months and median OS of 3.9 months.[89] Experience with the combination of doxorubicin and gemcitabine given every 2 weeks with granulocyte- colony stimulating factor support in metastatic RCC was reported.[90] Among the 10 patients with sarcomatoid RCC treated in that series, 2 had complete responses and 1 had a partial response. Two of the patients with complete responses were subsequently reported to have survived 6 years and 8 years; both of these patients initially had a local tumor recurrence in the renal bed.[91] Based on these preliminary observations, a phase 2 clinical trial (ECOG 8802; NCT00068393) of doxorubicin and gemcitabine in metastatic sarcomatoid RCC is in progress. Preliminary results from ECOG 8802, reported in abstract form, suggested an overall response rate of 16%, median OS 8.8 months, and PFS 3.5 months.[92] Single-arm phase 2 trials are currently evaluating the role of chemotherapy and VEGF-targeted agents given in combination.[93,94]

SUMMARY

Recently, there have been considerable advances in the understanding of CCRCC. This progress has been translated into the development of several drugs with improved efficacy, of which the kinase inhibitors have demonstrated the most significant activity. Initial studies of these drugs have shown promising activity in metastatic NCCRCC, and additional prospective studies of these and other agents are needed. Several such studies are open to recruitment or are planned, and their results will help to define the role of these drugs in the management of NCCRCC. Further work is being done to understand the pathogenesis of NCCRCC, and it is hoped that this will lead to a situation whereby treatment can be optimized for each individual patient.

REFERENCES

1. Jemal A, Siegel R, Ward E, et al. Cancer statistics, 2008. CA Cancer J Clin 2008; 58:71–96.
2. Beck SD, Patel MI, Snyder ME, et al. Effect of papillary and chromophobe cell type on disease-free survival after nephrectomy for renal cell carcinoma. Ann Surg Oncol 2004;11:71–7.
3. Cheville JC, Lohse CM, Zincke H, et al. Comparisons of outcome and prognostic features among histologic subtypes of renal cell carcinoma. Am J Surg Pathol 2003;27:612–24.
4. Patard JJ, Leray E, Rioux-Leclercq N, et al. Prognostic value of histologic subtypes in renal cell carcinoma: a multicenter experience. J Clin Oncol 2005; 23:2763–71.
5. Reuter VE. The pathology of renal epithelial neoplasms. Semin Oncol 2006;33: 534–43.
6. Motzer RJ, Mazumdar M, Bacik J, et al. Survival and prognostic stratification of 670 patients with advanced renal cell carcinoma. J Clin Oncol 1999;17:2530–40.
7. Ronnen EA, Kondagunta GV, Ishill N, et al. Treatment outcome for metastatic papillary renal cell carcinoma patients. Cancer 2006;107:2617–21.
8. Escudier B, Eisen T, Stadler WM, et al. Sorafenib in advanced clear-cell renal-cell carcinoma. N Engl J Med 2007;356:125–34.
9. Motzer RJ, Hutson TE, Tomczak P, et al. Sunitinib versus interferon alfa in metastatic renal-cell carcinoma. N Engl J Med 2007;356:115–24.
10. Jacobsen J, Grankvist K, Rasmuson T, et al. Different isoform patterns for vascular endothelial growth factor between clear cell and papillary renal cell carcinoma. BJU Int 2006;97:1102–8.
11. Ljungberg BJ, Jacobsen J, Rudolfsson SH, et al. Different vascular endothelial growth factor (VEGF), VEGF-receptor 1 and -2 mRNA expression profiles between clear cell and papillary renal cell carcinoma. BJU Int 2006;98:661–7.

12. Preston RS, Philp A, Claessens T, et al. Absence of the Birt-Hogg-Dube gene product is associated with increased hypoxia-inducible factor transcriptional activity and a loss of metabolic flexibility. Oncogene 2011;30:1159–73.

13. Swartz MA, Karth J, Schneider DT, et al. Renal medullary carcinoma: clinical, pathologic, immunohistochemical, and genetic analysis with pathogenetic implications. Urology 2002;60:1083–9.

14. Krause DS, Van Etten RA. Tyrosine kinases as targets for cancer therapy. N Engl J Med 2005;353:172–87.

15. Schlessinger J. Cell signaling by receptor tyrosine kinases. Cell 2000;103:211–25.

16. Hudson CC, Liu M, Chiang GG, et al. Regulation of hypoxia-inducible factor 1alpha expression and function by the mammalian target of rapamycin. Mol Cell Biol 2002;22:7004–14.

17. Hara S, Oya M, Mizuno R, et al. Akt activation in renal cell carcinoma: contribution of a decreased PTEN expression and the induction of apoptosis by an Akt inhibitor. Ann Oncol 2005;16:928–33.

18. Shin Lee J, Seok Kim H, Bok Kim Y, et al. Expression of PTEN in renal cell carcinoma and its relation to tumor behavior and growth. J Surg Oncol 2003;84:166–72.

19. Vignot S, Faivre S, Aguirre D, et al. mTOR-targeted therapy of cancer with rapamycin derivatives. Ann Oncol 2005;16:525–37.

20. Delahunt B, Eble JN, McCredie MR, et al. Morphologic typing of papillary renal cell carcinoma: comparison of growth kinetics and patient survival in 66 cases. Hum Pathol 2001;32:590–5.

21. Yang XJ, Tan MH, Kim HL, et al. A molecular classification of papillary renal cell carcinoma. Cancer Res 2005;65:5628–37.

22. Kosaka T, Mikami S, Miyajima A, et al. Papillary renal cell carcinoma: clinicopathological characteristics in 40 patients. Clin Exp Nephrol 2008;12:195–9.

23. Schmidt L, Junker K, Nakaigawa N, et al. Novel mutations of the MET proto-oncogene in papillary renal carcinomas. Oncogene 1999;18:2343–50.

24. van den Berg E, van der Hout AH, Oosterhuis JW, et al. Cytogenetic analysis of epithelial renal-cell tumors: relationship with a new histopathological classification. Int J Cancer 1993;55(2):223–7.

25. Linehan WM, Walther MM, Zbar B. The genetic basis of cancer of the kidney. J Urol 2003;170:2163–72.

26. Mendel DB, Laird AD, Xin X, et al. In vivo antitumor activity of SU11248, a novel tyrosine kinase inhibitor targeting vascular endothelial growth factor and platelet-derived growth factor receptors: determination of a pharmacokinetic/pharmacodynamic relationship. Clin Cancer Res 2003;9:327–37.

27. O'Farrell AM, Abrams TJ, Yuen HA, et al. SU11248 is a novel FLT3 tyrosine kinase inhibitor with potent activity in vitro and in vivo. Blood 2003;101:3597–605.

28. Faivre S, Delbaldo C, Vera K, et al. Safety, pharmacokinetic, and antitumor activity of SU11248, a novel oral multitarget tyrosine kinase inhibitor, in patients with cancer. J Clin Oncol 2006;24:25–35.

29. O'Farrell AM, Foran JM, Fiedler W, et al. An innovative phase I clinical study demonstrates inhibition of FLT3 phosphorylation by SU11248 in acute myeloid leukemia patients. Clin Cancer Res 2003;9:5465–76.

30. Gore ME, Porta C, Oudard S, et al. Sunitinib in metastatic renal cell carcinoma (mRCC): preliminary assessment of toxicity in an expanded access trial with subpopulation analysis [abstract]. J Clin Oncol 2007;25(20 Suppl):5010.

31. Plimack ER, Jonash E, Bekele BN, et al. Sunitinib in non-clear cell renal cell carcinoma (ncc-RCC): a phase II study [abstract]. J Clin Oncol 2008;26(20 Suppl): 5112.

32. Plimack ER, Jonash E, Bekele BN, et al. Sunitinib in papillary renal cell carcinoma (pRCC): results from a single-arm phase II study [abstract]. J Clin Oncol 2010; 28(Suppl):4604.

33. Ravaud A, Oudard S, Gravis-Mescam G, et al. First-line sunitinib in type I and II papillary renal cell carcinoma (PRCC): SUPAP, a phase II study of the French Genito-Urinary Group (GETUG) and the Group of Early Phase trials (GEP) [abstract]. J Clin Oncol 2009;27(Suppl):5146.

34. Molina AM, Feldman DR, Ginsberg MS, et al. Phase II trial of sunitinib in patients with metastatic non-clear cell renal cell carcinoma. Invest New Drugs 2010. [Epub ahead of print].

35. Lee J, Ahn J, Lim S, et al. Multicenter prospective phase II study of sunitinib in non-clear cell type renal cell carcinoma. J Clin Oncol 2011;29(Suppl 7) [abstract: 325].

36. Wilhelm SM, Carter C, Tang L, et al. BAY 43-9006 exhibits broad spectrum oral antitumor activity and targets the RAF/MEK/ERK pathway and receptor tyrosine kinases involved in tumor progression and angiogenesis. Cancer Res 2004;64: 7099–109.

37. Sridhar SS, Hedley D, Siu LL. Raf kinase as a target for anticancer therapeutics. Mol Cancer Ther 2005;4:677–85.

38. Ratain MJ, Eisen T, Stadler WM, et al. Phase II placebo-controlled randomized discontinuation trial of sorafenib in patients with metastatic renal cell carcinoma. J Clin Oncol 2006;24:2505–12.

39. Choueiri TK, Plantade A, Elson P, et al. Efficacy of sunitinib and sorafenib in meta-static papillary and chromophobe renal cell carcinoma. J Clin Oncol 2008;26: 127–31.

40. Stadler WM, Figlin RA, McDermott DF, et al. Safety and efficacy results of the advanced renal cell carcinoma sorafenib expanded access program in North America. Cancer 2010;116:1272–80.

41. Beck J, Bajata E, Escudier B, et al. A large open-label, non-comparative phase III study of the multi-targeted kinase inhibitor sorafenib in European patients with advanced renal cell carcinoma. Eur J Cancer 2007;(Suppl 7):244 [abstract: 4506].

42. Unnithan J, Vaziri S, Wood D, et al. Characterization of type II papillary renal cell carcinoma and efficacy of sorafenib. Genitourinary Cancers Symposium 2008 [abstract: 409].

43. Hudes G, Carducci M, Tomczak P, et al. Temsirolimus, interferon alfa, or both for advanced renal-cell carcinoma. N Engl J Med 2007;356:2271–81.

44. Dutcher JP, de Souza P, McDermott D, et al. Effect of temsirolimus versus interferon-alpha on outcome of patients with advanced renal cell carcinoma of different tumor histologies. Med Oncol 2009;26:202–9.

45. Yang S, de Souza P, Alemao E, et al. Quality of life in patients with advanced renal cell carcinoma treated with temsirolimus or interferon-alpha. Br J Cancer 2010; 102:1456–60.

46. Perera AD, Kleymenova EV, Walker CL. Requirement for the von Hippel-Lindau tumor suppressor gene for functional epidermal growth factor receptor blockade by monoclonal antibody C225 in renal cell carcinoma. Clin Cancer Res 2000;6: 1518–23.

47. Gordon MS, Hussey M, Nagle RB, et al. Phase II study of erlotinib in patients with locally advanced or metastatic papillary histology renal cell cancer: SWOG S0317. J Clin Oncol 2009;27:5788–93.

48. Eder JP, Shapiro GI, Appleman LJ, et al. A phase I study of foretinib, a multi-targeted inhibitor of c-Met and vascular endothelial growth factor receptor 2. Clin Cancer Res 2010;16:3507–16.

49. Srinivasan R, Choueiri TK, Vaishampayan U, et al. A phase II study of the dual MET/VEGFR2 inhibitor XL880 in patients (pts) with papillary renal carcinoma (PRC) [abstract]. J Clin Oncol 2008;26(20 Suppl):5103.

50. Srinivasan R, Linehan W, Vaishampayan U, et al. A phase II study of two dosing regimens of GSK 1363089 (GSK089), a dual MET/VEGFR2 inhibitor, in patients (pts) with papillary renal carcinoma (PRC). J Clin Oncol 2009;27(Suppl) [abstract: 5103].

51. Bannasch P, Schacht U, Storch E. Morphogenese undhobe Mikromorphologie epithelialer Nierentumoren bei Nitrosomorpholine-vergifteten Ratten. I. Induktion und Histologie der Tumon. Z Krebsforsch Klin Onkol Cancer Res Clin Oncol 1974;81:311–31 [in German].

52. Thoenes W, Storkel S, Rumpelt HJ. Human chromophobe cell renal carcinoma. Virchows Arch B Cell Pathol Incl Mol Pathol 1985;48:207–17.

53. Crotty TB, Farrow GM, Lieber MM. Chromophobe cell renal carcinoma: clinico-pathological features of 50 cases. J Urol 1995;154:964–7.

54. Stec R, Grala B, Maczewski M, et al. Chromophobe renal cell cancer—review of the literature and potential methods of treating metastatic disease. J Exp Clin Cancer Res 2009;28:134.

55. Gad S, Lefevre SH, Khoo SK, et al. Mutations in BHD and TP53 genes, but not in HNF1beta gene, in a large series of sporadic chromophobe renal cell carcinoma. Br J Cancer 2007;96:336–40.

56. Yamazaki K, Sakamoto M, Ohta T, et al. Overexpression of KIT in chromophobe renal cell carcinoma. Oncogene 2003;22:847–52.

57. Kovacs A, Störkel S, Thoenes W, et al. Mitochondrial and chromosomal DNA alterations in human chromophobe renal cell carcinomas. J Pathol 1992;167:273–7.

58. Marur S, Eliason J, Heilbrun LK, et al. Phase II trial of capecitabine and weekly docetaxel in metastatic renal cell carcinoma. Urology 2008;72:898–902.

59. Davis CJ, Mostofi FK, Sesterhenn IA. Renal medullary carcinoma: the seventh sickle cell nephropathy. Am J Surg Pathol 1995;19:1–11.

60. Berman LB. Sickle cell nephropathy. JAMA 1974;228:1279.

61. Sathyamoorthy K, Teo A, Atallah M. Renal medullary carcinoma in a patient with sickle-cell disease. Nat Clin Pract Urol 2006;3:279–83.

62. Patel K, Livni N, Macdonald D. Renal medullary carcinoma, a rare cause of hematuria in sickle cell trait. Br J Haematol 2006;132:1.

63. Yan BC, Mackinnon AC, Al-Ahmadie HA. Recent developments in the pathology of renal tumors: morphology and molecular characteristics of select entities. Arch Pathol Lab Med 2009;133:1026–32.

64. Srigley JR, Delahunt B. Uncommon and recently described renal carcinomas. Mod Pathol 2009;22(Suppl 2):S2–23.

65. Tannir NM, Lim ZD, Rao P, et al. Outcome of patients with renal medullary carcinoma (RMC) treated in the era of targeted therapies (TT): a multicenter experience. GU ASCO Symposium. Orlando (FL), February 18, 2011.

66. Albadine R, Wang W, Brownlee NA, et al. Topoisomerase II alpha status in renal medullary carcinoma: immuno-expression and gene copy alterations of a potential target of therapy. J Urol 2009;182(2):735–40.

67. Schaeffer EM, Guzzo TJ, Furge KA, et al. Renal medullary carcinoma: molecular, pathological and clinical evidence for treatment with topoisomerase-inhibiting therapy. BJU Int 2010;106(1):62–5.

68. Cheng JX, Tretiakova M, Gong C, et al. Renal medullary carcinoma: rhabdoid features and the absence of INI1 expression as markers of aggressive behavior. Mod Pathol 2008;21(6):647–52.

69. Mariño-Enríquez A, Ou WB, Weldon CB, et al. ALK rearrangement in sickle cell trait-associated renal medullary carcinoma. Genes Chromosomes Cancer 2011;50(3): 146–53.

70. Heng DY, Choueiri TK. Non-clear cell renal cancer: features and medical management. J Natl Compr Canc Netw 2009;7:659–65.

71. Aghajanian C, Soignet S, Dizon DS, et al. A phase I trial of the novel proteasome inhibitor PS341 in advanced solid tumor malignancies. Clin Cancer Res 2002;8: 2505–11.

72. Kondagunta GV, Drucker B, Schwartz L, et al. Phase II trial of bortezomib for patients with advanced renal cell carcinoma. J Clin Oncol 2004;22:3720–5.

73. Ronnen EA, Kondagunta GV, Motzer RJ. Medullary renal cell carcinoma and response to therapy with bortezomib. J Clin Oncol 2006;24:e14.

74. Ansari J, Fatima A, Chaudhri S, et al. Sorafenib induces therapeutic response in a patient with metastatic collecting duct carcinoma of kidney. Onkologie 2009;32: 44–6.

75. MacLennan GT, Farrow GM, Bostwick DG. Low-grade collecting duct carcinoma of the kidney: report of 13 cases of low-grade mucinous tubulocystic renal carcinoma of possible collecting duct origin. Urology 1997;50:679–84.

76. Cossu-Rocca P, Eble JN, Delahunt B, et al. Renal mucinous tubular and spindle carcinoma lacks the gains of chromosomes 7 and 17 and losses of chromosome Y that are prevalent in papillary renal cell carcinoma. Mod Pathol 2006;19:488–93.

77. Amin MB, MacLennan GT, Gupta R, et al. Tubulocystic carcinoma of the kidney clinicopathologic analysis of 31 cases of a distinctive rare subtype of renal cell carcinoma. Am J Surg Pathol 2009;33:384–92.

78. Mego M, Sycova-Mila Z, Rejlekova K, et al. Expand+sunitinib in the treatment of tubulocystic carcinoma of the kidney. A case report. Ann Oncol 2008;19(9):1655–6.

79. Argani P, Ladanyi M. Translocation carcinoma of the kidney. Clin Lab Med 2005; 25:363–78.

80. Camparo P, Vasiliu V, Molinie V, et al. Renal translocation carcinomas—clinicopathologic, immunohistochemical and gene expression profiling analysis of 31 cases with a review of the literature. Am J Surg Pathol 2008;35:656–70.

81. Argani P, Lal P, Hutchinson B, et al. Aberrant nuclear immunoreactivity for TFE3 in neoplasms with TFE3 gene fusions: a sensitive and specific immunohistochemical assay. Am J Surg Pathol 2003;27:750–61.

82. Choueiri TK, Lim ZD, Hirsch MS, et al. Vascular endothelial growth factor-targeted therapy for the treatment of adult metastatic Xp11.2 translocation renal cell carcinoma. Cancer 2010;116:5219–25.

83. Malouf GG, Camparo P, Oudard S, et al. Targeted agents in metastatic Xp11 translocation/TFE3 gene fusion renal cell carcinoma (RCC): a report from the Juvenile RCC Network. Ann Oncol 2010;21:1834–8.

84. Dhillon J, Tannir NM, Matin SF, et al. Thyroid-like follicular carcinoma of the kidney with metastases to the lungs and retroperitoneal lymph nodes. Hum Pathol 2011; 42:146–50.

85. Mian BM, Bhadkamkar N, Slaton JW, et al. Prognostic factors and survival of patients with sarcomatoid renal cell carcinoma. J Urol 2002;167:65–70.

86. Abel EJ, Culp SH, Matin SF, et al. Percutaneous biopsy of primary tumor in metastatic renal cell carcinoma to predict high risk pathological features: comparison with nephrectomy assessment. J Urol 2010;184:1877–81.

87. Shuch B, Said J, La Rochelle JC, et al. Cytoreductive nephrectomy for kidney cancer with sarcomatoid histology—is up-front resection indicated and, if not, is it avoidable? J Urol 2009;182:2164–71.

88. Golshayan AR, George S, Heng DY, et al. Metastatic sarcomatoid renal cell carcinoma treated with vascular endothelial growth factor-targeted therapy. J Clin Oncol 2009;27:235–41.
89. Escudier B, Droz JP, Rolland F, et al. Doxorubicin and ifosfamide in patients with metastatic sarcomatoid renal cell carcinoma: a phase II study of the Genitourinary Group of the French Federation of Cancer Centers. J Urol 2002;168:959–61.
90. Nanus DM, Garino A, Milowsky MI, et al. Active chemotherapy for sarcomatoid and rapidly progressing renal cell carcinoma. Cancer 2004;101:1545–51.
91. Dutcher JP, Nanus D. Long-term survival of patients with sarcomatoid renal cell cancer treated with chemotherapy. Med Oncol 2010. [Epub ahead of print].
92. Haas N, Manola J, Pins M. ECOG 8802: Phase II trial of doxorubicin and gemcitabine in metastatic renal cell carcinoma with sarcomatoid features. 2009 ASCO Genitourinary Cancers Symposium. Orlando (FL) [abstract: 285].
93. Michaelson M. Combination sunitinib and gemcitabine in sarcomatoid and/or poor-risk patients with metastatic renal cell carcinoma. NCT00556049.
94. Pagliaro L. Capecitabine, gemcitabine, and bevacizumab in combination for patients with sarcomatoid renal cell carcinoma. NCT00496587.

Clinical and Molecular Prognostic Factors in Renal Cell Carcinoma: What We Know So Far

Patricia A. Tang, MD, FRCPC, Michael M. Vickers, MD, FRCPC,
Daniel Y.C. Heng, MD, MPH, FRCPC*

KEYWORDS

- Renal cell carcinoma • Prognostic factors • Predictive factors
- Biomarkers

Before the advent of molecular targeted therapy, treatment of metastatic renal cell carcinoma (mRCC) involved immunotherapy with high-dose interleukin (IL)-2 in selected patients, interferon-α, and cytoreductive nephrectomy.[1–5] Current standard therapies focus on inhibiting angiogenesis via the vascular endothelial growth factor (VEGF) pathway (sorafenib, sunitinib, pazopanib, and bevacizumab)[6–10] or the mammalian target of rapamycin (mTOR) pathway (temsirolimus and everolimus).[11–13] The treatment landscape of mRCC is rapidly evolving, thus predictive and prognostic factors must be continuously evaluated to reflect advances in systemic therapy.

A prognostic factor provides information about the patient's overall disease outcome independent of any specific intervention.[14] A predictive factor provides information about the probability of benefit or toxicity from a specific intervention.[14] Many clinical prognostic factors remain unchanged; however, a myriad of biomarkers surrounding angiogenesis is emerging. Although most require prospective validation, they offer promising insights into diagnosis, predicting response to therapy, and prognostication of overall survival. These biomarkers are key elements that allow clinicians to potentially individualize cancer therapy, compare and risk-stratify patients in clinical trials, and accurately counsel patients on the status of their disease. This review discusses important findings in the realm of predictive and prognostic factors that are both clinical and laboratory based.

The authors have nothing to disclose.
Department of Oncology, Tom Baker Cancer Center, University of Calgary, 1331-29th Street North West, Calgary, AB, Canada T2N 4N2
* Corresponding author.
E-mail address: daniel.heng@albertahealthservices.ca

Hematol Oncol Clin N Am 25 (2011) 871–891
doi:10.1016/j.hoc.2011.04.003
0889-8588/11/$ – see front matter © 2011 Elsevier Inc. All rights reserved.

CLINICAL PROGNOSTIC FACTORS

Prognostic factors have been derived from patients treated in clinical trials as well as retrospective population-based databases, with survival as the primary end point. There are 4 general groups of prognostic factors: those associated with patient status, tumor burden, proinflammatory markers, and treatment-related factors (**Table 1**). Many of these have been combined in multivariable analysis to enable discrimination between those who have a favorable, intermediate, and poor prognosis (**Tables 2** and **3**).

Patient Factors

In a review of mRCC patients treated with IL-2–based immunotherapy after nephrectomy, survival was negatively affected by the presence of constitutional symptoms such as weight loss, decreased appetite, musculoskeletal pain, sweats, rashes, and respiratory and gastrointestinal symptoms.[15] Poor performance status, as assessed by Eastern Cooperative Oncology Group (ECOG) or Karnofsky Performance Status (KPS) scales, is consistently associated with shortened overall survival for patients after nephrectomy, as well as in the metastatic setting.[16–21]

Tumor Burden

Patients with greater than one site of metastases,[17,20,22] no prior nephrectomy,[19,22] and bone metastases have an associated poorer prognosis.[20,23] Other markers of increased tumor burden are also associated with worse overall survival. These markers include elevated lactate dehydrogenase (LDH) due to high cell turnover, anemia, hypercalcemia due to bone metastases or paraneoplastic syndromes,[16–20,22] and hyponatremia due to syndrome of inappropriate antidiuretic hormone secretion (eg, due to brain or pulmonary metastases) or paraneoplastic syndromes.[24,25] The interval between diagnosis and the development or treatment of metastatic disease, also known as the disease-free interval (DFI), is inversely linked to prognosis, as it is an indirect measure of indolent versus aggressive disease.[17,18,26–28]

Proinflammatory Markers

Markers of inflammation such as elevated erythrocyte sedimentation rate (ESR) and C-reactive protein (CRP) have been linked to decreased overall survival in retrospective

Table 1	
Prognostic factors in advanced renal cell carcinoma	
Category	**Prognostic Factor**
Patient-related factors	Symptoms Performance status
Tumor burden	Site and or number of metastatic sites Alkaline phosphatase Hyponatremia Lactate dehydrogenase Anemia Hypercalcemia Disease-free interval
Proinflammatory markers	Erythrocyte sedimentation rate C reactive protein Neutrophilia Thrombocytosis
Treatment	Cytoreductive nephrectomy

Table 2
Comparison of multivariate prognostic-factor models in renal cell carcinoma

Model	MSKCC Motzer et al[18]	UISS Zisman et al[21]	Groupe Français d'Immunothérapie[28]	Heng et al[16]	Patil et al[20]	Choueiri et al[26]
Patient population	463 patients treated with interferon-α on prospective clinical trials	Prospective cohort of 814 patients who underwent nephrectomy (Stage I–IV patients)	782 patients treated with immunotherapy on trials	645 patients treated with sunitinib, sorafenib, or bevacizumab at multiple North American centers	375 patients treated with sunitinib from an RCT	120 patients treated with bevacizumab, sorafenib, sunitinib, or axitinib on prospective clinical trials at a single center
Common prognostic factors compared with Motzer criteria	KPS <80% LDH >1.5× ULN Corrected calcium >10 mg/dL (2.5 mmol/L) Hemoglobin < LLN Disease-free interval <1 y	ECOG PS	ECOG PS Hemoglobin < LLN Disease-free-interval <1 y	KPS <80% Corrected calcium > ULN Hemoglobin < LLN Disease-free interval <1 y	ECOG status LDH > ULN Corrected calcium > ULN Hemoglobin < LLN Disease-free-interval <1 y	ECOG status Corrected calcium <8.5 mg/dL or >10 mg/dL Disease-free-interval <2 y
Significant prognostic factors specific to model		Fuhrman histologic grade 1997 TNM staging	Number of metastatic sites SR ≥100 or CRP ≥50	Neutrophils > ULN Platelets > ULN	Bone metastases	Neutrophils >4500/µL Platelets >300,000/µL

Abbreviations: CRP, C-reactive protein; ECOG PS, Eastern Cooperative Group performance status; KPS, Karnofsky performance status; LDH, lactate dehydrogenase; LLN, lower limit of normal; MSKCC, Memorial Sloan Kettering Cancer Center; SR, sedimentation rate; TNM, Tumor Node Metastasis; ULN, upper limit of normal.

Table 3
Summary of evidence for selected molecular biomarkers in renal cell carcinoma

Biomarker	Method	Role in Renal Cell Cancer	Comments
VHL alterations	Mutations: PCR, SSCP, sequencing Promoter hypermethylation: methylation-specific PCR	Conflicting evidence regarding role as prognostic factor Conflicting evidence regarding role as a predictive of response to targeted therapies	Larger studies focusing on VHL mutations with functional significance required to clarify prognostic and predictive role
HIF-1α	IHC	Conflicting evidence regarding role as prognostic factor Not predictive of response to interferon-α or temsirolimus	Nuclear and cytoplasmic staining should be assessed
	Western blot	Predictive: high levels of HIF-1α or HIF-2α associated with increased response rate to sunitinib (n = 43)	Larger studies needed
VEGF-A	ELISA	Potentially prognostic: high VEGF associated with poor OS Baseline levels not predictive of response to sunitinib, sorafenib, pazopanib, or bevacizumab plus interferon	Further work is required to define cut point between high and low VEGF and significant changes in VEGF
	SNP	Predictive: VEGFA −1154 AA genotype (vs GG) associated with poor OS for patients treated with pazopanib (n = 241) but not for sunitinib (n = 63)	Confirmatory prospective trials needed
CAIX	IHC	Prognostic role unclear in patients who had nephrectomy Predictive role not established for targeted therapy	Cutpoint of ≤85% for low versus >85% for high, established using survival tree analysis[75] Caveat: CAIX expression in metastatic lesions may not be representative of primary tumors Larger studies needed

mTOR pathway	IHC	PTEN not predictive, prognostic role unclear PS6 expression predictive of response to temsirolimus in one small study	pAkt difficult to measure from paraffin-embedded tissue
B7-H1	IHC	Prognostic: positive expression associated with shorter survival in patients who had nephrectomy for clear cell RCC	Predictive studies needed, especially in patients receiving PD-1 inhibitors
STAT3	SNP	Polymorphism in 5' region of STAT3, rs4796793, predictive of response to interferon-α in one small study	Larger studies needed in different ethnic populations
NGAL	N/A	High NGAL levels associated with worse PFS for patients on sunitinib (unclear if prognostic or predictive)	NGAL threshold of 110 ng/mL needs to be validated in larger studies
IMP3	IHC	Prognostic: positive expression associated with shorter survival	Predictive studies needed
Thymidylate synthetase expression	mRNA	Predictive: low expression associated with improved PFS in cytokine refractory Japanese mRCC patients treated with S-1 (n = 45)	Should be evaluated as a predictive marker in future trials of S-1

Abbreviations: CAIX, carbonic anhydrase IX; ELISA, enzyme-linked immunosorbent assay; IHC, immunohistochemistry; N/A, not available; OS, overall survival; PFS, progression-free survival; PCR, polymerase chain reaction; PD-1, programmed death-1; PTEN, phosphatase and tensin homolog; RCC, renal cell cancer; SSCP, single-strand conformation polymorphism; SNP, single-nucleotide polymorphism; VHL, Von Hippel-Lindau; VEGF, vascular endothelial growth factor.

and prospective series.[28–31] ESR and CRP have yet to be evaluated as prognostic factors in patients treated with targeted therapy. Neutrophilia is a poor prognostic factor for patients treated with antiangiogenic drugs in two multivariable prognostic-factor models [16,26] but not in immunotherapy models.[17,18,28] Although thrombocytosis is rare in patients with mRCC, its presence is associated with worse outcomes in some series.[16,26,32] Thrombocytosis may be related to production of interleukin-6 and other growth factors by the tumor.[33] In addition, platelet granules contain proangiogenic factors, which may promote tumor growth.[34,35]

Treatment-Related Factors

For patients who present with metastatic disease and good performance status, performing cytoreductive nephrectomy prior to interferon-α therapy improves survival compared with interferon-α alone in two randomized studies.[2,5]

Multivariable Prognostic Models

In light of the plethora of prognostic factors, multivariable models have been created to classify patients into poor, intermediate, and favorable risk groups for use in the clinic as well as in clinical trials (see **Table 2**). For Stage I to IV patients, the University of California Los Angeles integrated staging system (UISS) is the most widely studied prognostic model[21] that correlates with postnephrectomy outcomes. The Mayo Clinic metastases-free survival score (SSIGN) was derived from analysis of 1671 patients who had a nephrectomy for clear-cell RCC (ccRCC),[15] and subsequently was externally validated.[36,37] Multivariate analysis revealed development of metastases was significantly associated with tumor stage, regional lymph node status, tumor size, nuclear grade, and histologic tumor necrosis ($P<.001$ for all).[15]

In the era of immunotherapy, the most well known and used prognostic model for mRCC was developed at the Memorial Sloan-Kettering Cancer Center (MSKCC) by Motzer and colleagues[18,19] (see **Table 2**). This model stratified patients based on the number of risk factors: favorable risk (no risk factors), intermediate risk (1 risk factor), and poor risk (2–3 risk factors), with median overall survival times of 22.1 months, 12 months, and 5 months, respectively. The Groupe Français d'Immunotherapie derived a slightly different model based on 782 patients treated with immunotherapy on clinical trials (see **Table 2**).[28] The MSKCC prognostic criteria were externally validated and expanded at the Cleveland Clinic[17]; thus it became the standard prognostic-factor model for patients with metastatic disease.

Additional prognostic-factor models have been created, based on mRCC patients treated with angiogenesis inhibitors and internally validated (see **Table 2**).[16,20,26] These models are similar to the original MSKCC criteria. Two of the models did not observe an association between overall survival and LDH, and both these models found that neutrophilia and thrombocytosis were prognostic.[16,26] The Heng criteria were derived from a large population-based database that segregated patients into 3 risk categories: favorable risk (no risk factors, median overall survival not reached), intermediate risk (1–2 risk factors, median overall survival 27 months), and poor risk (3 or more risk factors, median overall survival 8.8 months) (**Fig. 1**).[16] Formal comparison of these angiogenesis-era models are under way. In the phase 3 trial evaluating temsirolimus, Hudes and colleagues[11] defined poor-prognosis mRCC as the presence of at least 3 of the MSKCC criteria (see **Table 2**),[18] KPS of 60 to 70, or metastases in multiple organs. Thus, some patients in the trial would have been considered intermediate risk by strict MSKCC criteria.[18] At present, angiogenesis-era models are also used to classify patients treated with mTOR inhibitors.

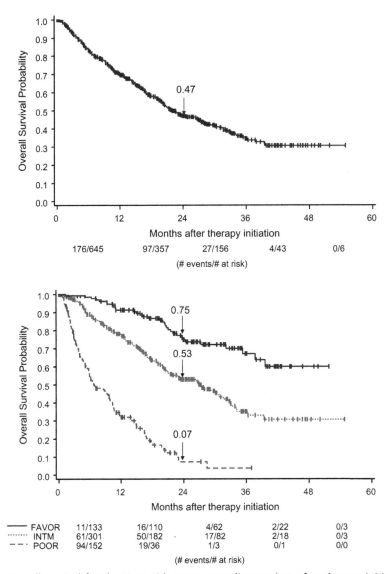

Fig. 1. Overall survival for the Heng risk group according to time after therapy initiation. FAVOR, favorable risk; INTM, intermediate risk; POOR, poor risk. (*Modified from* Heng D, Xie W, Regan M, et al. Prognostic factors for overall survival with metastatic renal cell carcinoma treated with vascular endothelial growth factor-targeted agents: results form a large, multicentre study. J Clin Oncol 2009;27:5794. Copyright © 2009 American Society of Clinical Oncology; with permission.)

These multivariable models are often used to analyze outcomes from clinical trials to determine the magnitude of benefit from novel therapies across the favorable, intermediate, and poor prognosis risk groups. It appears that all risk groups benefit from targeted therapies in prospective trials and retrospective population-based analyses.[6–8,11–13,38] In the pivotal trial that demonstrated the superiority of sunitinib compared with interferon-α in mRCC, subgroup analyses revealed a significant benefit in progression-free survival (PFS) in the favorable and intermediate MSKCC risk groups.[8] The poor risk group had too few patients to detect a difference in this phase 3 trial[8]; however, in a retrospective population-based analysis there appeared to be benefit in all risk groups.[38] Thus, these prognostic-factor models are useful in estimating overall survival but may not be predictive of treatment benefit.

BIOMARKERS IN RENAL CELL CARCINOMA

A biomarker is a characteristic that can be objectively measured and evaluated as an indicator of a normal biological process, pathogenic process, or pharmacologic response to treatment.[39] A variety of biomarkers has been evaluated in patients with RCC with the goal of individualizing cancer care and improving on the clinical prognostic-factor models. Markers associated with hypoxia and angiogenesis have been evaluated, for example, the Von Hippel-Lindau (VHL) pathway, hypoxia-inducible factor (HIF), VEGF family, carbonic anhydrase IX (CAIX), and the mammalian target of rapamycin (mTOR) pathway. Other promising markers include immune regulators, neutrophil gelatinase-associated lipocalin (NGAL), IMP3, thymidylate synthetase, and molecular expression profiling.

Von Hippel-Lindau Pathway

VHL is a tumor-suppressor gene located on chromosome 3p25 that encodes a gene product (pVHL).[40] The VHL pathway plays a crucial role in adaptation to hypoxia (**Fig. 2**), and functional loss of pVHL has been implicated in hereditary and sporadic ccRCC.[40] In the absence of VHL, HIF is able to activate many downstream signaling pathways associated with angiogenesis, as detailed in **Fig. 2**.

Von Hippel-Lindau Alterations

The frequency of VHL mutations in sporadic RCC has been estimated to be more than 42%.[41–46] VHL mutations can occur via frameshift deletions/insertions, missense and nonsense mutations, loss of heterozygosity (LOH), and VHL promoter methylation.[47] Exploration into the prognostic role of VHL gene mutation has produced conflicting results. Several groups have failed to demonstrate a relationship between VHL genetic alterations and survival.[44,48,49] Others have suggested that VHL inactivation is associated with a more favorable outcome.[50,51] Conversely, other studies found that loss of function mutations were associated with worse clinical outcomes.[45,52] Thus the prognostic value of VHL gene mutation is not clear. Loss of function of pVHL is thought to be an early step in the carcinogenesis that is followed by further genetic alterations[53]; this may account for the lack of impact on prognosis. This area of study is limited by the available technology able to identify mutations or alterations in promoter methylation, as well as the possible influence of missense mutations that may not have functional significance.

Investigation into VHL mutation as a predictive factor has lagged behind the development of targeted therapy. In the realm of immunotherapy, a small study of patients with VHL alteration (n = 16) did not reveal any association with response to immunotherapy.[52] Choueiri and colleagues[54] evaluated VHL gene status in 123 patients with metastatic ccRCC who were treated with antiangiogenic therapies. Patients with loss-of-function mutations had higher response rates than those with wild-type VHL (relative risk [RR] 52% vs 31%, respectively; $P = .04$) and loss-of-function mutation was validated on multivariate analysis as an independent predictor of response. PFS and overall survival were not significantly influenced by VHL gene status or loss-of-function mutations, although at the time of publication only 40% of patients had died, making the survival data somewhat immature. VHL alterations were not associated with benefit from treatment with axitinib (n = 13),[55] pazopanib (n = 63),[56] or temsirolimus (n = 16).[57] Prospective studies involving large, well-defined patient cohorts with standardized laboratory analysis are needed to further clarify this issue.

Hypoxia-Inducible Factor

HIF has been evaluated as a prognostic factor using immunohistochemistry (IHC) on tissue microarrays (TMAs). High cytoplasmic HIF-1α expression was associated with a trend toward improved survival by Lidgren and colleagues[58] (n = 176 ccRCC); conversely, it was associated with significantly shorter survival in a smaller series analyzed by Dorevic and colleagues[59] (n = 94). High nuclear HIF-1α expression (>35%) was associated with worse survival by Klatte and colleagues[60] (n = 357), whereas Dorevic and colleagues found that it was associated with better survival. Patel and colleagues[61] evaluated pretreatment HIF levels by Western analysis in 43 mRCC patients treated with sunitinib. The presence of high levels of HIF-1α ($P = .003$) or HIF-2α ($P = .001$) was associated with a higher likelihood of response. Figlin and colleagues[62] analyzed IHC expression of HIF-1α and HIF-2α in a subset of patients with available archival paraffin-embedded tumor samples from Hudes' randomized phase 3 trial of temsirolimus, interferon-α, or the combination, in advanced RCC with poor prognostic factors.[11] Results for HIF-2α were not analyzed due to heterogeneous HIF-2α staining.[62] There was no correlation between baseline HIF-1α levels with survival or response. At this time, the prognostic value of HIF-1α remains unclear.

Vascular Endothelial Growth Factor Family

The VEGF family includes multiple ligands (VEGF-A, B, C, D, and platelet-derived growth factor) as well as 3 tyrosine kinase receptors (VEGFR-1, 2, 3), which are part of the signaling pathways for angiogenesis and/or lymphangiogenesis. Given the intrinsic role of angiogenesis in the pathophysiology of RCC, a better understanding of these markers is expected to reveal important information about outcomes and therapeutic efficacy.

Patients with RCC have higher serum VEGF levels compared with healthy controls.[63] On multivariate analysis, VEGF levels are not associated with overall survival in RCC patients treated with nephrectomy (n = 164).[63]

For metastatic patients treated with immunotherapy, the results are conflicting. A study of 138 patients found no association (n = 138)[64]; however, serum VEGF was an independent prognostic factor in a larger study of 302 patients.[65] The TARGET phase 3 trial, which randomized patients with mRCC to sorafenib or placebo, analyzed baseline VEGF levels in 712 patients.[66] Higher VEGF levels significantly correlated with worse MSKCC score ($P<.0001$) and worse ECOG performance status ($P<.0001$). On multivariate analysis, higher baseline VEGF was an independent poor prognostic factor for PFS in the placebo arm, as well as overall survival for patients treated with placebo and sorafenib.

Baseline VEGF levels were not predictive of response from sorafenib in the TARGET trial,[66] bevacizumab in the phase 3 AVOREN trial,[67] the phase 2 trial of pazopanib,[56] or patients treated with sunitinib.[68,69]

Multiplatform Analysis

In a larger set of patients treated with pazopanib (n = 215), plasma levels of candidate markers (HGF, IL-6, IL-8, E-selectin, and VEGF) were assessed using 3 different platforms.[70] Results from the 3 platforms were highly correlated and VEGF levels

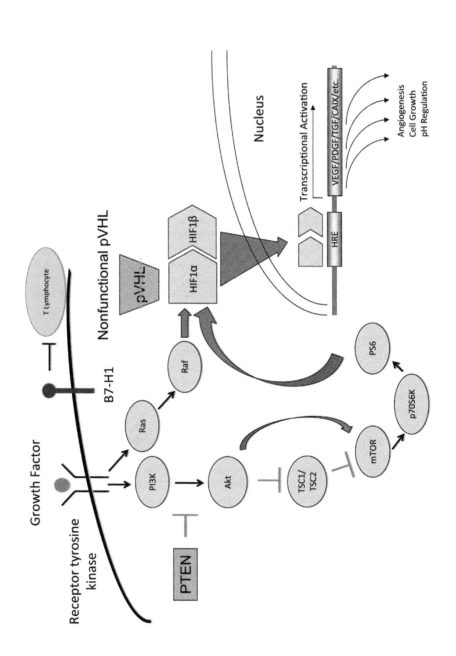

were not predictive. Lower baseline levels of HGF, IL-8, and IL-6 were significantly correlated with tumor shrinkage. Elevated levels of E-selectin, and lower levels of IL-6 and HGF were correlated with longer PFS. Large prospective trials are required to clarify the predictive role of these biomarkers.

Single-Nucleotide Polymorphism Analysis

Genomic DNA from 63 patients treated with sunitinib was analyzed by Kim and colleagues for single-nucleotide polymorphisms (SNPs) in VEGF (−2578, −1154, 936, −634) and VEGFR2 (889 and 1416). VEGF SNP 936 was associated with tumor shrinkage, and VEGFR2 SNPs were correlated with survival.[71,72] Recently, Xu and colleagues[73] analyzed 27 functional polymorphisms in angiogenesis and exposure-related genes from 241 patients treated with pazopanib. Polymorphisms in IL-8, FGFR2, VEGF (1154), FLT4, and NR112 were associated with overall survival ($P \leq .05$). SNPs show promising potential as predictive and prognostic biomarkers, and further studies with larger numbers of patients are warranted.

Carbonic Anhydrase IX

CAIX is a transmembrane enzyme that might maintain a normal pH in hypoxic tumor cells, thereby fostering cancer growth and metastasis.[74] CAIX expression, as assessed by IHC, is present in 94% to 97% of ccRCC.[75,76] Bui and colleagues[75] found that low CAIX expression ($\leq$85%) was associated with worse overall survival for mRCC, but not for patients with localized disease using tissue microarrays (TMAs). Conversely, Sandlund and colleagues[77] found that low CAIX expression was associated with poor prognosis in patients with Stage I to III disease, but not in patients with mRCC. Leibovich and colleagues[76] conducted the largest retrospective study to date (n = 730) and found that low CAIX expression ($\leq$85%) was not a significant prognostic factor on multivariate analysis. Leibovich's group analyzed CAIX expression from whole tissue sections and noted significant intratumoral heterogeneity. Bui and colleagues[75] observed that metastatic lesions had significantly lower CAIX staining levels compared with matched primary specimens; however, only 15 cases were analyzed. Thus, metastatic lesions may not be representative of the primary tumor. It is uncertain whether CAIX is a prognostic factor for RCC.

Tumor CAIX expression has also been evaluated as a predictive factor for patients with mRCC. Retrospective analyses suggested that high CAIX expression (>85%) was predictive of response to IL-2.[75,78] A small study evaluated the impact of CAIX expression (IHC) and SNPs on outcomes of patients treated with IL-2 (n = 54).[79] There was no association between SNPs and CAIX expression. The C allele variant of CA9 SNP rs12553173 and high CAIX expression (>85%) were both associated with increased response rates to IL-2, and were independent prognostic factors for overall survival.[79]

Fig. 2. Molecular pathways evaluated as biomarkers in renal cell cancer. Receptor tyrosine kinases are activated through ligand binding, leading to recruitment of phosphoinositol-3-kinase (PI3K) and activation of Akt. This step is inhibited by phosphatase and tensin homolog (PTEN). Akt inactivates tuberous sclerosis complex (TSC)1/2, resulting in constitutive activation of mammalian target of rapamycin (mTOR). This leads to activation of p70S6 kinase (p70S6K), which phosphorylates the 40S ribosomal S6 protein (PS6). PS6 leads to upregulation of hypoxia inducible factor (HIF)-1α. Loss of function of the von Hippel-Lindau gene product (pVHL) allows HIF-1α to bind to HIF-1β. This complex translocates to the nucleus to activate HIF-responsive elements (HRE). This leads to transcription of genes important in angiogenesis, growth, and pH regulation. B7-H1 is a negative regulator of anti-tumoral T-cell mediated immunity.

Conversely, in the prospective phase 2 SELECT trial, there was a trend toward higher response rates to IL-2 in patients with low CAIX ($\leq$85%) compared with high CAIX (RR 38% vs 23%, $P = .13$).[80]

Choueiri and colleagues[81] evaluated tumor CAIX expression (IHC) in 94 patients treated with antiangiogenic therapies. CAIX expression was neither prognostic nor predictive of response to sunitinib. For sorafenib-treated patients, high CAIX expression (>85%) was associated with more tumor shrinkage compared with low CAIX expression (mean difference -22%). An analysis of 20 patients from a randomized phase 2 trial of temsirolimus in mRCC showed that CAIX expression (IHC) was not predictive of response.[57] Further studies are required to evaluate CAIX as a predictive factor.

VHL Pathway Analysis

Analysis of VHL mutation status as well as plasma CAIX, VEGF, sVEGFR2, tissue inhibitor of metalloproteinase 1 (TIMP-1), and Ras p21 was performed in the TARGET trial of sorafenib versus placebo in advanced RCC.[82] On multivariate analysis that included ECOG performance status, MSKCC score, and the biomarkers assayed, only baseline TIMP-1 levels were prognostic for survival ($P = .002$). However, baseline TIMP-1 levels were available for only 123 patients. No predictive markers were identified.

Mammalian Target of Rapamycin Pathway

The mTOR pathway is downstream of the phosphoinositide-3-kinase (PI3K) and Akt pathway that is regulated by the phosphatase and tensin homolog (PTEN) tumor suppressor gene (see **Fig. 2**). Mutations in PTEN have not been found in RCC; however, diminished protein expression with increased levels of phosphoAkt (pAkt) have been observed.[83] Activation of the mTOR pathway leads to activation of p70 S6 kinase (p70S6K), which phosphorylates the 40S ribosomal S6 protein (PS6) and upregulates HIF-1 gene expression. In patients with VHL mutations, mTOR activation can potentiate expression of HIF-inducible genes and promote cancer progression.[84] PTEN, p70SK, and PS6 have been evaluated as pharmacodynamic markers of mTOR inhibition with temsirolimus (CCI-779) and everolimus (RAD001).

In vivo experiments have demonstrated that p70S6K inhibition by temsirolimus[85] and everolimus[86] are similar in peripheral blood mononuclear cells (PBMC) and tumor tissue. In 9 RCC patients treated with temsirolimus, there was a significant linear association between p70S6K activity inhibition in PBMCs (24 hours after treatment) and time to progression.[85] The recommended phase 2 dose of everolimus was based on a pharmacokinetic/pharmacodynamic model using PBMC p70S6K inhibition.[86] As mentioned previously, Cho and colleagues[57] examined expression of CAIX, PS6, pAkt, and PTEN in paraffin-embedded tissue sections from 20 patients with advanced RCC treated with temsirolimus in a phase 2 clinical trial. These investigators found a positive association between PS6 expression ($P = .02$) and a trend toward positive expression of pAkt ($P = .07$) with objective response to temsirolimus. These results are early and require further evaluation.

Immune Regulators

Inhibition of T-cell mediated immunity has been shown to impair a host's ability to generate a productive immune response against cancer. The B7 family consists of coregulatory molecules that inhibit T-cell mediated immunity.[87] These molecules are normally present on monocyte-derived cells; however, aberrant expression has been linked to poor prognosis in RCC (see **Table 3**).[88,89] Tumoral B7-H1 expression, as determined by IHC, has been evaluated in patients who underwent nephrectomy for ccRCC in a series of 196 fresh-frozen as well as 306 paraffin-embedded specimens.[89,90] Positive expression of B7-H1 was associated with increased risk of death on multivariate analysis in both studies.[89] Krambeck and colleagues[88] analyzed tumoral B7-H4 expression using IHC on 259 fresh-frozen RCC nephrectomy specimens. Positive tumor B7-H4 expression was associated with an increased risk of cancer-related mortality on univariate analysis; however, this was not statistically significant after adjusting for SSIGN score.[15] Cancer-specific survival rates were significantly lower for patients with coexpression of B7-H1 and B7-H4 on multivariate analysis after adjusting for SSIGN score ($P<.001$). This result suggests that B7-H1 and B7-H4 may abrogate immune responses against RCC and that therapies that stimulate T-cell mediated immunity may be beneficial in RCC.

Signal transducer and activator 3 (STAT3) is a ligand-induced transcription factor[91] that is activated in response to growth factors and cytokines, and is an important contributor to impaired antitumor immunity.[92] Ito and colleagues[93] analyzed 463 SNPs in 33 candidate genes from 75 Japanese patients treated with interferon-α for mRCC, and found that a STAT3 polymorphism was the most significant predictor of response (odds ratio 2.73). This work underscores the importance of the immune system in cytokine-based therapy for RCC, but has not been validated in other ethnic populations.

Neutrophil Gelatinase-Associated Lipocalin

Another potential predictive biomarker for patients with mRCC treated with sunitinib is NGAL. NGAL is an acute-phase protein linked to metalloproteinase-9 (MMP-9), which is involved in the degradation of the extracellular matrix, invasion, and metastasis.[94] This protein induces a survival response[95] and is upregulated in several human cancers (for a recent review see Ref.[96]). NGAL expression is present in clear-cell, papillary, and chromophobe RCCs.[97] Porta and colleagues[98] evaluated MSKCC score,[18] baseline plasma VEGF, and NGAL titers in 85 patients with advanced RCC treated with sunitinib. On univariate analysis, baseline VEGF and NGAL were significant predictors of PFS, whereas MSKCC score was not. Patients with NGAL levels above 177 ng/mL had an RR of progressing of 1.86 (95% confidence interval [CI]: 1.142–3.019; $P = .03$) and a median PFS of 3.35 months (95% CI: 2.3–10.9) compared with 8.15 months (95% CI: 5.5–11.6) in patients with NGAL levels below this threshold. After adjusting the NGAL threshold to 110 ng/mL, both VEGF and NGAL maintained significance on bivariate and multivariate analysis. This study is another showing that baseline VEGF levels have prognostic potential and that molecular markers can outperform a clinical score (MSKCC score). The NGAL threshold established by this study requires external validation.

IMP3

IMP3 is a member of the insulin-like growth factor II (IGF-II) mRNA-binding protein family that is thought to regulate the production of IGF-II. It is expressed during embryogenesis, but its expression is virtually absent in normal adult tissues. Jiang and colleagues[99] analyzed IMP3 IHC expression in 371 patients with localized primary RCC tumors. IMP3 status (positive vs negative) was a significant independent prognostic factor for overall survival, hazard ratio 4.01 (95% CI: 2.66–6.05; $P<.0001$), after multivariate adjustment for age, sex, tumor size, stage, grade, and histology. Using the same criteria for IMP3 assessment, the prognostic value of IMP3 was externally validated by Hoffmann and colleagues.[100] IMP3 expression was present in 29.8% of ccRCC specimens (213/716). On multivariate analysis, positive IMP3 expression was associated with an increase in the risk of death from RCC (hazard ratio 1.42, $P<.024$). IMP3 has not been evaluated as a predictive marker.

Thymidylate Synthetase

S-1 is an oral combination of tegafur, a prodrug of fluorouracil (FU), and 2 other agents that act to maintain effective concentrations of FU in plasma and tumor while inhibiting the phosphorylation of FU in the gastrointestinal tract, minimizing gastrointestinal toxicity from FU.[101] S-1 is widely used in Asia. A phase 2 study of 45 Japanese patients with cytokine refractory mRCC demonstrated a 24.4% objective response rate.[102] Pharmacogenetic analysis of FU-related enzymes revealed that thymidylate synthetase (TS) expression was significantly lower in patients who responded to treatment ($P = .048$), and PFS was significantly longer in patients with TS mRNA levels below the median level ($P = .006$). There was no significant difference in response rate and overall survival between the low versus high TS group. No significant association was observed for the other FU-related enzymes that were analyzed. Intratumoral expression of TS mRNA is a promising predictive marker for benefit from S-1. FU-related gene polymorphisms should be evaluated prospectively in future randomized controlled trials of S-1 and in different ethnic populations.

Molecular Expression Profiling

Analysis of molecular expression profiles permits simultaneous measurement of thousands of genes to create a global picture of cellular function. Multiple groups have evaluated gene expression profiling in RCC, with variable results.[103–107] Rini and colleagues.[104] conducted the largest genomic study of 931 patients who underwent nephrectomy for localized ccRCC using reverse transcriptase quantitative polymerase chain reaction. From the 732 genes examined, they identified 16 genes significantly associated with relapse-free survival after adjustments for clinicopathological covariates and false discovery (hazard ratio 0.68–0.80). External validation of this promising prognostic multigene algorithm is warranted. Given the clinical utility of the 21-gene recurrence score for hormone receptor–positive, node-negative breast cancer (OncotypeDx),[108] gene expression profiling has the potential to aid in risk stratification in localized RCC as well. It is essential that investigators adhere to rigorous statistical methodology to control for multiple testing and to minimize bias.[109]

Biomarker Prognostic Models

The integration of multiple biomarkers and clinical variables into nomograms has the potential to provide more meaningful information on outcomes than either alone. Ki-67 is a marker of cell proliferation that has been associated with risk of cancer progression in multivariate ccRCC models.[110–112] Kim and colleagues[113] constructed a TMA from samples of 150 ccRCC patients and assessed IHC expression of 8 molecular markers: Ki67, p53, gelsolin, vimentin, epithelial cell adhesion molecule, CAIX, carbonic anhydrase XII, and PTEN. A prognostic model including CAIX, PTEN, vimentin, p53, tumor stage, and performance status was significantly more accurate than the UISS.[21] Thus, analysis of several biomarkers permits evaluation of their relative prognostic utility. Parker and colleagues[114] derived another biomarker-based scoring system from 634 patients with ccRCC. This weighted algorithm (BioScore) integrated dichotomized expression of B7-H1, Ki-67, and survivin. Patients with high BioScores (>4) were 5 times more likely to die from RCC than those with low scores. In addition, the sequential use (as opposed to integration into a new model) of BioScore with existing clinicopathologic scoring systems (TNM, UISS, SSIGN) further enhanced the predictive ability compared with each of these scoring systems alone. Prospective validation of these biomarker prognostic models is required before routine clinical use can come about.

SUMMARY

Elucidation of prognostic and predictive molecular markers is the future challenge for improving outcomes of patients with mRCC. The additional obstacles for molecular markers are the development of a reproducible assay, assessment of baseline inter-patient and intrapatient variability, and derivation of threshold values that separate normal from abnormal.[14] Future prognostic biomarker studies should compare the performance of the putative marker with clinical prognostic models, such as the Heng criteria.[16] Incorporation of clinical and molecular models into prognostic models provides an unparalleled potential to provide information regarding a patient's disease trajectory. External validation is paramount for generalizability, due to the presence of biases that are difficult to quantify in study populations from single institutions.[115]

REFERENCES

1. Coppin C, Porzsolt F, Awa A, et al. Immunotherapy for advanced renal cell cancer. Cochrane Database Syst Rev 2005;1:CD001425.
2. Flanigan RC, Salmon SE, Blumenstein BA, et al. Nephrectomy followed by interferon alfa-2b compared with interferon alfa-2b alone for metastatic renal-cell cancer. N Engl J Med 2001;345:1655.
3. Fyfe G, Fisher RI, Rosenberg SA, et al. Results of treatment of 255 patients with metastatic renal cell carcinoma who received high-dose recombinant interleukin-2 therapy. J Clin Oncol 1995;13:688.
4. Klapper JA, Downey SG, Smith FO, et al. High-dose interleukin-2 for the treatment of metastatic renal cell carcinoma: a retrospective analysis of response and survival in patients treated in the surgery branch at the National Cancer Institute between 1986 and 2006. Cancer 2008;113:293.
5. Mickisch GH, Garin A, van Poppel H, et al. Radical nephrectomy plus interferon-alfa-based immunotherapy compared with interferon alfa alone in metastatic renal-cell carcinoma: a randomised trial. Lancet 2001;358:966.
6. Escudier B, Eisen T, Stadler WM, et al. Sorafenib in advanced clear-cell renal-cell carcinoma. N Engl J Med 2007;356:125.
7. Escudier B, Pluzanska A, Koralewski P, et al. Bevacizumab plus interferon alfa-2a for treatment of metastatic renal cell carcinoma: a randomised, double-blind phase III trial. Lancet 2007;370:2103.
8. Motzer RJ, Hutson TE, Tomczak P, et al. Sunitinib versus interferon alfa in metastatic renal-cell carcinoma. N Engl J Med 2007;356:115.
9. Rini BI, Halabi S, Rosenberg JE, et al. Phase III trial of bevacizumab plus interferon alfa versus interferon alfa monotherapy in patients with metastatic renal cell carcinoma: final results of CALGB 90206. J Clin Oncol 2010;28:2137.
10. Sternberg CN, Davis ID, Mardiak J, et al. Pazopanib in locally advanced or metastatic renal cell carcinoma: results of a randomized phase III trial. J Clin Oncol 2010;28:1061.
11. Hudes G, Carducci M, Tomczak P, et al. Temsirolimus, interferon alfa, or both for advanced renal-cell carcinoma. N Engl J Med 2007;356:2271.
12. Motzer RJ, Escudier B, Oudard S, et al. Phase 3 trial of everolimus for metastatic renal cell carcinoma: final results and analysis of prognostic factors. Cancer 2010;116:4256.

13. Motzer RJ, Escudier B, Oudard S, et al. Efficacy of everolimus in advanced renal cell carcinoma: a double-blind, randomised, placebo-controlled phase III trial. Lancet 2008;372:449.

14. Dancey JE, Dobbin KK, Groshen S, et al. Guidelines for the development and incorporation of biomarker studies in early clinical trials of novel agents. Clin Cancer Res 2010;16:1745.

15. Leibovich BC, Han KR, Bui MH, et al. Scoring algorithm to predict survival after nephrectomy and immunotherapy in patients with metastatic renal cell carcinoma. Cancer 2003;98:2566.

16. Heng DY, Xie W, Regan MM, et al. Prognostic factors for overall survival in patients with metastatic renal cell carcinoma treated with vascular endothelial growth factor-targeted agents: results from a large, multicenter study. J Clin Oncol 2009;27:5794.

17. Mekhail TM, Abou-Jawde RM, Boumerhi G, et al. Validation and extension of the Memorial Sloan-Kettering prognostic factors model for survival in patients with previously untreated metastatic renal cell carcinoma. J Clin Oncol 2005;23:832.

18. Motzer RJ, Bacik J, Murphy BA, et al. Interferon-alfa as a comparative treatment for clinical trials of new therapies against advanced renal cell carcinoma. J Clin Oncol 2002;20:289.

19. Motzer RJ, Mazumdar M, Bacik J, et al. Survival and prognostic stratification of 670 patients with advanced renal cell carcinoma. J Clin Oncol 1999;17:2530.

20. Patil S, Figlin RA, Hutson TE, et al. Prognostic factors for progression-free and overall survival with sunitinib targeted therapy and with cytokine as first-line therapy in patients with metastatic renal cell carcinoma. Ann Oncol 2011; 22:295.

21. Zisman A, Pantuck AJ, Dorey F, et al. Improved prognostication of renal cell carcinoma using an integrated staging system. J Clin Oncol 2001;19:1649.

22. Motzer RJ, Bukowski RM, Figlin RA, et al. Prognostic nomogram for sunitinib in patients with metastatic renal cell carcinoma. Cancer 2008;113:1552.

23. Royston P, Reitz M, Atzpodien J. An approach to estimating prognosis using fractional polynomials in metastatic renal carcinoma. Br J Cancer 2006;94:1785.

24. Jeppesen AN, Jensen HK, Donskov F, et al. Hyponatremia as a prognostic and predictive factor in metastatic renal cell carcinoma. Br J Cancer 2010;102:867.

25. Schutz FA, Xie W, Heng DY, et al. The effect of low serum sodium on treatment outcome to vascular endothelial growth factor (VEGF)-targeted therapy in metastatic renal cell carcinoma: results from a large international collaboration. J Clin Oncol 2011;29 [abstract: 322].

26. Choueiri TK, Garcia JA, Elson P, et al. Clinical factors associated with outcome in patients with metastatic clear-cell renal cell carcinoma treated with vascular endothelial growth factor-targeted therapy. Cancer 2007;110:543.

27. Elson PJ, Witte RS, Trump DL. Prognostic factors for survival in patients with recurrent or metastatic renal cell carcinoma. Cancer Res 1988;48:7310.

28. Negrier S, Escudier B, Gomez F, et al. Prognostic factors of survival and rapid progression in 782 patients with metastatic renal carcinomas treated by cytokines: a report from the Groupe Francais d'Immunotherapie. Ann Oncol 2002; 13:1460.

29. Atzpodien J, Royston P, Wandert T, et al. Metastatic renal carcinoma comprehensive prognostic system. Br J Cancer 2003;88:348.

30. Ljungberg B, Grankvist K, Rasmuson T. Serum acute phase reactants and prognosis in renal cell carcinoma. Cancer 1995;76:1435.

31. Ljungberg B, Landberg G, Alamdari FI. Factors of importance for prediction of survival in patients with metastatic renal cell carcinoma, treated with or without nephrectomy. Scand J Urol Nephrol 2000;34:246.
32. Suppiah R, Shaheen PE, Elson P, et al. Thrombocytosis as a prognostic factor for survival in patients with metastatic renal cell carcinoma. Cancer 2006;107:1793.
33. Hollen CW, Henthorn J, Koziol JA, et al. Serum interleukin-6 levels in patients with thrombocytosis. Leuk Lymphoma 1992;8:235.
34. Mohle R, Green D, Moore MA, et al. Constitutive production and thrombin-induced release of vascular endothelial growth factor by human megakaryo-cytes and platelets. Proc Natl Acad Sci U S A 1997;94:663.
35. O'Byrne KJ, Dobbs N, Propper D, et al. Vascular endothelial growth factor platelet counts, and prognosis in renal cancer. Lancet 1999;353:1494.
36. Ficarra V, Martignoni G, Lohse C, et al. External validation of the Mayo Clinic Stage, Size, Grade and Necrosis (SSIGN) score to predict cancer specific survival using a European series of conventional renal cell carcinoma. J Urol 2006;175:1235.
37. Fujii Y, Saito K, Iimura Y, et al. External validation of the Mayo Clinic cancer specific survival score in a Japanese series of clear cell renal cell carcinoma. J Urol 2008;180:1290.
38. Heng DY, Chi KN, Murray N, et al. A population-based study evaluating the impact of sunitinib on overall survival in the treatment of patients with metastatic renal cell cancer. Cancer 2009;115:776.
39. Biomarkers Definitions Working Group. Biomarkers and surrogate endpoints: preferred definitions and conceptual framework. Clin Pharmacol Ther 2001;69:89.
40. Seizinger BR, Rouleau GA, Ozelius LJ, et al. Von Hippel-Lindau disease maps to the region of chromosome 3 associated with renal cell carcinoma. Nature 1988;332:268.
41. Brauch H, Weirich G, Brieger J, et al. VHL alterations in human clear cell renal cell carcinoma: association with advanced tumor stage and a novel hot spot mutation. Cancer Res 1942;60:2000.
42. Gnarra JR, Tory K, Weng Y, et al. Mutations of the VHL tumour suppressor gene in renal carcinoma. Nat Genet 1994;7:85.
43. Herman JG, Latif F, Weng Y, et al. Silencing of the VHL tumor-suppressor gene by DNA methylation in renal carcinoma. Proc Natl Acad Sci U S A 1994;91:9700.
44. Kondo K, Yao M, Yoshida M, et al. Comprehensive mutational analysis of the VHL gene in sporadic renal cell carcinoma: relationship to clinicopathological parameters. Genes Chromosomes Cancer 2002;34:58.
45. Schraml P, Struckmann K, Hatz F, et al. VHL mutations and their correlation with tumour cell proliferation, microvessel density, and patient prognosis in clear cell renal cell carcinoma. J Pathol 2002;196:186.
46. Shuin T, Kondo K, Torigoe S, et al. Frequent somatic mutations and loss of heterozygosity of the von Hippel-Lindau tumor suppressor gene in primary human renal cell carcinomas. Cancer Res 1994;54:2852.
47. Kaelin WG Jr. The von Hippel-Lindau tumor suppressor protein and clear cell renal cell carcinoma. Clin Cancer Res 2007;13:680s.
48. Baldewijns MM, van Vlodrop IJ, Smits KM, et al. Different angiogenic potential in low and high grade sporadic clear cell renal cell carcinoma is not related to alterations in the von Hippel-Lindau gene. Cell Oncol 2009;31:371.

49. Smits KM, Schouten LJ, van Dijk BA, et al. Genetic and epigenetic alterations in the von Hippel-Lindau gene: the influence on renal cancer prognosis. Clin Cancer Res 2008;14:782.

50. Patard JJ, Fergelot P, Karakiewicz PI, et al. Low CAIX expression and absence of VHL gene mutation are associated with tumor aggressiveness and poor survival of clear cell renal cell carcinoma. Int J Cancer 2008;123:395.

51. Yao M, Yoshida M, Kishida T, et al. VHL tumor suppressor gene alterations associated with good prognosis in sporadic clear-cell renal carcinoma. J Natl Cancer Inst 2002;94:1569.

52. Kim JH, Jung CW, Cho YH, et al. Somatic VHL alteration and its impact on prognosis in patients with clear cell renal cell carcinoma. Oncol Rep 2005; 13:859.

53. Mandriota SJ, Turner KJ, Davies DR, et al. HIF activation identifies early lesions in VHL kidneys: evidence for site-specific tumor suppressor function in the nephron. Cancer Cell 2002;1:459.

54. Choueiri TK, Vaziri SA, Jaeger E, et al. von Hippel-Lindau gene status and response to vascular endothelial growth factor targeted therapy for metastatic clear cell renal cell carcinoma. J Urol 2008;180:860.

55. Gad S, Sultan-Amar V, Meric J, et al. Somatic von Hippel-Lindau (VHL) gene analysis and clinical outcome under antiangiogenic treatment in metastatic renal cell carcinoma: preliminary results. Target Oncol 2007;2:3.

56. Hutson TE, Davis ID, Machiels JH, et al. Biomarker analysis and final efficacy and safety results of a phase II renal cell carcinoma trial with pazopanib (GW786034), a multi-kinase angiogenesis inhibitor. J Clin Oncol 2008;26 [abstract: 5046].

57. Cho D, Signoretti S, Dabora S, et al. Potential histologic and molecular predictors of response to temsirolimus in patients with advanced renal cell carcinoma. Clin Genitourin Cancer 2007;5:379.

58. Lidgren A, Hedberg Y, Grankvist K, et al. Hypoxia-inducible factor 1alpha expression in renal cell carcinoma analyzed by tissue microarray. Eur Urol 2006;50:1272.

59. Dorevic G, Matusan-Ilijas K, Babarovic E, et al. Hypoxia inducible factor-1alpha correlates with vascular endothelial growth factor A and C indicating worse prognosis in clear cell renal cell carcinoma. J Exp Clin Cancer Res 2009;28:40.

60. Klatte T, Seligson DB, Riggs SB, et al. Hypoxia-inducible factor 1 alpha in clear cell renal cell carcinoma. Clin Cancer Res 2007;13:7388.

61. Patel PH, Chadalavada RS, Ishill NM, et al. Hypoxia-inducible factor (HIF) 1 and 2 levels in cell lines and human tumor predicts response to sunitinib in renal cell carcinoma (RCC). J Clin Oncol 2008;26 [abstract: 5008].

62. Figlin RA, de Souza P, McDermott D, et al. Analysis of PTEN and HIF-1alpha and correlation with efficacy in patients with advanced renal cell carcinoma treated with temsirolimus versus interferon-alpha. Cancer 2009;115:3651.

63. Jacobsen J, Rasmuson T, Grankvist K, et al. Vascular endothelial growth factor as prognostic factor in renal cell carcinoma. J Urol 2000;163:343.

64. Negrier S, Perol D, Menetrier-Caux C, et al. Interleukin-6, interleukin-10, and vascular endothelial growth factor in metastatic renal cell carcinoma: prognostic value of interleukin-6—from the Groupe Francais d'Immunotherapie. J Clin Oncol 2004;22:2371.

65. Negrier S, Chabaud S, Escudier B, et al. Serum level of vascular endothelial growth factor (VEGF) as an independent prognostic factor in metastatic renal cell carcinoma (MRCC). J Clin Oncol 2007;25 [abstract: 5044].

66. Escudier B, Eisen T, Stadler WM, et al. Sorafenib for treatment of renal cell carcinoma: Final efficacy and safety results of the phase III treatment approaches in renal cancer global evaluation trial. J Clin Oncol 2009;27:3312.
67. Escudier B, Ravaud A, Negrier S, et al. Update on AVOREN trial in metastatic renal cell carcinoma (mRCC): efficacy and safety in subgroups of patients (pts) and pharmacokinetic (PK) analysis. J Clin Oncol 2008;26 [abstract: 5025].
68. Deprimo SE, Bello CL, Smeraglia J, et al. Circulating protein biomarkers of pharmacodynamic activity of sunitinib in patients with metastatic renal cell carcinoma: modulation of VEGF and VEGF-related proteins. J Transl Med 2007;5:32.
69. Rini BI, Michaelson MD, Rosenberg JE, et al. Antitumor activity and biomarker analysis of sunitinib in patients with bevacizumab-refractory metastatic renal cell carcinoma. J Clin Oncol 2008;26:3743.
70. Tran HT, Liu Y, Lin Y, et al. Use of a multiplatform analysis of plasma cytokines and angiogenic factors (CAFs) to identify baseline CAFs associated with pazopanib response and tumor burden in renal cell carcinoma (RCC) patients. J Clin Oncol 2010;28 [abstract: 4522].
71. Kim JJ, Vaziri SA, Elson P, et al. Role of VEGF and VEGFR2 single nucleotide polymorphisms (SNPs) in predicting treatment-induced hypertension and clinical outcome in metastatic clear cell RCC patients treated with sunitinib. J Clin Oncol 2010;28 [abstract: 4629].
72. Kim JJ, Vaziri SA, Elson P, et al. VEGF single nucleotide polymorphisms (SNPs) and correlation to sunitinib-induced hypertension (HTN) in metastatic renal cell carcinoma (mRCC) patients (pts). J Clin Oncol 2009;27 [abstract: 5005].
73. Xu C, Ball HA, Bing N, et al. Association of genetic markers in angiogenesis- or exposure-related genes with overall survival in pazopanib (P) treated patients (Pts) with advanced renal cell carcinoma. J Clin Oncol 2011;29 [abstract: 303].
74. Ivanov S, Liao SY, Ivanova A, et al. Expression of hypoxia-inducible cell-surface transmembrane carbonic anhydrases in human cancer. Am J Pathol 2001;158: 905.
75. Bui MH, Seligson D, Han KR, et al. Carbonic anhydrase IX is an independent predictor of survival in advanced renal clear cell carcinoma: implications for prognosis and therapy. Clin Cancer Res 2003;9:802.
76. Leibovich BC, Sheinin Y, Lohse CM, et al. Carbonic anhydrase IX is not an independent predictor of outcome for patients with clear cell renal cell carcinoma. J Clin Oncol 2007;25:4757.
77. Sandlund J, Oosterwijk E, Grankvist K, et al. Prognostic impact of carbonic anhydrase IX expression in human renal cell carcinoma. BJU Int 2007;100:556.
78. Atkins M, Regan M, McDermott D, et al. Carbonic anhydrase IX expression predicts outcome of interleukin 2 therapy for renal cancer. Clin Cancer Res 2005;11:3714.
79. de Martino M, Klatte T, Seligson DB, et al. CA9 gene: single nucleotide polymorphism predicts metastatic renal cell carcinoma prognosis. J Urol 2009;182:728.
80. McDermott DF, Ghebremichael MS, Signoretti S, et al. The high-dose aldesleukin (HD IL-2) "SELECT" trial in patients with metastatic renal cell carcinoma (mRCC). J Clin Oncol 2010;28 [abstract: 4514].
81. Choueiri TK, Regan MM, Rosenberg JE, et al. Carbonic anhydrase IX and pathological features as predictors of outcome in patients with metastatic clear-cell renal cell carcinoma receiving vascular endothelial growth factor-targeted therapy. BJU Int 2010;106:772.
82. Pena C, Lathia C, Shan M, et al. Biomarkers predicting outcome in patients with advanced renal cell carcinoma: results from sorafenib phase III Treatment

Approaches in Renal Cancer Global Evaluation Trial. Clin Cancer Res 2010;16: 4853.

83. Kondo K, Yao M, Kobayashi K, et al. PTEN/MMAC1/TEP1 mutations in human primary renal-cell carcinomas and renal carcinoma cell lines. Int J Cancer 2001;91:219.

84. Turner KJ, Moore JW, Jones A, et al. Expression of hypoxia-inducible factors in human renal cancer: relationship to angiogenesis and to the von Hippel-Lindau gene mutation. Cancer Res 2002;62:2957.

85. Peralba JM, DeGraffenried L, Friedrichs W, et al. Pharmacodynamic evaluation of CCI-779, an inhibitor of mTOR, in Cancer Patients. Clin Cancer Res 2003;9: 2887.

86. Tanaka C, O'Reilly T, Kovarik JM, et al. Identifying optimal biologic doses of everolimus (RAD001) in patients with cancer based on the modeling of preclinical and clinical pharmacokinetic and pharmacodynamic data. J Clin Oncol 2008;26:1596.

87. Carreno BM, Collins M. BTLA: a new inhibitory receptor with a B7-like ligand. Trends Immunol 2003;24:524.

88. Krambeck AE, Thompson RH, Dong H, et al. B7-H4 expression in renal cell carcinoma and tumor vasculature: associations with cancer progression and survival. Proc Natl Acad Sci U S A 2006;103:10391.

89. Thompson RH, Kuntz SM, Leibovich BC, et al. Tumor B7-H1 is associated with poor prognosis in renal cell carcinoma patients with long-term follow-up. Cancer Res 2006;66:3381.

90. Thompson RH, Gillett MD, Cheville JC, et al. Costimulatory B7-H1 in renal cell carcinoma patients: Indicator of tumor aggressiveness and potential therapeutic target. Proc Natl Acad Sci U S A 2004;101:17174.

91. Darnell JE Jr. STATs and gene regulation. Science 1997;277:1630.

92. Kortylewski M, Kujawski M, Wang T, et al. Inhibiting Stat3 signaling in the hematopoietic system elicits multicomponent antitumor immunity. Nat Med 2005;11:1314.

93. Ito N, Eto M, Nakamura E, et al. STAT3 polymorphism predicts interferon-alfa response in patients with metastatic renal cell carcinoma. J Clin Oncol 2007; 25:2785.

94. Matthaeus T, Schulze-Lohoff E, Ichimura T, et al. Co-regulation of neutrophil gelatinase-associated lipocalin and matrix metalloproteinase-9 in the postischemic rat kidney. J Am Soc Nephrol 2001;12:787A.

95. Tong Z, Wu X, Ovcharenko D, et al. Neutrophil gelatinase-associated lipocalin as a survival factor. Biochem J 2005;391:441.

96. Bolignano D, Donato V, Lacquaniti A, et al. Neutrophil gelatinase-associated lipocalin (NGAL) in human neoplasias: a new protein enters the scene. Cancer Lett 2010;288:10.

97. Barresi V, Ieni A, Bolignano D, et al. Neutrophil gelatinase-associated lipocalin immunoexpression in renal tumors: correlation with histotype and histological grade. Oncol Rep 2010;24:305.

98. Porta C, Paglino C, De Amici M, et al. Predictive value of baseline serum vascular endothelial growth factor and neutrophil gelatinase-associated lipocalin in advanced kidney cancer patients receiving sunitinib. Kidney Int 2010; 77:809.

99. Jiang Z, Chu PG, Woda BA, et al. Analysis of RNA-binding protein IMP3 to predict metastasis and prognosis of renal-cell carcinoma: a retrospective study. Lancet Oncol 2006;7:556.

100. Hoffmann NE, Sheinin Y, Lohse CM, et al. External validation of IMP3 expression as an independent prognostic marker for metastatic progression and death for patients with clear cell renal cell carcinoma. Cancer 2008;112:1471.

101. Shirasaka T, Shimamato Y, Ohshimo H, et al. Development of a novel form of an oral 5-fluorouracil derivative (S-1) directed to the potentiation of the tumor selective cytotoxicity of 5-fluorouracil by two biochemical modulators. Anticancer Drugs 1996;7:548.

102. Naito S, Eto M, Shinohara N, et al. Multicenter phase II trial of S-1 in patients with cytokine-refractory metastatic renal cell carcinoma. J Clin Oncol 2010;28:5022.

103. Kosari F, Parker AS, Kube DM, et al. Clear cell renal cell carcinoma: gene expression analyses identify a potential signature for tumor aggressiveness. Clin Cancer Res 2005;11:5128.

104. Rini BI, Zhou M, Aydin H, et al. Identification of prognostic genomic markers in patients with localized clear cell renal cell carcinoma (ccRCC). J Clin Oncol 2010;28 [abstract: 4501].

105. Takahashi M, Rhodes DR, Furge KA, et al. Gene expression profiling of clear cell renal cell carcinoma: gene identification and prognostic classification. Proc Natl Acad Sci U S A 2001;98:9754.

106. Vasselli JR, Shih JH, Iyengar SR, et al. Predicting survival in patients with metastatic kidney cancer by gene-expression profiling in the primary tumor. Proc Natl Acad Sci U S A 2003;100:6958.

107. Zhao H, Ljungberg B, Grankvist K, et al. Gene expression profiling predicts survival in conventional renal cell carcinoma. PLoS Med 2006;3:e13.

108. Paik S, Shak S, Tang G, et al. A multigene assay to predict recurrence of tamoxifen-treated, node-negative breast cancer. N Engl J Med 2004;351:2817.

109. Dupuy A, Simon RM. Critical review of published microarray studies for cancer outcome and guidelines on statistical analysis and reporting. J Natl Cancer Inst 2007;99:147.

110. Bui MH, Visapaa H, Seligson D, et al. Prognostic value of carbonic anhydrase IX and KI67 as predictors of survival for renal clear cell carcinoma. J Urol 2004; 171:2461.

111. Dudderidge TJ, Stoeber K, Loddo M, et al. Mcm2, Geminin, and KI67 define proliferative state and are prognostic markers in renal cell carcinoma. Clin Cancer Res 2005;11:2510.

112. Tollefson MK, Thompson RH, Sheinin Y, et al. Ki-67 and coagulative tumor necrosis are independent predictors of poor outcome for patients with clear cell renal cell carcinoma and not surrogates for each other. Cancer 2007;110: 783.

113. Kim HL, Seligson D, Liu X, et al. Using tumor markers to predict the survival of patients with metastatic renal cell carcinoma. J Urol 2005;173:1496.

114. Parker AS, Leibovich BC, Lohse CM, et al. Development and evaluation of BioScore: a biomarker panel to enhance prognostic algorithms for clear cell renal cell carcinoma. Cancer 2009;115:2092.

115. Justice AC, Covinsky KE, Berlin JA. Assessing the generalizability of prognostic information. Ann Intern Med 1999;130:515.

Management of Treatment-Related Toxicity with Targeted Therapies for Renal Cell Carcinoma: Evidence-Based Practice and Best Practices

Laurie Appleby, APRN, MS[a], Stephanie Morrissey, RN, BSN[a],
Joaquim Bellmunt, MD, PhD[b], Jonathan Rosenberg, MD[a],*

KEYWORDS

- Renal cell carcinoma • Treatment-related toxicity
- Evidence-based practice • Tyrosine kinase inhibitor
- mTOR inhibitor

The advent of targeted agents for the treatment of advanced renal cell carcinoma has led to dramatic improvements in therapy. However, the chronic use of these medications has also led to the identification of new toxicities that require long-term management. The vascular endothelial growth factor (VEGF) receptor inhibitors (sunitinib, sorafenib, and pazopanib), VEGF-ligand inhibitor (bevacizumab), and mTOR inhibitors (temsirolimus and everolimus) each present different challenges for patient management. Quality of life for patients on chronic therapy has become increasingly important, and effective management of toxicity is needed to maximize the benefits of treatment. In addition, toxicity from these agents may affect treatment compliance, particularly with daily oral agents.

Despite being "targeted" agents, these drugs affect multiple organ systems that have the potential to impair quality of life and function. Nearly every organ system is affected to some degree. This review delineates the toxicities that require monitoring, the underlying pathophysiology (when known), and treatments that may have benefits in relieving symptoms and side effects.

[a] The Lank Center for Genitourinary Oncology, Dana-Farber Cancer Institute, Harvard Medical School, 450 Brookline Avenue, D1230, Boston, MA 02215, USA
[b] Hospital del Mar, Passeig Marítim 25-29, Barcelona 08003, Spain
* Corresponding author.
E-mail address: jonathan_rosenberg@dfci.harvard.edu

Hematol Oncol Clin N Am 25 (2011) 893–915
doi:10.1016/j.hoc.2011.05.004
0889-8588/11/$ – see front matter © 2011 Elsevier Inc. All rights reserved.

CARDIOVASCULAR TOXICITIES

VEGF inhibition by the approved anti-VEGF therapies has differential effects on the VEGF-VEGF receptor axis in tumor cells and normal tissues. In noncancer tissues, endothelial dysfunction and microvascular rarefaction set the stage for the development of hypertension (HTN), cardiomyopathy, thrombotic microangiopathy, and proteinuria.

Hypertension: The Problem

The most relevant cardiovascular side effect in clinical practice is HTN.[1,2] The recognition of this side effect is an important issue because poorly controlled HTN can lead to serious cardiovascular events. HTN is an established risk factor for coronary heart disease, stroke, heart failure, and end-stage renal disease.[3] Anticipation of HTN complications with anti-VEGF therapies, early detection, and personalized management may improve clinical outcomes and tolerance.

HTN de novo or worsening control of a preexisting diagnosis after the introduction of antiangiogenic treatment may indicate underlying mechanisms such as renal thrombotic microangiopathy[4] or glomerular lesions, but more commonly it is isolated HTN secondary to treatment itself. HTN induced by antiangiogenic drugs is probably related to an increase in systemic vascular resistance (SVR). It is thought that decreased production of nitric oxide (NO) in the wall of arterioles and other resistance vessels is one of the main involved mechanisms. VEGF increases NO synthesis through upregulation of endothelial NO synthase, and VEGF inhibition diminishes NO synthesis.[5,6] Measurements of urinary nitrate levels suggest that they decline with anti-VEGF tyrosine kinase inhibitors (TKIs), supporting this hypothesis.[7] In anticipation of cardiovascular complications with anti-VEGF therapies, early detection and personalized management may improve clinical outcomes and tolerance.[8]

The incidence of hypertension of any grade was reported to range from 9% to 30% in a recent review of randomized controlled trials,[9] but this incidence could be even higher if a more strict definition and classification of HTN were used such as the Seventh Report of the Joint National Committee on Prevention, Detection, Evaluation, and Treatment of High Blood Pressure (JNC7),[10] rather than the National Cancer Institute Common Terminology Criteria for Adverse Events. Three meta-analyses of phase 1, phase 2, and phase 4 trials conducted in various types of cancer found a respective incidence of high-grade hypertension of 8.3% (95% confidence interval [CI] 5.6–12.1) for sunitinib,[11] 6.5% (95% CI 1.8–21.1) for sorafenib,[12] and 7.1% (95% CI 3.4–14.1) for bevacizumab[13] in the subgroup of metastatic renal cell carcinoma (mRCC) patients.

On the other hand, HTN induced by anti-VEGF agents may be a predictive factor of oncologic response. In a retrospective analysis of 544 mRCC patients treated with sunitinib, the 441 patients presenting high systolic blood pressure had a statistically significantly improved progression-free survival (PFS) (12.5 vs 2.5 months) and overall survival (OS) (30.5 vs 7.8 months) with respect to other patients. Similarly, the 362 patients presenting high diastolic blood pressure had a statistically significantly improved PFS (13.4 vs 5.3 months) and OS (32.1 vs 15.0 months) with respect to other patients.[14,15] Similar observations are reported for axitinib.[14] In fact, the importance of hypertension as a potential clinical biomarker is prospectively being explored in the dose titration trial of axitinib (NCT00835978).

Hypertension Management

The proper management of hypertension is of fundamental importance in mRCC patients, but it can only be extrapolated from guidelines available for the general population.[16] Lifestyle modifications should be encouraged, but these nonpharmacologic strategies are not always suitable for patients with altered performance status related to metastatic cancer necessitating early drug intervention.

No clear recommendation for an antihypertensive agent can be made in this context because of a lack of controlled studies addressing the subject. Only one randomized study showed a beneficial effect of use of a calcium channel blocker (CCB) to prevent or minimize HTN secondary to antiangiogenic therapy.[17] Nitrates seem as effective as well.[16] Blood pressure (BP)-lowering drugs should be individualized to the patient's clinical circumstances, and angiogenic inhibitors should be dose reduced and sometimes withheld in patients who have experienced hypertensive crisis.[8,16] Treatment suspension is mandatory in the case of life-threatening events.

The medical literature gives no indication that cancer-affected patients with HTN or pre-HTN should be managed in a way other than that recommended in the JNC7 guidelines. For patients with stage 1 or 2 uncomplicated HTN, the target BP level is less than 140/90 mm Hg. Current guidelines from the National Kidney Foundation, which have not been specifically validated in patients with cancer-related kidney diseases, recommend a target BP of 125/75 mm Hg or less, as tolerated, for patients with diabetes mellitus, proteinuria, or reduced kidney function; alternatively, the recommended BP goal is 130/80 mm Hg.[18] Indeed, in cancer patients with comorbidities such as chronic kidney disease, a target BP level of less than 135/85 mm Hg may be acceptable.[19] BP monitoring while receiving angiogenic inhibitors should be undergone at least weekly for the first 8 weeks and before any infusion or cycle thereafter.

Antihypertensive agents should be selected according to patient's comorbidities, drug interactions, and contraindications. Given the efficacy of angiotensin-converting enzyme (ACE) inhibitors and angiotensin-2 receptor antagonist (ARA), clinicians may consider using one as a first-line agent when a patient's plasma creatinine is less than 2 mg/dL and there is no evidence of hyperkalemia or renal artery stenosis. ACE inhibitors or ARA may be preferred for those patients with proteinuria, chronic kidney disease risks, or metabolic syndrome. The nondihydropyridine CCBs, such as verapamil and diltiazem, are cytochrome P450 3A4 (CYP3A4) inhibitors, and nifedipine, a dihydropyridine CCB, has been shown to induce VEGF secretion.[20] In the absence of available data from clinical studies, CCB dihydropyridines, such as amlodipine and felodipine, are the preferred class of CCB, and the nondihydropyridine CCB should be contraindicated or used cautiously in conjunction with angiogenic inhibitors metabolized by CYP3A4. Dihydropyridine CCB should be preferred in elderly or black patients.[16] A general guideline on the use of antihypertensive agents is shown in **Table 1**.

Table 1	
Interactions between antihypertensive agents and angiogenic inhibitors	
Antihypertensive Class	**Interaction**
ACE, ARB, diuretics, β-blockers, α-blockers, nitrate derivatives	Minor degree of interaction
Nifedipine, calcium channel blockers	Some degree of interaction
Verapamil and diltiazem	Not recommended for use with oral drugs using CYP3A4 pathway (only with bevacizumab)

Abbreviations: ACE, angiotensin-converting enzyme inhibitor; ARB, angiotensin receptor blocker; CYP3A4, cytochrome P450 3A4.

ARTERIAL THROMBOEMBOLIC EVENTS

VEGF-directed agents can alter the hemostatic balance by interfering with the integrity of the endothelial cells, decreasing the production of nitric oxide, and altering membrane lipids. These agents have been associated with both coagulative and bleeding disorders. Meta-analyses have shown that bevacizumab was significantly associated with an increased risk of arterial thromboembolism (relative risk [RR], 2.08 (95% CI 1.28–3.40, P = .003)).[21] A subsequent report confirmed an overall RR for arterial thromboembolic events (ATEs) with bevacizumab-based therapy versus controls of 1.46 (95% CI 1.11–1.93, P = .007)[22] as well as an increased risk of venous thromboembolism (RR for all grades, 3.0; 95% CI, 1.23–7.33; RR for grade 3–4 events, 2.86; 95% CI, 0.62–13.24).[23]

Similarly, treatment with the VEGF receptor TKIs sunitinib and sorafenib is associated with a significant increase in the risk of ATEs. The RR of ATEs associated with sorafenib and sunitinib was 3.03 (95% CI, 1.25–7.37; P = .015) compared with control patients with an overall incidence of 1.4%.[24] This risk did not depend on the type of TKI used or type of malignancy (renal cell carcinoma [RCC] vs non-RCC).

CARDIOTOXICITY

Cardiac damage from TKI treatment may be a largely underestimated phenomenon. VEGF may play a critical role in coordinated tissue growth and angiogenesis in the heart.[25,26] Blocking this pathway may lead to a disruption in cardiac remodeling and consequently induce heart failure. Careful cardiovascular monitoring as well as prophylactic cardiovascular treatment is essential, and may allow continuation of aggressive therapy for the underlying cancer.[27]

In the phase 2 clinical trials of sunitinib in RCC, 8.9% of patients developed a reduction in left ventricular ejection fraction (LVEF).[28,29] The incidence of left ventricular cardiac dysfunction (LVCD) reported with sunitinib in the phase 3 trial was 13%, with 3% of patients experiencing grade 3 events, but the incidence was not different between the sunitinib and interferon groups.[30] Interferon, however, may cause cardiomyopathy as well.[31] The sunitinib expanded access trial reported cardiac failure of any grade in less than 1% of patients, although a baseline cardiac evaluation was not performed per protocol.[32]

In a retrospective analysis, a decline in cardiac function was noted in 3% of patients treated with sunitinib.[33] Heart failure was preceded by hypertension in all patients, and the resultant left ventricular dysfunction was not completely reversible, even on discontinuation of sunitinib.[33] A single-center analysis of patients receiving sunitinib for renal cell cancer or gastrointestinal stromal tumor described 15% with symptomatic congestive heart failure (CHF); importantly, in this report cardiac function appeared to improve with discontinuation of sunitinib and introduction of CHF medication.[34] There is no general consensus on the frequency required for the LVEF monitoring. Patients presenting a history of coronary artery disease and/or hypertension can have their ejection fraction monitored every 2 or 3 cycles. Treatment should be suspended for grade 3 to 4 LVCD and the patient referred to a specialist.

Serious cardiotoxicity was infrequent in the prospective trials of sorafenib. In one phase 3 trial, the rates of cardiac ischemia/myocardial infarction were not statistically different in the sorafenib and placebo arms.[35] In another phase 3 study, the incidences of cardiac ischemia and infarction were significantly higher in the sorafenib arm (RCC: 3% vs 1%; P<.01).[36] An independent review of two studies by the Food and Drug Administration indicated that the incidence of ischemia/infarction was higher in the sorafenib group (2.9%) than in the placebo group (0.4%).[37] A prospective evaluation of 74 patients with renal cell cancer receiving sorafenib or sunitinib with detailed cardiovascular monitoring observed up to a 34% incidence of cardiac toxicity; half were symptomatic, with significant decreases in LVEF in 12% of patients. Other important cardiac toxicities (eg, arrhythmias, electrocardiographic [ECG] changes, cardiac enzymes elevations, acute coronary artery syndrome) were also seen, with ECG changes in 16% of cases.[27]

CHF has been occasionally reported for bevacizumab. A meta-analysis assessing the risk of serious CHF in patients with breast cancer receiving bevacizumab revealed an overall incidence of 1.6% with an RR of CHF in bevacizumab-treated patients of 4.74 (95% CI 1.66–11.18; $P<.001$) compared with placebo.[38]

Experience with the VEGF receptor antagonists suggests related cardiac toxicities may be reversible on withdrawal of those agents and/or initiation of cardiovascular treatment, and that the VEGF receptor TKIs can be safely resumed, sometimes with a lower dose.[27,34] It is not known if this treatment paradigm applies to bevacizumab-treated patients, as the pharmacokinetics of bevacizumab are different and the half-life (approximately 21 days) is prolonged.

Better cooperation among clinical and translational cardiologists and oncologists will be required from the early phases of drug development and for daily management of patients. It will be essential to identify effective strategies to address the cardiovascular on-target toxicity. Prospective studies specifically conducted in mRCC patients treated with targeted agents (eg, VEGF receptor TKIs) are presently lacking and are urgently needed.

BLEEDING

A meta-analysis has shown that bevacizumab was significantly associated with an increased risk of bleeding (RR for high-grade events, 3.7; 95% CI 2.6–5.5) in mRCC patients, compared with controls.[39] Sunitinib and sorafenib are also associated with an increased risk of bleeding (RR for all grades, 2·74; 95% CI 1·32–5·69; RR for high grade, 5.14; 95% CI 1.35–19.64) in patients with mRCC.[40] A higher incidence of intracerebral hemorrhage has been recently reported in patients with metastatic RCC treated with TKIs targeting the VEGF receptors sorafenib and sunitinib.[41] This retrospective study showed an incidence of 7% (5 of 67) of fatal intracerebral hemorrhage, with 4 out of 5 patients presenting with brain metastasis. This result was probably related to uncontrolled HTN at diagnosis.[42]

This increased risk should be managed with a thorough medical history, frequent clinical examinations, and thorough investigation of suspicious symptoms. Grade 2 to 4 thrombotic or bleeding events require treatment suspension and appropriate treatment until recovery to grade 1.

METABOLIC EFFECTS OF TARGETED THERAPIES

Use of mTOR inhibitors is associated with alteration in glucose and lipid homeostasis, reflective of the central role of the mTOR protein in these processes. TKIs have been implicated in thyroid dysfunction.

Hyperglycemia

Grade 3 to 4 hyperglycemia occurs in up to 15% of patients treated with mTOR inhibitors.[43,44] In patients with diabetes mellitus treated with these agents, frequent monitoring of blood sugar and adjustment of medications is necessary to prevent hyperglycemic crises. For patients without diabetes mellitus, frequent screening of blood sugar is required to monitor for the emergence of hyperglycemia. Because patients with RCC frequently have impaired renal function, the use of certain oral hypoglycemic agents may be contraindicated. Biguanides such as metformin are contraindicated in patients with a creatinine clearance of less than 60 mL/min, due to the risk of lactic acidosis. Of interest, treatment with TKIs such as sunitinib and sorafenib have been observed to improve glycemic control in patients with diabetes mellitus.[45]

Hyperlipidemia

Hyperlipidemia is frequently observed with mTOR inhibitors. Three percent of patients treated with temsirolimus or everolimus experienced grade 3 or 4 hyperlipidemia in phase 3 testing.[43,44] Although patients who are treated with these agents may have limited life expectancies due to their underlying malignancy, many will live for at least several years, and may be at high risk from complications due to lipid abnormalities. Evaluation of lipids should occur at baseline and every 6 weeks if they are above recommended levels. Statins and bile-acid sequestering agents are first-line therapy for hypercholesterolemia, and for significant hypertriglyceridemia nicotinic acid or fibrates are indicated. Treatment of hypercholesterolemia and hyperlipidemia should follow standard guidelines.[46] Caution should be used when considering agents to manage these metabolic toxicities, and certain statins are substrates of CYP3A4, so drug metabolism may be altered.

Thyroid Dysfunction

Hypothyroidism was reported in 14% of patients treated with sunitinib in the RCC phase 3 trial,[30] though reported less frequently with pazopanib,[47] and not reported with sorafenib[36] in phase 3 testing. Retrospective evaluations of sorafenib and sunitinib suggest that the incidence of hypothyroidism is significant in certain populations.[48,49] Hypothyroidism may contribute to other adverse effects, including fatigue and anemia. Evaluation of thyroid-stimulating hormone (TSH) and T4 at the initiation of therapy will provide a baseline. Thyroid dysfunction with sunitinib may result in changes between days 1 and 28 of each cycle, so monitoring at the beginning and end of 4-week cycles may be required in patients with symptoms consistent with hypothyroidism. Monitoring of TSH every 6 to 8 weeks during VEGF receptor–targeted therapy is necessary to monitor for treatment-related thyroid dysfunction. Thyroid replacement should be initiated for patients with TSH greater than 10 IU on day 1 of two consecutive cycles.[50] The underlying pathophysiology of thyroid dysfunction remains somewhat unclear; many patients experience a brief mild drug-induced thyrotoxicosis, but an autoimmune etiology does not appear to be involved.

RENAL EFFECTS

Renal dysfunction has been observed with sunitinib therapy, although in general renal toxicity has been mild. In a meta-analysis of 13 clinical trials with sunitinib, 65.6% of patients with kidney cancer experienced an increase in creatinine, with an RR of 1.35 (P<.001), although the frequency of severe renal toxicity was low (<1%).[11] Proteinuria, however, is observed in many patients receiving antiangiogenic agents, bevacizumab in particular.[51] High-grade proteinuria was observed in 2.2% of patients (more common in patients with kidney cancer than other cancers [11.9%]) and may lead to nephrotic syndrome in some patients.[52,53] In general, bevacizumab therapy is recommended to be held back when more than 2 g of protein are excreted in 24 hours, and potentially reinstituted when proteinuria has lessened. Use of an ACE inhibitor or an ARA may be appropriate, depending on the underlying kidney function, to reduce proteinuria and prevent progression of renal dysfunction, although there are limited data to support this with targeted therapy–induced proteinuria.

DERMATOLOGIC EFFECTS

Among the most common adverse events seen with these agents are cutaneous adverse events.[54,55] Visible dermatologic toxicities can affect the patient physically, psychologically, and socially.[56] These toxicities are particularly important to monitor because their manifestation can lead to poor adherence, suboptimal dosing, and discontinuation of an effective therapy.[54–57]

The potential cutaneous toxicities seen with targeted therapies include hand-foot skin reaction (HFSR), rash, xerosis, pruritus, alopecia, erythema, skin discoloration, hair depigmentation, and subungual hemorrhages (**Table 2**).[54–58] HFSR is the most clinically significant of these dermatologic side effects. It is primarily seen with the multitargeted TKIs sorafenib and sunitinib, though less so with pazopanib.[59] HFSR has not been described with the mTOR inhibitors temsirolimus and everolimus.[60]

HFSR is distinct from the hand-foot syndrome seen in patients receiving more conventional chemotherapy, such as, capecitabine or parenteral 5-fluorouracil.[56–58,61,62] Classic hand-foot skin syndrome or palmar-plantar erythrodysesthesia (PPE) presents as symmetric, painful, red, edematous areas on the palms and soles. The HFSR associated with TKIs is more localized, and well-defined hyperkeratotic lesions are present. The pathogenesis of HFSR remains unknown. Platelet-derived growth factor (PDGF) and c-kit are present in epithelium of sweat ducts. Inhibitory effects of sunitinib and sorafenib on PDGF and of sunitinib on c-kit may play a role.[55]

Symptoms of HFSR include tingling, burning, paresthesia, and/or dysesthesia on the palms and/or soles, and generally occur during the first 2 to 4 weeks of TKI therapy.[56–59] Callous-like blisters (which usually do not contain fluid), erythema, dry or cracked skin, edema, desquamation, and hyperkeratosis are usually seen at pressure and flexor areas of the palms and/or soles.[56,58,59] Severe and painful calluses can significantly affect a patient's quality of life leading to a decline in function that may require discontinuation of therapy (**Fig. 1**). In patients receiving sunitinib, symptoms of HFSR usually resolve during the 2-week break period.[54,60]

To date, there are no evidence-based treatment guidelines on various topical remedies for HFSR. The management of side effects is based largely on clinical experience and advice from specialists.[63] Prophylactic and supportive measures should begin

Table 2	
Cutaneous adverse events associated with targeted therapies in the treatment of RCC	
Adverse Event	**Overall Incidence (%)**
Hand-foot skin reaction	9–62
Rash	19–76
Pruritus	19–38
Erythema	16
Alopecia	27–53
Hair depigmentation	10–38
Skin discoloration	16–41 (sunitinib)
Subungual splinter hemorrhages	25
Xerosis	16–31

Data from Refs.[54–57]

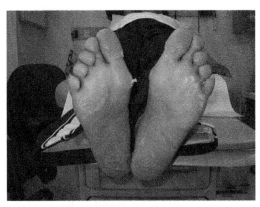

Fig. 1. Hand-foot syndrome during sorafenib therapy.

before treatment starts. A full skin examination should be done prior to the start of therapy and at each visit.[56] Patients with preexisting calluses may be predisposed to HFSR, and a pedicure is recommended.[56,58] Application of an emollient-based moisturizer twice daily should begin before or at the beginning of treatment. If HFSR does develop, switching to a urea-based moisturizer may be helpful.[62] Urea is a keratolytic that helps break down hyperkeratosis, and decreases epidermal thickness.[57,62] Topical steroids, for example, clobetasol propionate cream, can be an effective palliative measure given its anti-inflammatory properties.[57,58] Patients should be cautioned to avoid excess pressure or friction on affected areas. Avoidance of restrictive footwear and the wearing of gel insoles are advised. Wearing of cotton socks has been recommended.[56,58] However, in their practice the authors recommend woolen socks, for example, SmartWool socks (SmartWool, Steamboat Springs, CO, USA), which can wick away sweat and reduce friction. Use of analgesics may be indicated to control pain.[56] Some patients may be required to temporarily discontinue therapy or undergo dose reduction to alleviate symptoms. Once symptoms have resolved, the drug should be restarted at 50% of the starting dose. If, after careful monitoring, the toxicity does not recur, titration to full dose may be possible.[56]

Of interest is a recent abstract presented at the 2011 Genitourinary Symposium. Michaelson and colleagues[64] retrospectively evaluated 770 patients on sunitinib from 5 clinical trials to investigate correlations between the development of HFSR and efficacy end points. The investigators found that there was a strong correlation between the development of sunitinib-associated HFSR and improved clinical outcomes. If this finding is validated, patients and clinicians may be reluctant to reduce dose or temporarily halt therapy for fear of affecting efficacy.

The rash associated with targeted therapies can range from a mild erythematous flushing of the face to a more severe exfoliative dermatitis. The rash associated with the mTOR inhibitors tends to be milder than that seen with the TKIs, and is more maculopapular in appearance.[60,65] Pruritus may or may not be present. Frequently the rash involves the face, scalp, and upper torso.[57,58] Unlike the rash seen with endothelial growth factor receptor inhibitors, there is no known correlation with development of the rash and response to treatment.[56,58]

As with HFSR, the absence of hard clinical data in the treatment of skin toxicities leads to a reliance on empirical evidence for treatment strategies. Papulopustular rashes can be treated with topical antibiotics, although in more severe cases systemic antibiotics may be required.[57,58] Treatment with colloidal oatmeal lotion has been effective in treating acneform eruptions.[66] If pruritus is present, antihistamines or "anti-itch" lotions, for example, Sarna, may be indicated. With sorafenib, these pruritic rashes frequently appear on the scalp, and betamethasone lotion may provide relief. Xerosis, with or without associated pruritus, can be relieved by the use of emollient-based moisturizers, such as, Aveeno and Eucerin. Again, the authors recommend patients begin using these moisturizers at the beginning of treatment with a targeted therapy. Patients should be educated to refrain from exposing the affected areas to hot water, as this may exacerbate symptoms.[57,58]

Photosensitivity has been described with sunitinib,[57] and patients should be advised to avoid prolonged sun exposure and use sunscreen. The skin discoloration seen in patients taking sunitinib usually presents as a yellowing or hypopigmentation of the skin.[57,58] These changes may be distressful to the patient, who should be made aware of their potential appearance. Sunitinib and pazopanib have also been associated with hair depigmentation (gray or white).[47,57,59] These changes resolve after discontinuation of the offending agent.

The appearance of subungual hemorrhage is unique to sunitinib and sorafenib. This condition is not associated with pain or change in nail integrity, and requires no treatment.[67]

PULMONARY TOXICITY

Noninfectious pneumonitis a class effect of mTOR inhibition.[68–70] Radiographically it appears as ground-glass opacities and nonmalignant lung consolidations. Patients may be asymptomatic or present with cough, dyspnea, or fatigue.[70] To date, pneumonitis has been seen more often with everolimus.[69] In the RECORD-1 trial of everolimus, an incidence of 13% was reported.[44] White and colleagues[70] presented data from an independent, blinded, retrospective radiological review of the same study and found an incidence of clinical pneumonitis of 13.5%. However, 38.9% of patients without clinical pneumonitis had new radiographic findings, compatible with pneumonitis. There are similar data with temsirolimus. The Global Advanced Renal Cell Carcinoma trial did not distinguish pneumonitis as an adverse event, although 26% of subjects developed a cough.[43] These early data lead the authors to believe that the prevalence of noninfectious pneumonitis may be higher than is appreciated. At present the etiology of pneumonitis and mTOR inhibition is unknown.

Careful clinical monitoring for this adverse event should be done at each visit (**Box 1**). Pretreatment pulmonary function tests (PFT) may be needed, especially if the patient has a history of pulmonary disease. A chest computed tomography scan should be performed on any patient exhibiting new respiratory symptoms. Recommended management is outlined in **Table 3**.

GASTROINTESTINAL TOXICITY

Gastrointestinal symptoms are associated with sunitinib, sorafenib, pazopanib, and the mTOR inhibitors, and less often with bevacizumab.[24,55,71] Prevention of gastrointestinal symptoms or early intervention can lead to better quality of life for patients with RCC. Similar to other toxicities, there are no prospective data to guide toxicity management with these therapies.

Gastrointestinal toxicities include anorexia, nausea, vomiting, diarrhea, dyspepsia, mucositis/stomatitis, and taste alteration.[63] Impairment of the alimentary system can interrupt daily oral dosing of oral agents, resulting in weight loss, dehydration, and electrolyte imbalance, and can potentiate the risk of renal failure. There are several pharmacologic and nonpharmacologic interventions that will control and often prevent

---

Box 1
Examples of CYP3A4 inhibitors and inducers[a]

CYP3A4 Inhibitors

Amiodarone

Aprepitant

Atazanavir

Clarithromycin

Cyclosporin

Darunavir

Diltiazem

Fluconazole

Grapefruit juice

Indinavir

Itraconazole

Ritonavir

Saquinavir

Telithromycin

Verapamil

Voriconazole

CYP3A4 Inducers

Carbamazepine

Dexamethasone

Efavirenz

Nafcillin

Oxcabazepine

Phenobarbital

Phenytoin

Primidone

Rifampin

[a] List is not inclusive. Available at: http://medicine.iupui.edu/clinpharm/ddis/table.asp. Accessed January 22, 2011.

---

moderate gastrointestinal symptoms in patients receiving multitargeted therapies (**Table 4**).

Anorexia

Anorexia can occur as a lone toxicity or in combination with nausea and/or vomiting, and may lead to weight loss and dehydration. It is often difficult for patients who experience anorexia to increase their oral intake. To combat this, changing eating habits may be helpful. Patients should be encouraged to eat small, frequent meals, and meals should include foods that are high in protein and calories. Spicy foods or foods that have strong odors are not recommended, as they can trigger nausea.

Table 3
Management of pulmonary toxicity

Grade	Symptoms	Management	Dose Modification
1	Asymptomatic	No specific therapy	None
2	Clinical symptoms not interfering with ADL	CT scan and PFT	Hold or reduce dose If no recovery to grade 1 or less within 3 weeks, discontinue
3	Clinical symptoms interfering with ADL, and/or O_2 indicated	CT scan and PFT Rule out infectious etiology Prescribe corticosteroids Pulmonary consultation for bronchoscopy	Hold drug until recovery to grade 1 or less If no recovery within 3 weeks, or no clinical benefit, discontinue treatment Restart drug at within 3 weeks at reduced dose if evidence of clinical benefit
4	Life-threatening, ventilatory support required	CT scan and PFT Rule out infectious etiology Prescribe corticosteroids Pulmonary consultation for bronchoscopy	Discontinue treatment

Abbreviations: ADL, activities of daily living; CT, computed tomography; PFT, pulmonary function testing (including spirometry, room air oxygen saturation, and diffusion capacity of carbon monoxide).

Data from White DA, Camus P, Endo M, et al. Noninfectious pneumonitis after everolimus therapy for advanced renal cell carcinoma. Am J Respir Crit Care Med 2010;182:396.

Temperature and textures of foods can exacerbate symptoms; patients often prefer foods served at room temperature.[63] A nutrition consultation may help in identifying foods that are more palatable for the patient receiving a targeted therapy. Pharmacologic interventions include the use of megestrol acetate or low-dose corticosteroids.[72] Caution must be used with these medications, as there may be drug interactions with the targeted agents the patient is receiving. Properly addressing anorexia will help prevent weight loss, dehydration, and electrolyte imbalance in the patient receiving a TKI. Dose interruption and dose modification may be avoided and quality of life improved if interventions are initiated early.

Nausea and Vomiting

Nausea and vomiting are frequent occurrences in patients receiving mTOR inhibitors and TKIs.[69,73] Although the incidence of nausea is less than with cytotoxic chemotherapy, patients receiving multitargeted therapies do experience moderate symptoms of nausea.[74–78] Prevention of nausea/vomiting should be a primary goal when treating patients receiving multitargeted therapies for RCC. Early intervention of antiemetic regimens may limit dose interruptions of drug treatment as well as potentially prevent weight loss, dehydration, malnutrition, and electrolyte abnormalities. While nausea/vomiting often can lead to anorexia, symptoms may present independently. As with all toxicities associated with TKIs, it is important to rule out underlying causes. Patients with metastatic RCC are at risk for brain metastases; therefore, new onset of nausea/vomiting may warrant follow-up with neurologic examination and/or imaging of the brain. Similarly, electrolyte abnormalities such as hypercalcemia, hyponatremia,

Table 4
Interventions for control and prevention of moderate gastrointestinal symptoms in patients receiving multitargeted therapies

Toxicity	Nonpharmacologic Intervention	Pharmacologic Intervention
Anorexia	• Eat small, frequent meals • Eat foods high in protein, calories • Avoid foods that are spicy, or have strong odors • Eat foods that are room temperature, bland in flavor and texture • Drink plenty of fluids to avoid dehydration • Supplement with protein shakes • Nutrition consult • Relaxation technique, exercise, acupuncture	• Megestrol • Low-dose corticoid • Steroids
Nausea/Vomiting (N/V)	• Rule out secondary cause for N/V • Eat small, frequent meals • Eat foods at room temperature • Eat bland foods that are easily digested • Relaxation technique: yoga, meditation, hypnosis, guided imagery, massage, acupuncture • Drink plenty of fluids	Dopamine receptor agonist • Metoclopramide • Prochlorperazine 5-HT$_3$ antagonist • Ondansetron • Granisetron Benzodiazapines • Lorazepam
Diarrhea	• Eat a bland diet (bananas, rice, apple sauce, toast) • Avoid spicy foods • Add fiber to diet to increase bulk • Substitute dairy with soy if lactose intolerance • Avoid high-fat foods • Avoid caffeine • Drink plenty of fluids • Avoid stress or stressful triggers • Relaxation techniques, guided imagery, yoga, meditation, acupuncture, massage	• Loperamide • Diphenoxlyate • Cholestyramine
Mucositis/ Stomatitis	• Eat soothing foods that are easy to chew • Drink fluids through a straw • Drink plenty of fluids • Have a dental evaluation before treatment • Continue oral care with gentle brushing with a soft toothbrush • Use alcohol-free oral products	Topical rinses • Mouthwashes containing viscous lidocaine Antifungal agents • Nystatin • Fluconazole • Clotrimazole troches

(continued on next page)

Table 4
(continued)

Toxicity	Nonpharmacologic Intervention	Pharmacologic Intervention
Dyspepsia	• Eat small, frequent meals • Limit snacks or meals late at night • Avoid caffeine, spicy foods, chocolate, or peppermint	H2 blockers • Famotidine • Ranitidine PPIs • Omeprazole • Pantoprazole
Altered taste	• Use plastic utensils • Eat foods at cooler than normal temperatures • Use additional spices, sauces, marinades, and fats to enhance flavor • Suck on hard candies before meals	

Abbreviation: PPI, proton pump inhibitor.

and hyperglycemia can produce nausea/vomiting. Pancreatitis, cholecystitis, and small bowel obstruction must also be ruled out. Underlying infection may also produce symptoms of nausea.

Management of nausea/vomiting is similar to management of anorexia. Eating small, frequent meals to avoid early satiety is recommended. Patients with nausea prefer foods served at room temperature, and foods that are bland and easily digestible. Nausea triggered by anxiety may be controlled by nonpharmacologic interventions such as relaxation techniques (yoga, guided imagery, meditation, and hypnosis). Patients have also benefited from acupuncture and massage.[79]

Because some targeted therapies involve oral agents that are taken daily, patients may require daily dosing of antiemetics, which is different from patients receiving cytotoxic chemotherapy whereby there are clearly defined cycles with peak periods of drug effect. Pharmacologic interventions for nausea/vomiting related to TKIs include the use of the dopamine receptor antagonists metoclopramide and prochlorperazine.[73] The 5-HT$_3$ antagonist ondansetron can be effective in controlling nausea/vomiting if metoclopramide and prochlorperazine are not successful.[63,73] Benzodiazepine and corticosteroids have been effective as well.[63]

Diarrhea

Diarrhea is another symptom seen with many novel agents. More than 20% of patients receiving mTOR inhibitors and nearly 50% of patients receiving the VEGF inhibitors sunitinib, pazopanib, and sorafenib experience some degree of diarrhea. Diarrhea often can be controlled with dietary changes. Eating a bland diet and avoiding spicy foods may provide improvement of symptoms. Choosing foods like bananas, rice, apple sauce, and toast can be beneficial. The addition of fiber to the diet either by dietary choices or with bulk laxatives may decrease the amount of loose stools by slowing gastrointestinal motility. Small, frequent meals are often better tolerated than large meals. Diarrhea and cramping can be exacerbated by dairy intake. Avoidance of dairy products and replacing them with soy-based or lactose-free choices may improve symptoms. Avoiding foods that are high in fat and maintaining a caffeine-free diet can decrease symptoms of diarrhea. In addition to avoiding foods that can trigger cramping and diarrhea, patients should also be aggressive with oral rehydration and drink plenty of fluids.

If dietary or behavior modifications are not successful, pharmacologic interventions may alleviate diarrhea. Patients are encouraged to initiate treatment with antidiarrheal agents at the first signs of loose stools. The use of loperamide and diphenoxylate can be helpful.[80] Cholestyramine may also be used 30 minutes before meals.[73]

Mucositis

Mucositis can occur anywhere along the gastrointestinal tract from the oral cavity to the rectum. Oral mucositis/stomatitis has been seen with sunitinib, sorafenib, pazopanib, and the mTOR inhibitors. Oral mucositis has been associated with painful canker sores that can appear on the lips, tongue, and soft palate. Eating foods that are soothing such as watermelon, sherbet, pudding, bananas, yogurt, and popsicles are recommended. These foods are gentle on the oral mucosa and also provide fluid and nutrition. Drinking fluids through a straw can be helpful when sores are located in the mouth or on the tongue. Mouthwashes that contain viscous lidocaine or are alcohol free are helpful in maintaining good oral hygiene as well as providing relief for oral discomfort. Toothpastes that are alcohol free are recommended. Patients should use a soft toothbrush and perform gentle brushing.[81] If possible, a dental evaluation is recommended for patients before initiating systemic treatment. Patients may need an antifungal mouthwash such as nystatin if oral candidiasis is suspected, and treatment with fluconazole or clotrimazole troches may be added as well. Severe mucositis/stomatitis can lead to difficulty in swallowing, and may interfere with continuous dosing of treatment regimens; it is essential that patients experiencing mucositis/stomatitis stay well hydrated and nourished.

Dyspepsia

Dyspepsia can occur alone or in conjunction with nausea/vomiting. Small, frequent meals, the avoidance of caffeine-containing foods, spicy foods, and foods containing peppermint or chocolate may limit the incidence of symptoms. Patients may require pharmacologic interventions if dietary modifications are unsuccessful. Aluminum and magnesium hydroxide, famotidine, ranitidine or omeprazole, and pantoprazole are agents that may lessen the incidence of dyspepsia associated with targeted therapies.

Altered Taste

Altered taste is also seen with some of the novel agents used to treat RCC. There are several recommendations that may enhance taste or, at a minimum, decrease the amount of taste alteration reported by patients. Little research has been conducted that determines the standard of care for treatment, and most patients report trial-and-error interventions to be most successful. Patients receiving anticancer medications often complain of a metallic taste to their food. Use of plastic utensils may decrease the incidence of metallic taste. Patients also report that eating foods at colder than normal temperatures and eating small, frequent meals can limit taste changes. The use of additional spices, marinades, fats, and sauces may also enhance the flavor of food. Sucking on sour hard candies before meals can also decrease taste alterations experienced by patients.

FATIGUE

Fatigue is a common side effect of cancer treatment, affecting more than 70% of cancer patients at some point during their treatment.[82] Treatment-related fatigue has also been reported with hormonal and biologic therapy, particularly cytokines such as interleukin-2 and interferon.[83] Fatigue is a frequent side effect of the VEGF-targeted therapies sunitinib, sorafenib, and pazopanib, but is less common in the mTOR inhibitor temsirolimus. With multiple targeted agents available today, addressing fatigue early in treatment is important to ensure the best outcome for patients.

Fatigue is a subjective symptom that can be attributed to cancer treatment, underlying malignancy, or comorbid conditions (eg, anemia, cachexia, and depression). While fatigue is a known toxicity of novel agents, evaluation for alternative causes, such as anemia and hypothyroidism, is important. Fatigue may also manifest in patients secondary to psychosocial issues and depression, requiring social work and psychiatric intervention. In addition, cancer patients often experience disturbance in sleep pattern. Recommendations may include limiting caffeinated beverages at night, limiting naps during the day, and increasing physical activity level. Exercise may beneficial in certain populations of cancer patients.[84] Low levels of activity that are gradually increased over time may improve symptoms, although patients should consult with their physicians before initiating an exercise regimen. Alternative therapies such as acupuncture, massage therapy, and guided imagery may be beneficial to patients.[85]

Pharmacologic interventions may also be successful in minimizing complaints of fatigue. Cancer patients are often prescribed multiple medications that can cause drowsiness. Antiemetics, narcotics, and medications for insomnia could have lethal interactions if combined in improper doses. Psychostimulants may be prescribed for patients with moderate to severe levels of fatigue. Methylphenidate and modafinil have been used, with reports of success.[86]

Ultimately, dose reduction of the agent may be necessary to ensure uninterrupted treatment while minimizing symptoms.

DRUG INTERACTIONS AND TARGETED THERAPIES

Sunitinib is metabolized by CYP3A4 to produce its active metabolite. That metabolite is further degraded by the CYP3A4 isoenzyme to produce an inactive metabolite.[87] Coadministration of strong inhibitors of CYP3A4 may increase plasma concentrations of sunitinib (see **Box 1**). Conversely, coadministration of strong inducers of CYP3A4 may decrease plasma concentrations to subtherapeutic levels (see **Box 1**). If the concomitant use of a CYP3A4 inducer or inhibitor cannot be avoided, sunitinib dose modification may be required.[77] Pazopanib and temsirolimus metabolism are both mediated by the CYP3A4 isoenzyme, and the same precautions should be taken.[75,78]

It is interesting that although sorafenib metabolism is also mediated by CYP3A4, plasma concentration does not seem to be affected by concomitant administration of CYP3A4 inhibitors, in part because sorafenib is partly metabolized by glucuronidation pathways. However, plasma concentration does appear to be affected by coadministration of strong CYP3A4 inducers, and dose modification is recommended.[60,88] Everolimus is a substrate of CYP3A4 and efflux pump P-glycoprotein (PgP). Concomitant administration of drugs or agents that affect either of these pathways can alter the plasma concentration of everolimus.[74] **Table 5** contains guidelines for dose modification of these drugs.

MEDICATION ADHERENCE

Keep a watch also on the faults of the patients, which also make them lie about the taking of things prescribed.
                                                                    —*Hippocrates*

At present, there are more than 40 oral anticancer agents in use.[89] It is that estimated 25% of antineoplastic drugs currently in development are oral drugs.[90] Historically

Table 5
Dose modifications for drug interactions

	Sorafenib	Sunitinib	Temsirolimus	Everolimus	Pazopanib
Strong CYP3A4 inhibitors	No dose modification necessary	Reduce sunitinib dose to a minimum of 37.5 mg daily	Reduce dose of temsirolimus to 12.5 mg/wk. If strong inhibitor is discontinued allow 1 week washout period before escalating to the previous dose used before coadministration of the inhibitor	Do not coadminister with everolimus	Reduce pazopanib dose to 400 mg daily
Strong CYP3A4 inducers	Consider dose increase. Monitor for adverse events	Consider increasing sunitinib dose, may increase to a maximum of 82.5 mg daily. Monitor for adverse events	Consider increasing the temsirolimus dose to 50 mg/wk. Monitor for adverse events. If the strong inducer is discontinued, allow 1 week washout period before reducing to the previous dose used before coadministration of the inhibitor	Consider increasing the everolimus dose using 5-mg increments up to a maximum dose of 20 mg daily	Pazopanib should not be used if chronic use of CYP3A4 inducers cannot be avoided
Other interactions	Avoid coadministration with UGT1A1 and UGT1A9 substrates			PgP inhibitors should not be coadministered with everolimus PgP inducers: consider increasing the everolimus dose using 5-mg increments up to a maximum dose of 20 mg daily	

Abbreviation: PgP, P-glycoprotein.
Data from Refs.[60,74–78]

patients have been treated almost exclusively with parenteral agents. Hence, the administration of a particular treatment regimen was within the control of the clinician.

However, with oral chemotherapeutic agents responsibility for proper dosing and monitoring for side effects shifts from the clinician to the patient and his or her family.[90] Clinicians may lose faith in a particular treatment regimen if there is disease progression when the culprit is in poor adherence rather than as the result of a drug being ineffective. In a study of 2378 patients with primary breast cancer being treated with adjuvant tamoxifen; adherence during the first year of treatment was 87%; however, by year 4 adherence rates had fallen to 50%.[91]

Although there have been no exact links identified, there are certain factors that seem to influence adherence (**Box 2**). However, even though these risks may be missing from a patient's profile, it does not follow that the patient is not at risk for poor adherence to his or her treatment regimen.[92] For example, patients taking oral targeted therapeutic drugs have probably experienced some form of temporary regimen modification because of side effects or drug holidays built into the treatment program. This pattern may lead patients to believe that intermittent adherence is routine and acceptable.[93]

Oncologists and oncology nurses play a key role in optimizing patient adherence. Establishing a trusting and collaborative relationship, improved communication, provision of education and counseling, close follow-up, and optimizing convenience of clinic scheduling have been identified as effective interventions (**Table 6**).[71,89,90,92,93] In their practice the authors carry out "proactive calling," which involves calling the patient within the first week of the prescribed regimen to assess proper dosing, side effects, and the patient's overall understanding of the regimen. Patients are seen back in clinic at the 2-week and 4-week mark for assessment. At every call and clinic visit the patient is asked in an open-ended fashion about their dosing practices. These techniques build trust between patient and caregiver, and may improve adherence and lead to improved outcomes.

Box 2
Potential risk factors for nonadherence
Complex dosing regimen
Side effects
Cost, copayment
Cognitive and/or physical impairment
Depression
Comorbid conditions
Polypharmacy
Lack of belief in treatment
Hectic lifestyle
Dissatisfaction with care
Poor patient-provider relationship
Illiteracy
Inadequate social support
Data from Refs.[89,92,94]

Table 6
Interventions to improve medication adherence

Patient Education	Counseling	Follow-Up
Side effects and management	Emphasize the value of the regimen	Timely and convenient clinic visits
Benefits/risks of treatment	Assess for barriers to adherence	Proactive calling
Drug regimen	Encourage use of pill boxes, medication diaries, and other aids	Contact patients who miss appointments
Disease	Listen to the patient	
Consequences of nonadherence		

Data from Refs.[92–96]

SUMMARY

While much progress has been made identifying effective management strategies for much toxicity from novel agents in RCC, there unfortunately remain few prospective data on optimal management of toxicity with these agents. The measures outlined in this article are often best practices but are not always evidence-based. As more of these agents are used in the clinic, our attention must turn toward prospective trials of supportive care and toxicity management in order to allow patients to experience the full benefits of RCC therapy.

REFERENCES

1. Bellmunt J, Eisen T, Fishman M, et al. Experience with sorafenib and adverse event management. Crit Rev Oncol Hematol 2011;78(1):24–32.
2. Bellmunt J, Montagut C, Albiol S, et al. Present strategies in the treatment of metastatic renal cell carcinoma: an update on molecular targeting agents. BJU Int 2007;99:274.
3. Canoy D, Luben R, Welch A, et al. Fat distribution, body mass index and blood pressure in 22,090 men and women in the Norfolk cohort of the European Prospective Investigation into Cancer and Nutrition (EPIC-Norfolk) study. J Hypertens 2004;22:2067.
4. Eremina V, Jefferson JA, Kowalewska J, et al. VEGF inhibition and renal thrombotic microangiopathy. N Engl J Med 2008;358:1129.
5. Hood JD, Meininger CJ, Ziche M, et al. VEGF upregulates ecNOS message, protein, and NO production in human endothelial cells. Am J Physiol 1998;274: H1054.
6. Horowitz JR, Rivard A, van der Zee R, et al. Vascular endothelial growth factor/ vascular permeability factor produces nitric oxide-dependent hypotension. Evidence for a maintenance role in quiescent adult endothelium. Arterioscler Thromb Vasc Biol 1997;17:2793.
7. Robinson ES, Khankin EV, Choueiri TK, et al. Suppression of the nitric oxide pathway in metastatic renal cell carcinoma patients receiving vascular endothelial growth factor-signaling inhibitors. Hypertension 2010;56:1131.
8. Vaklavas C, Lenihan D, Kurzrock R, et al. Anti-vascular endothelial growth factor therapies and cardiovascular toxicity: what are the important clinical markers to target? Oncologist 2010;15:130.

9. Di Lorenzo G, Autorino R, Bruni G, et al. Cardiovascular toxicity following sunitinib therapy in metastatic renal cell carcinoma: a multicenter analysis. Ann Oncol 2009;20:1535.

10. Chobanian AV, Bakris GL, Black HR, et al. Seventh report of the Joint National Committee on Prevention, Detection, Evaluation, and Treatment of High Blood Pressure. Hypertension 2003;42:1206.

11. Zhu X, Stergiopoulos K, Wu S. Risk of hypertension and renal dysfunction with an angiogenesis inhibitor sunitinib: systematic review and meta-analysis. Acta Oncol 2009;48:9.

12. Wu S, Chen JJ, Kudelka A, et al. Incidence and risk of hypertension with sorafenib in patients with cancer: a systematic review and meta-analysis. Lancet Oncol 2008;9:117.

13. Ranpura V, Pulipati B, Chu D, et al. Increased risk of high-grade hypertension with bevacizumab in cancer patients: a meta-analysis. Am J Hypertens 2010;23:460.

14. Rini BI. Biomarkers: hypertension following anti-angiogenesis therapy. Clin Adv Hematol Oncol 2010;8:415.

15. Rixe O, Billemont B, Izzedine H. Hypertension as a predictive factor of sunitinib activity. Ann Oncol 2007;18:1117.

16. Izzedine H, Ederhy S, Goldwasser F, et al. Management of hypertension in angiogenesis inhibitor-treated patients. Ann Oncol 2009;20:807.

17. Langenberg MH, van Herpen CML, De Bono J, et al. Effective strategies for management of hypertension after vascular endothelial growth factor signaling inhibition therapy: results from a phase II randomized, factorial, double-blind study of cediranib in patients with advanced solid tumors. J Clin Oncol 2009;27:6152.

18. National Kidney Foundation. K/DOQI clinical practice guidelines for chronic kidney disease: evaluation, classification, and stratification. Am J Kidney Dis 2002;39:S1.

19. Chobanian AV, Bakris GL, Black HR, et al. The seventh report of the joint national committee on prevention, detection, evaluation, and treatment of high blood pressure: the JNC 7 report. JAMA 2003;289:2560.

20. Miura S, Fujino M, Matsuo Y, et al. Nifedipine-induced vascular endothelial growth factor secretion from coronary smooth muscle cells promotes endothelial tube formation via the kinase insert domain-containing receptor/fetal liver kinase-1/NO pathway. Hypertens Res 2005;28:147.

21. Ranpura V, Hapani S, Chuang J, et al. Risk of cardiac ischemia and arterial thromboembolic events with the angiogenesis inhibitor bevacizumab in cancer patients: a meta-analysis of randomized controlled trials. Acta Oncol 2010;49:287.

22. Schutz FA, Je Y, Azzi GR, et al. Bevacizumab increases the risk of arterial ischemia: a large study in cancer patients with a focus on different subgroup outcomes. Ann Oncol 2011;22(6):1404–12.

23. Nalluri SR, Chu D, Keresztes R, et al. Risk of venous thromboembolism with the angiogenesis inhibitor bevacizumab in cancer patients: a meta-analysis. JAMA 2008;300:2277.

24. Choueiri TK, Schutz FA, Je Y, et al. Risk of arterial thromboembolic events with sunitinib and sorafenib: a systematic review and meta-analysis of clinical trials. J Clin Oncol 2010;28:2280.

25. Deuse T, Peter C, Fedak PW, et al. Hepatocyte growth factor or vascular endothelial growth factor gene transfer maximizes mesenchymal stem cell-based myocardial salvage after acute myocardial infarction. Circulation 2009;120:S247.

26. Giordano FJ, Gerber HP, Williams SP, et al. A cardiac myocyte vascular endothelial growth factor paracrine pathway is required to maintain cardiac function. Proc Natl Acad Sci U S A 2001;98:5780.

27. Schmidinger M, Zielinski CC, Vogl UM, et al. Cardiac toxicity of sunitinib and sorafenib in patients with metastatic renal cell carcinoma. J Clin Oncol 2008;26:5204.

28. Motzer RJ, Michaelson MD, Redman BG, et al. Activity of SU11248, a multitargeted inhibitor of vascular endothelial growth factor receptor and platelet-derived growth factor receptor, in patients with metastatic renal cell carcinoma. J Clin Oncol 2006;24:16.

29. Motzer RJ, Rini BI, Bukowski RM, et al. Sunitinib in patients with metastatic renal cell carcinoma. JAMA 2006;295:2516.

30. Motzer RJ, Hutson TE, Tomczak P, et al. Sunitinib versus interferon alfa in metastatic renal-cell carcinoma. N Engl J Med 2007;356:115.

31. Khakoo AY, Halushka MK, Rame JE, et al. Reversible cardiomyopathy caused by administration of interferon alpha. Nat Clin Pract Cardiovasc Med 2005;2:53.

32. Gore ME, Szczylik C, Porta C, et al. Safety and efficacy of sunitinib for metastatic renal-cell carcinoma: an expanded-access trial. Lancet Oncol 2009;10:757.

33. Khakoo AY, Kassiotis CM, Tannir N, et al. Heart failure associated with sunitinib malate: a multitargeted receptor tyrosine kinase inhibitor. Cancer 2008;112:2500.

34. Telli ML, Witteles RM, Fisher GA, et al. Cardiotoxicity associated with the cancer therapeutic agent sunitinib malate. Ann Oncol 2008;19:1613.

35. Llovet JM, Ricci S, Mazzaferro V, et al. Sorafenib in advanced hepatocellular carcinoma. N Engl J Med 2008;359:378.

36. Escudier B, Eisen T, Stadler WM, et al. Sorafenib in advanced clear-cell renal-cell carcinoma. N Engl J Med 2007;356:125.

37. Kane RC, Farrell AT, Saber H, et al. Sorafenib for the treatment of advanced renal cell carcinoma. Clin Cancer Res 2006;12:7271.

38. Choueiri TK, Mayer EL, Je Y, et al. Congestive heart failure risk in patients with breast cancer treated with bevacizumab. J Clin Oncol 2011;29(6):632–8.

39. Hapani S, Sher A, Chu D, et al. Increased risk of serious hemorrhage with bevacizumab in cancer patients: a meta-analysis. Oncology 2010;79:27.

40. Je Y, Schutz FA, Choueiri TK. Risk of bleeding with vascular endothelial growth factor receptor tyrosine-kinase inhibitors sunitinib and sorafenib: a systematic review and meta-analysis of clinical trials. Lancet Oncol 2009;10:967.

41. Pouessel D, Culine S. High frequency of intracerebral hemorrhage in metastatic renal carcinoma patients with brain metastases treated with tyrosine kinase inhibitors targeting the vascular endothelial growth factor receptor. Eur Urol 2008;53:376.

42. Porta C, Imarisio I, Paglino C. Re: Damien Pouessel, Stephane Culine. High frequency of intracerebral hemorrhage in metastatic renal carcinoma patients with brain metastases treated with tyrosine kinase inhibitors targeting the vascular endothelial growth factor receptor. Eur Urol 2008;53:1092.

43. Hudes G, Carducci M, Tomczak P, et al. Temsirolimus, interferon alfa, or both for advanced renal-cell carcinoma. N Engl J Med 2007;356:2271.

44. Motzer RJ, Escudier B, Oudard S, et al. Efficacy of everolimus in advanced renal cell carcinoma: a double-blind, randomised, placebo-controlled phase III trial. Lancet 2008;372:449.

45. Agostino N, Chinchilli VM, Lynch CJ, et al. Effect of the tyrosine kinase inhibitors (sunitinib, sorafenib, dasatinib, and imatinib) on blood glucose levels in diabetic and nondiabetic patients in general clinical practice. J Oncol Pharm Pract 2010. [Epub ahead of print]. DOI: 10.1177/1078155210378913.

46. Grundy SM, Cleeman JI, Merz CNB, et al. Implications of recent clinical trials for the national cholesterol education program adult treatment panel III guidelines. Circulation 2004;110:227.

47. Sternberg CN, Davis ID, Mardiak J, et al. Pazopanib in locally advanced or metastatic renal cell carcinoma: results of a randomized phase III trial. J Clin Oncol 2010;28:1061.

48. Miyake H, Kurahashi T, Yamanaka K, et al. Abnormalities of thyroid function in Japanese patients with metastatic renal cell carcinoma treated with sorafenib: a prospective evaluation. Urol Oncol 2010;28:515.

49. Rini BI, Tamaskar I, Shaheen P, et al. Hypothyroidism in patients with metastatic renal cell carcinoma treated with sunitinib. J Natl Cancer Inst 2007;99:81.

50. Wolter P, Stefan C, Decallonne B, et al. The clinical implications of sunitinib-induced hypothyroidism: a prospective evaluation. Br J Cancer 2008;99:448.

51. Zhu X, Wu S, Dahut WL, et al. Risks of proteinuria and hypertension with bevacizumab, an antibody against vascular endothelial growth factor: systematic review and meta-analysis. Am J Kidney Dis 2007;49:186.

52. Rini BI, Halabi S, Rosenberg JE, et al. Bevacizumab plus interferon alfa compared with interferon alfa monotherapy in patients with metastatic renal cell carcinoma: CALGB 90206. J Clin Oncol 2008;26:5422.

53. Wu S, Kim C, Baer L, et al. Bevacizumab increases risk for severe proteinuria in cancer patients. J Am Soc Nephrol 2010;21:1381.

54. Autier J, Escudier B, Wechsler J, et al. Prospective study of the cutaneous adverse effects of sorafenib, a novel multikinase inhibitor. Arch Dermatol 2008; 144:886.

55. Chu D, Lacouture ME, Weiner E, et al. Risk of hand-foot skin reaction with the multitargeted kinase inhibitor sunitinib in patients with renal cell and non-renal cell carcinoma: a meta-analysis. Clin Genitourin Cancer 2009;7:11.

56. Lacouture ME, Wu S, Robert C, et al. Evolving strategies for the management of hand-foot skin reaction associated with the multitargeted kinase inhibitors sorafenib and sunitinib. Oncologist 2008;13:1001.

57. Rosenbaum SE, Wu S, Newman MA, et al. Dermatological reactions to the multitargeted tyrosine kinase inhibitor sunitinib. Support Care Cancer 2008;16:557.

58. Porta C, Paglino C, Imarisio I, et al. Uncovering Pandora's vase: the growing problem of new toxicities from novel anticancer agents. The case of sorafenib and sunitinib. Clin Exp Med 2007;7:127.

59. Lee WJ, Lee JL, Chang SE, et al. Cutaneous adverse effects in patients treated with the multitargeted kinase inhibitors sorafenib and sunitinib. Br J Dermatol 2009;161:1045.

60. Hutson TE, Figlin RA, Kuhn JG, et al. Targeted therapies for metastatic renal cell carcinoma: an overview of toxicity and dosing strategies. Oncologist 2008; 13(10):1084–96.

61. Beldner M, Jacobson M, Burges GE, et al. Localized palmar-plantar epidermal hyperplasia: a previously undefined dermatologic toxicity to sorafenib. Oncologist 2007;12:1178.

62. Lacouture ME, Reilly LM, Gerami P, et al. Hand foot skin reaction in cancer patients treated with the multikinase inhibitors sorafenib and sunitinib. Ann Oncol 2008;19:1955.

63. Schwandt A, Wood LS, Rini B, et al. Management of side effects associated with sunitinib therapy for patients with renal cell carcinoma. Onco Targets Ther 2009; 2:51.

64. Michaelson M, Cohen D, Li S, et al. Hand-foot syndrome (HFS) as a potential biomarker of efficacy in patients (pts) with metastatic renal cell carcinoma (mRCC) treated with sunitinib (SU). In American Society of Clinical Oncology: Genitourinary Cancers Symposium. Orlando (FL), February 17–19, 2011.

65. Bellmunt J, Szczylik C, Feingold J, et al. Temsirolimus safety profile and management of toxic effects in patients with advanced renal cell carcinoma and poor prognostic features. Ann Oncol 2008;19:1387.
66. Alexandrescu DT, Vaillant JG, Dasanu CA. Effect of treatment with a colloidal oatmeal lotion on the acneform eruption induced by epidermal growth factor receptor and multiple tyrosine-kinase inhibitors. Clin Exp Dermatol 2007;32:71.
67. Wood L. Managing the side effects of sunitinib and sorafenib. Community Oncol 2006;3:558.
68. Rodriguez-Pascual J, Cheng E, Maroto P, et al. Emergent toxicities associated with the use of mTOR inhibitors in patients with advanced renal carcinoma. Anticancer Drugs 2010;21:478.
69. Schmidinger M, Bellmunt J. Plethora of agents, plethora of targets, plethora of side effects in metastatic renal cell carcinoma. Cancer Treat Rev 2010;36:416.
70. White DA, Camus P, Endo M, et al. Noninfectious pneumonitis after everolimus therapy for advanced renal cell carcinoma. Am J Respir Crit Care Med 2010; 182:396.
71. Cramer J, Roy A, Burrell A, et al. Medication compliance and persistence: terminology and definitions. Value Health 2008;11:44.
72. Yavuzsen T, Davis MP, Walsh D, et al. Systematic review of the treatment of cancer-associated anorexia and weight loss. J Clin Oncol 2005;23:8500.
73. Bhojani N, Jeldres C, Patard J-J, et al. Toxicities associated with the administration of sorafenib, sunitinib, and temsirolimus and their management in patients with metastatic renal cell carcinoma. Eur Urol 2008;53:917.
74. Everolimus [package insert]. East Hanover, NJ: Novartis Pharmaceuticals; 2009.
75. Pazopanib [package insert]. Research Triangle Park, NC: GlaxoSmithKline; 2009.
76. Sorafenib [package insert]. West Haven, CT and Emeryville, CA; Bayer Pharmaceutical Corporation and Onyx Pharmaceuticals, Inc.; 2006.
77. Sunitinib [package insert]. New York, NY: Pfizer Labs; 2006.
78. Temsirolimus [package insert]. Philadelphia, PA: Wyeth Pharmaceuticals, Inc.; 2010.
79. Mansky PJ, Wallerstedt DB. Complementary medicine in palliative care and cancer symptom management. Cancer J 2006;12:425.
80. Wood LS. Management of vascular endothelial growth factor and multikinase inhibitor side effects. Clin J Oncol Nurs 2009;13(Suppl):13.
81. Peterson DE, Bensadoun RJ, Roila F, et al, On behalf of the EGWG. Management of oral and gastrointestinal mucositis: ESMO clinical recommendations. Ann Oncol 2009;20:174.
82. Larkin JM, Pyle LM, Gore ME. Fatigue in renal cell carcinoma: the hidden burden of current targeted therapies. Oncologist 2010;15:1135.
83. Wang XS. Pathophysiology of cancer-related fatigue. Clin J Oncol Nurs 2008; 12:11.
84. McNeely ML, Courneya KS. Exercise programs for cancer-related fatigue: evidence and clinical guidelines. J Natl Compr Canc Netw 2010;8:945.
85. Ernst E. Massage therapy for cancer palliation and supportive care: a systematic review of randomised clinical trials. Support Care Cancer 2009;17:333.
86. Minton O, Richardson A, Sharpe M, et al. Psychostimulants for the management of cancer-related fatigue: a systematic review and meta-analysis. J Pain Symptom Manage 2011;41(4):761–7.
87. Haoualaa A, Widmer N, Buclin T, et al. Cardiovascular drug interactions with tyrosine kinase inhibitors. Cardiovasc Med 2010;13:147.

88. Horn J, Hansten P. Drug interactions with tyrosine kinase inhibitors. 2010. Available at: www.PharmacyTimes.com. Accessed February 5, 2011.

89. Moore S. Adherence to oral therapies for cancer: barriers and models for change. Journal of the Advanced Practitioner in Oncology 2010;1:155.

90. Weingart S, Brown E, Bach P, et al. NCCN task force report: oral chemotherapy. J Natl Compr Canc Netw 2008;6:s1.

91. Partridge AW, Winer PS, Avorn EP. Nonadherence to adjuvant tamoxifen therapy in women with primary breast cancer. J Clin Oncol 2003;21:602.

92. Osterberg L, Blaschke T. Adherence to medication. N Engl J Med 2005;353:487.

93. Blasdel C, Bubalo J. Adherence to oral cancer therapies: meeting the challenge of new patient care needs. 2006. Available at: www.clinicaloncology.com/download/563SR-Novartis.pdf. Accessed February 5, 2011.

94. Moore S. Facilitating oral chemotherapy treatment and compliance through patient/family-focused education. Cancer Nurs 2007;30:112.

95. Ruddy K, Mayer E, Partridge A. Patient adherence and persistence with oral anti-cancer treatment. CA Cancer J Clin 2009;59:56.

96. Viele C. Managing oral chemotherapy: the healthcare practitioner's role. Am J Health Syst Pharm 2007;64:S25.

Future Directions in Renal Cell Carcinoma: 2011 and Beyond

Daniel C. Cho, MD[a,b,*], Michael B. Atkins, MD[a,b]

KEYWORDS

• Renal cell carcinoma • Future directions
• Therapeutic outcomes

NOVEL THERAPEUTIC STRATEGIES INCORPORATING APPROVED AGENTS

In 2010, an estimated 58,000 new cases of renal cell carcinoma (RCC) were diagnosed in the United States and approximately 13,000 individuals died of this disease.[1] Renal cancer is made up of several different types of cancer, each of which has distinct molecular underpinnings and a different response to treatment. For clear cell RCC (the most common variant), 3 potentially distinct targets and related therapeutic approaches are available: immunotherapy, vascular endothelial growth factor (VEGF) (antiangiogenic therapy), and mTOR (mammalian target of rapamycin) (targeted therapy). Several therapies have received approval for the treatment of advanced RCC. **Table 1** displays an algorithm for the current use of the agents. Application of these treatment options has improved the overall survival (OS) for patients with advanced RCC from a median of 10 months in 1999[2] to in excess of 2 years.[3] Nonetheless, for patients who either present with or develop metastatic disease the expected 5-year survival rate is still only approximately 10%. Although there are ongoing efforts to further clarify what can be expected therapeutically from these existing agents, much effort will be focused on identifying potential opportunities to enhance the efficacy of approved therapies either through: (1) use of novel dosing or scheduling strategies; (2) defining optimal treatment sequencing; (3) identifying opportunities for successful application of combination therapy; and (4) developing predictive biomarkers of response to particular therapies. It is hoped that such efforts will not only lead to

This work was partially supported by grant P50 CA101942 from the National Cancer Institute.
Disclosures: DC has served as a consultant to Novartis and Genentech MBA- has served as a consultant to Pfizer, Genentech, BMS, Aveo, Bayer, Novartis and Prometheus.
[a] Division of Hematology/Oncology, Beth Israel Deaconess Medical Center, Harvard Medical School, 330 Brookline Avenue, Boston, MA 02215, USA
[b] Kidney Cancer Program, Dana-Farber/Harvard Cancer Center, 375 Longwood Avenue, Boston, MA 02215, USA
* Corresponding author. Division of Hematology/Oncology, Beth Israel Deaconess Medical Center and Harvard Medical School, 330 Brookline Avenue, Boston, MA 02215.
E-mail address: dcho1@bidmc.harvard.edu

Hematol Oncol Clin N Am 25 (2011) 917–935
doi:10.1016/j.hoc.2011.05.001
0889-8588/11/$ – see front matter © 2011 Elsevier Inc. All rights reserved.

Table 1
Current therapeutic options for clear cell RCC therapy

Setting	Phase III Trials	Alternatives
First-line therapy		
Good or intermediate risk[a]	Sunitinib or bevacizumab plus IFN or pazopanib	High-dose IL-2, IFN-α
Poor risk[a]	Temsirolimus	Sunitinib
Second-line therapy		
Previous cytokine	Sorafenib	Sunitinib or bevacizumab
Previous VEGFR inhibitor	Everolimus	Other VEGF-targeted therapy
Previous mTOR inhibitor	Clinical trials	Clinical trials

[a] Memorial Sloan-Kettering Cancer Center risk status.

improved clinical outcomes using currently available therapies but will also highlight obstacles that can be overcome only with the identification of novel therapeutic targets and strategies.

Novel Dosing or Scheduling Strategies

The determination of optimal dose for VEGF pathway inhibitors has been based on phase I trials. However, the optimal dose derived from dose-limiting toxicities observed in a handful of patients may not be the optimal dose for each individual patient. For example, studies with sorafenib have suggested that some patients at time of resistance may respond to an increase in sorafenib dose from 400 to 600 mg twice a day[4] and that in patients in whom sorafenib dose is routinely escalated every 4 weeks, if tolerated, tumor response rates may be considerably higher.[5] Thus, it is conceivable that some patients who experience disease progression on currently available agents may be receiving less than their optimum dose.

This conclusion is supported by investigations into the relationship between sunitinib exposure and efficacy end points in patients with advanced solid tumors including metastatic RCC.[6] Houk and colleagues[6] determined that higher steady-state area under the curve (AUC) of total drug (sunitinib and its active metabolite SU12662) was significantly associated with longer time to tumor progression (TTP) and improved OS; as well as higher probability of tumor response. These results suggest that maintaining the highest tolerable dose of sunitinib may be important for maximum efficacy. Furthermore, because there is likely wide pharmacokinetic variation between individuals, to maintain optimal drug exposure, it is conceivable that dosing patients based on blood levels similar to antibiotics or anticonvulsants may prove more efficacious than using the current standard daily dose of 50 mg for all patients. Studies aimed at dosing patients based on drug concentration (AUC) are being planned and may ultimately alter the dosing paradigm for sunitinib and other VEGF pathway blockers.

The development of either systolic or diastolic hypertension has also been shown to correlate with response to VEGF pathway inhibitor therapy.[7] Houk and colleagues[6] also established a correlation with total drug concentration (sunitinib and its metabolite) and diastolic blood pressure, which suggests that hypertension might represent a surrogate marker for VEGF receptor (VEGFR) tyrosine kinase inhibitor (TKI) blood levels and that escalating drug dose until hypertension is observed might represent an alternative means of ensuring sufficient dosing. However, this pharmacodynamic parameter may be confounded by the additional variable of VEGF/VEGFR polymorphisms which might decouple the direct correlation between blood level and pharmacodynamic effect (hypertension and/or response). The clinical usefulness of this strategy is being investigated in a trial in which patients without hypertension after an initial 4 weeks of axitinib therapy are randomly assigned to receive either additional axitinib or placebo (NCT00835978). This trial will also provide the opportunity to further establish any linkage between axitinib blood levels, hypertension (a potential pharmacodynamic marker), and tumor response.

An alternative strategy for achieving higher peak drug concentrations and minimizing toxicity is to use an intermittent treatment schedule. The effect of sunitinib treatment schedule was recently examined in a phase III trial. The standard sunitinib treatment schedule (50 mg/d for 4 weeks followed by 2 weeks off treatment) was compared with continuous daily treatment (37.5 mg/d) in 292 patients with advanced RCC.[8] Preliminary results showed a trend toward inferior TTP with the continuous dosing schedule (median 7.1 vs 9.9 months, hazard ratio 0.77, 95% confidence interval 0.57–1.04). OS and adverse event profiles were similar for the 2 regimens. Whether this finding represents a dose (pharmacokinetic) effect or a schedule effect (delaying resistance development by providing frequent treatment breaks), and how these results might influence treatment schedule considerations for other VEGFR inhibitors in patients with RCC, is an area of potential future investigation.

The Role of Sequential Versus Combination Therapy

The availability of multiple treatment strategies for patients with advanced RCC has engendered considerable interest in treatment sequencing approaches and combination regimens. Early data supported the notion that both VEGF pathway inhibitors[9,10] and mTOR-targeted therapies[11] were active after disease progression on cytokine-based therapy. The RECORD1 trial firmly established that everolimus was more active than placebo in patients whose disease had progressed after VEGFR TKI (sunitinib, sorafenib, or both) therapy.[12] However, a small retrospective analysis suggested that high-dose (HD) IL-2 administered after sunitinib or sorafenib resulted in an unexpectedly high rate of cardiac toxicity and produced no tumor responses, suggesting that if HD interleukin 2 (IL-2)-based immunotherapy is to be considered, it might best be used as the initial treatment.[13] Furthermore, more recent data suggested that VEGF pathway inhibitors may have activity after disease progression on another VEGF (or even the same) pathway inhibitor. For example, sunitinib produced tumor responses in 23% of patients after progression on bevacizumab[14] and axitinib showed similar activity in patients showing disease progression after sorafenib.[15] Thus, the value of switching to an mTOR inhibitor after disease progression on a VEGF pathway inhibitor versus switching to another (perhaps more potent) VEGF pathway inhibitor remains to be determined. Although this specific question is being partially studied in a randomized phase III trial comparing temsirolimus with sorafenib in patients whose disease has progressed on sunitinib, such decisions will likely need to be individualized. For example, in patients who show disease progression without significant toxicity on a particular VEGF pathway inhibitor, dose escalation may be indicated, whereas for patients who have experienced a response to a VEGF pathway blocker, but then show disease progression after dose reduction because of toxicity, switching to a different VEGF pathway blocker may restore disease sensitivity. Switching to an mTOR inhibitor might be the treatment of choice for patients whose disease is upfront resistant to VEGF pathway blockade or has progressed after multiple (or the most potent) VEGF pathway blocker(s). However, a retrospective study[16] showed that the institution of mTOR inhibitors may not be better than switching to alternate VEGF pathway inhibitors in patients with tumors that are primarily refractory to anti-VEGF therapy, suggesting that a different approach may be necessary for such patients.

An alternative strategy for maintaining disease control or enhancing treatment effect is to administer active treatments in combination. Combination therapy strategies could include the combining of molecularly targeted agents with immunotherapy (interferon [IFN] or HD IL-2), combining a VEGF blocking agent (bevacizumab) with a VEGFR TKI (vertical blockade) or combining a VEGF pathway inhibitor with an mTOR or other pathway inhibitor (horizontal blockade). All of these approaches have been tested clinically, with varying results.

Vertical blockade with either sorafenib or sunitinib combined with bevacizumab has shown impressive antitumor activity but disappointing toxicity. For example, the combination of sorafenib and bevacizumab produced tumor responses in 52% of patients with advanced RCC; however, the regimen also produced enhanced toxicity, necessitating drastic reductions in both agents to maintain its tolerability.[17] Similarly the combination of sunitinib and bevacizumab produced responses in more than 50% of patients but also produced a microangiopathic hemolytic anemia syndrome with associated kidney failure and neurologic toxicity in patients who received extended therapy.[18] This syndrome, which is similar to preeclampsia (a disease attributed to tissue VEGF starvation caused by high levels of circulating soluble VEGFR),[19] may show the limits of tolerability of prolonged and profound VEGF pathway blockade.

Compared with the vertical blockade, horizontal blockade strategies have in general been more tolerable. The combination of bevacizumab and erlotinib was well tolerated, but proved no more effective than bevacizumab alone.[20] In contrast, the combination of either temsirolimus or everolimus with bevacizumab was not only tolerable at the full doses of each agent[21,22] but also produced response rates that appeared to be superior to what would be anticipated with mTOR inhibition alone. The value of these mTOR + VEGF inhibitors combinations is being explored in a series of randomized phase II and III trials. However, the results of the initial trial were disappointing because the combination of bevacizumab and temsirolimus appeared more toxic, but not more efficacious than either sunitinib or bevacizumab plus IFN in treatment-naive patients with advanced RCC.[23]

Perhaps the most encouraging results have been seen with the combination of VEGF pathway inhibitors and immunotherapy. Both the AVOREN trial and the CALGB-led Intergroup Trial established a benefit for the addition of bevacizumab to IFN-α in terms of response rate and median progression-free survival (PFS).[10,24] The number of patients experiencing a complete or durable response remained small in the combination arm and lacking this or a bevacizumab alone arm, no information is available to firmly establish a contribution of IFN to the combination. Similar results were seen with the combination of bevacizumab and HD IL-2.[25] In this phase II trial, the activity of the combination appeared to be additive, with 8% of patients achieving a complete response (typical of HD IL-2) and a median PFS of 9 months similar to what is seen with bevacizumab alone.[20]

When considering the clinical usefulness of these combinations, one must keep in mind several principles: (1) lowering the dose of an active agent to accommodate the toxicity of a less active agent (as in the temsirolimus plus IFN combination) might diminish efficacy; (2) inhibition of additional pathways (at least in some tumors) may produce countervailing effects or just additional side effects for the patient; and (3) because of the additional toxicity and expense associated with the administration of 2 agents simultaneously, the results of horizontal blockade should be significantly better than the administration of the 2 component agents in sequence to be considered useful.

When viewed in their entirety, the results with combination regimens must be viewed as a major disappointment. Future approaches could be more fruitful by focusing on (1) combinations that might yield durable responses (ie, combinations with immuno-therapy); (2) studying combinations that involve the potential for maintenance of VEGF blockade at the time of resistance (eg, the CALGB trial comparing everolimus vs everolimus + bevacizumab in patients after disease progression on sunititinib or sorafenib); or (3) devising combinations based on understanding of mechanisms of resistance/escape that therefore have increased likelihood of delaying the onset of resistance. Several potential mechanisms for resistance and, therefore, promising pathways to be targeted in combination regimens are discussed in a later section of this review.

Patient Selection Strategies

The availability of approved agents with distinct mechanisms of action (immuno-therapy, mTOR, and VEGF pathway inhibitors) has complicated treatment decisions for patients with advanced RCC. Although randomized phase 3 trials can provide guidance for the average patient in a specific clinical situation, individual patients and tumors have distinct characteristics that may greatly influence their response to different treatments. Identifying the optimal treatment of an individual patient has become an important goal of current investigation. Many recent clinical trials have stratified patients by clinical prognostic factors developed by Motzer and colleagues[2] from analysis of patients treated with IFN-α. More recently, algorithms have been developed that identify prognostic factors for patients receiving VEGF pathway targeted therapies[3] (reviewed by Daniel Heng elsewhere in this issue). These novel algorithms have yet to be used prospectively and given that they overlap substantially with the prognostic factors identified for patients receiving IFN therapy, may be a better indicator of general tumor biology than the impact of specific treatment (or treatment approach) on a particular patient population. Although such algorithms may be useful, the goal remains to be able to choose treatment strategies based on models that take into consideration not just clinical factors but also the pathologic, molecular, and biologic features of the tumor.

Immunotherapy

Although recent phase 3 trials have established the superiority of VEGF-targeted and mTOR-targeted therapies over IFN-based immunotherapy in patients with advanced RCC,[10,11,26,27] a subset of patients clearly exist who develop significant clinical benefit from immunotherapy and for whom omitting this treatment option might greatly compromise their long-term treatment outcome. This situation is particularly true for HD IL-2 therapy, which has been shown in 2 randomized phase 3 trials to produce higher response rates and more durable complete responses than lower-dose cytokine regimens[28,29] and based on trial comparisons more off-treatment sustained responses than are seen with the VEGF and mTOR pathway inhibitors. Recent studies suggest that in the current era the response to HD IL-2 exceeds 25% with at least 10% of patients showing complete responses that last in excess of 2 years (see article by David F. McDermott elsewhere in this issue).[30] Thus, cytokine therapy, particularly HD IL-2, remains a reasonable initial treatment option for some patients with metastatic RCC. However, given the toxicity associated with HD IL-2, identifying predictors of response (or resistance) to this therapy and thus limiting its use to those most likely to benefit remains a high priority.

Efforts to identify predictive factors for response to HD IL-2 have focused on disease, immunohistochemistry (IHC), and gene expression patterns. Past data suggest that responses to immunotherapy are almost exclusively seen in patients with clear cell RCC.[31,32] Although initial efforts suggested that further subdivision of clear cell RCC based on percentage of granular or papillary features might be useful, this approach was not validated in a recently reported prospective trial.[30] Several retrospective analyses reported that IHC staining for carbonic anhydrase IX (CAIX), an enzyme the expression of which is mediated by the hypoxia-inducible factor (HIF) transcriptional complex, was associated with improved survival and a higher objective response rate in IL-2–treated patients[33,34]; however, this predictive biomarker has yet to be validated prospectively. More recent studies with array-based comparative genomic hybridization showed that tumors from complete responders to HD IL-2 had fewer whole chromosome losses than nonresponders.[35] The concentration of losses in sections of chromosome 9p (65% in nonresponders vs 0 in complete responders), which encompasses genes such as CAIX, pS6, and B7H1, adds some potential mechanistic significance to this observation. Studies in RCC and other tumors have suggested that immune cell infiltration (dendritic cells, natural killer cells, CD8 T cells) is associated with improved disease outcome as well as response rates to immunotherapy.[36–39] This research suggests that an extant, but blunted, immune recognition of the tumor may be a prerequisite for response to immunotherapy. Studies of patterns of tumor immune infiltrates using IHC, reverse transcription-polymerase chain reaction, and the examination of host DNA for polymorphisms associated with autoimmunity, are under way. Although the findings will likely require prospective validation, perhaps as part of the IL-2 Select trial, if confirmed they may provide powerful tools for clinicians in selecting patients not just for IL-2 therapy but also for novel immunotherapies in development. In addition, such biomarkers might provide clues to understanding the sensitivity of RCC, and possibly other tumor types, to immunotherapy.

mTOR inhibitors

Although the clinical benefit of HD IL-2 seems limited to patients with clear cell RCC, this may not be the case with inhibitors of the mTOR pathway. A subsequent analysis of the randomized phase 3 trial of temsirolimus versus IFN[26] showed that the median OS of patients with non–clear cell RCC (75% of whom had the papillary subtype) was 11.6 months in the temsirolimus group versus 4.3 months in the IFN group.[40] This differential contrasts with the minor improvement over IFN associated with temsirolimus therapy in patients with clear cell RCC. The preferential activity of temsirolimus in non–clear cell RCC also contrasts with what is seen with the VEGFR antagonists sorafenib and sunitinib, both of which have only limited activity against these RCC variants.[41] These observations suggest that the mechanism of action of mTOR inhibitors may be distinct from those of agents primarily inhibiting VEGFR signaling in the tumor endothelium. During the clinical development of mTOR inhibitors, the antagonism of HIF-1α expression by these drugs has often been proffered as a logical explanation for their clinical efficacy in RCC. However, these observations highlight the need for further investigation into the mechanism of action of mTOR inhibitors and the need to identify molecular features that may predict response to these agents.

Preliminary efforts to identify such predictive biomarkers have focused on pathologic surrogates of the basal activation status of the presumptive molecular targets of mTOR inhibitors. A small retrospective analysis of pretreatment tumor specimens from a subset of patients with RCC treated with temsirolimus as part of the randomized phase 2 trial[11] reported an association of high expression of either phospho-Akt or phospho-S6 ribosomal protein, substrates upstream and downstream of mTOR, respectively, with objective response to temsirolimus.[42] In contrast, no apparent correlation was found of CAIX or PTEN expression. A larger analysis of tumor specimens from patients treated with temsirolimus as part of the randomized phase 3 trial[26] also found no correlation between tumor PTEN expression and either tumor response or OS or PFS. In addition, no such correlations were observed with baseline HIF-1α expression.[43] Although the stability of certain phosphoproteins, in particular phospho-Akt, has been called into question, phospho-S6 seems to be a promising potential predictive biomarker for response to mTOR inhibitors. However, this marker still requires validation in larger retrospective analyses and/or prospective studies.

Future efforts to identify predictive biomarkers of response to mTOR inhibitors must be guided by insights into the mechanism of both response and resistance to mTOR inhibitors. For example, overexpression of eurokaryotic initiation factor 4E (eIF4E) would be expected to make a cell relatively resistant to growth inhibitory efforts of mTOR inhibition.[44] The frequency of basal overexpression of eIF4E in RCC remains to be investigated. Recent studies have also reported somatic activating mutations in mTOR in some RCC.[45] The extent to which such mutation or other mutations in regulators of the AKT/mTOR pathway (TSC1/TSC2; FOXO; PI3K, LKB1, or REDD1) occur needs to be determined along with the assessment of their potential impact on tumor responsiveness to mTOR-targeted therapy. Although the groups of patients deriving clinical benefit from mTOR inhibitors and VEGF-targeted therapies likely overlap to some degree, incorporation of molecular and pathologic features of the tumor into selection schemes will be important to help direct the use of mTOR inhibitors in the adjuvant, first-line, sequential, and combinational therapy for patients with RCC.

VEGF pathway inhibition

As noted earlier, clinical factors predictive of poor outcome with VEGF-targeted therapies tend to overlap those reported for IFN treatment. Heng and colleagues[3] report in a multivariable analysis that 4 of the 5 adverse prognostic factors in the Memorial Sloan Kettering Cancer Center model (time from diagnosis to current treatment less than 1 year, hemoglobin <lower limit of normal, corrected serum calcium > upper limit of normal, and Karnofsky performance scale score <80%), were also independent predictors of short survival in patients receiving VEGF pathway inhibitors. In addition, increased baseline platelet and neutrophil counts were associated with poor prognosis. From these factors, 3 prognostic subgroups were identified with a median OS of 27 months, 24 months, and 8.8 months, respectively. The clinical usefulness of these factors is compromised by the inability to sort out whether they are truly predictive or simply prognostic and because most patients show some degree of treatment shrinkage with VEGF pathway inhibition, making it harder to identify patients with upfront treatment resistance.

Efforts to identify molecular factors associated with poor outcome with VEGF pathway therapy have also begun. High baseline VEGF levels have been associated with poor outcome in both the TARGETs and Avoren trials[10,46]; however, patients with high and low baseline VEGF levels benefited from sorafenib and bevacizumab in terms of PFS. This finding suggests that serum VEGF, although having prognostic significance, is not a predictive biomarker for benefit from VEGF-targeted therapy. Rini and colleagues[14] suggested that lower baseline levels of sVEGFR-3 and VEGF-C were associated with longer PFS and better tumor response in patients receiving sunitinib after disease progression of bevacizumab. However, this work requires validation. Patel and colleagues[47] reported that the level of HIF-2α expression in pretreatment tumor specimens by Western analysis correlated directly with response to sunitinib treatment ($P<.0001$). Additional studies are needed to confirm the predictive value of HIF-2α for sunitinib and other VEGF-targeted agents in patients with metastatic RCC. However, given that HIF-2α expression seems to be a near universal feature of von Hippel-Lindau (VHL) null clear cell RCC, whereas HIF-1α expression is lost in up to 25% of tumors,[48] determining the differential effect of HIF-1α expression on treatment outcome may ultimately prove more useful.

Efforts to determine the predictive value of tumor *VHL* gene inactivation on response of patients with advanced RCC to VEGF-targeted agents have yielded conflicting data. Patients with tumors containing *VHL* inactivation (*VHL* mutated or methylated) had a response rate of 41% compared with 31% for patients with tumors with wild-type *VHL* (P = .34).[49] Patients treated with sorafenib and bevacizumab responded only if their *VHL* gene was inactivated in contrast to patients treated with sunitinib or axitinib who experienced responses irrespective of the *VHL* gene status of their tumor. In other studies, tumor *VHL* status did not seem to be predictive of response to axitinib (N = 13)[50] or pazopanib (N = 78).[51] Although data concerning the impact of tumor VHL gene status on PFS and OS in patients receiving VEGF-targeted therapy may be more clinically relevant, these results are nonetheless of potential therapeutic significance. They suggest either that sunitinib, axitinib, and possibly pazopanib have additional non–*VHL*-related antitumor effects in RCC or that the *VHL*/HIF/VEGF pathway remains an important target in *VHL* wild-type RCC but requires more potent inhibition for clinical activity to be manifest. More recent genotyping studies asserting that more than 90% of clear cell RCC have dysfunctional VHL[48,52] suggest that false-negative genotyping might contribute to the apparent lack of predictive value tumor VHL inactivation for response to VEGF pathway therapy. Alternatively, this lack of association might indicate that other molecular features (eg, baseline IL-8 expression, fibroblast growth factor [FGF] upregulation) may be more critical contributors to the resistance of clear cell RCC to VEGF pathway therapy.

Thus, the investigation of treatment selection factors for patients with advanced RCC remains a work in progress. Although some information is available, considerably more research is needed to identify and validate selection factors for particular treatment approaches. In the future, these approaches are likely to include not only clinical features and blood-based and tissue-based biomarkers but also sophisticated functional imaging studies and increasing assessment of both tumor and germline polymorphisms. Because identification of the optimal first-line treatment of a particular patient is a prerequisite to determining the optimal second-line therapy, treatment sequence, or, more importantly, determining those patients who need different treatment approaches altogether, initial treatment selection research remains a priority.

NOVEL THERAPEUTIC AGENTS

In addition to novel therapeutic strategies, the landscape of RCC will also be altered by the emergence of many novel therapeutic agents. Some of these new drugs represent the next generation of agents directed against already established therapeutic targets such VEGFR2 and mTOR. Others will be drugs with novel therapeutic targets in some cases identified through studies into the mechanisms of resistance and response to available therapies.

Novel Agents Targeting VEGF Signaling

As discussed earlier, the development of agents disrupting VEGF signaling has been a major therapeutic breakthrough for patients with advanced RCC. First-generation TKI with activity against VEGFR2, such as sunitinib and sorafenib, have emerged to form the backbone of advanced RCC therapy. However, these agents have certain limitations. Responses to these drugs are typically neither complete nor durable off therapy, and their usefulness is often limited to moderate disease regression and significant, but transient, prolongation of disease stability. Moreover, the continuous administration of these agents is limited in some patients by toxicity, requiring holding of medication, dose reduction, and even treatment cessation.[53]

The next generation of VEGF-targeted TKI may prove superior to first-generation TKI in terms of both efficacy and side effect profile. As shown in **Table 2**,[54,55] agents such as axitinib and tivozinib boast significantly greater potency against VEGFR compared with earlier-generation TKI. Moreover, the potency of these agents is relatively more focused on the VEGF receptors than other tyrosine kinase receptors such as C-Kit and platelet-derived growth factor receptors (PDGFRs). As these agents develop, the hope is that these molecular characteristics will lead to greater efficacy coupled with less toxicity compared with first-generation TKI.

Preliminary clinical results have been promising. In a phase II randomized discontinuation trial of tivozinib in patients with advanced RCC, the median PFS of all patients was 11.8 months and the objective response rate 27%.[56] However, in patients with clear cell RCC who had undergone nephrectomy, the PFS was 14.8 months and the objective response rate was 32%. Tivozinib is being studied in a randomized phase III trial versus sorafenib in patients with advanced RCC. Likewise, axitinib has shown robust clinical activity in patients with advanced RCC in multiple clinical settings. Axitinib was initially evaluated in a phase II trial in patients with cytokine-refractory RCC.[57] The median TTP of patients treated with axitinib was 15.7 months and the objective response rate 44.2%. Axitinib was subsequently studied in patients who had failed previous sorafenib and again it showed activity.[58] The median PFS of patients treated with axitinib was 7.1 months and the objective response rate 22.6%. Based on these results, axitinib is being assessed in a randomized phase III trial versus sorafenib in patients with advanced RCC who have failed sunitinib (Axis trial). Although the results from this trial have yet to be reported, preliminary press releases from Pfizer Pharmaceuticals indicate that the primary end point of this trial (superior PFS) has been met. Positive results from these 2 ongoing phase III trials will likely have an immediate impact on the second-line therapy for RCC and possibly change front-line therapy as well.

Novel Agents Targeting mTOR

Inhibitors of mTOR represent a second class of molecularly targeted agents that have shown activity in patients with advanced RCC, and 2 such agents, temsirolimus and everolimus, are now approved by the US Food and Drug Administration (FDA) for the treatment of patients with RCC.[12,26] Similar to VEGF-targeted TKI, significant responses to these agents are infrequent and typically short-lived and all patients treated with these drugs eventually develop progressive disease. The efficacy of these allosteric inhibitors of mTOR may be limited in part because they primarily inhibit the

Table 2
Potency of VEGFR TKIs

Agent	IC$_{50}$ (nM)				
	VEGFR-1	VEGFR-2	VEGFR-3	c-KitR	PDGFR-β
Tivozinib[54]	0.2	0.2	0.2	1.6	1.7
Axitinib[55]	1.2	0.3	0.3	1.6	1.7
Sunitinib[55]	2	10	17	10	8
Pazopanib[55]	15	8	10	2.4	14
Sorafenib[55]	NA	90	20	68	80

Abbreviations: IC$_{50}$, half maximal inhibitory concentration; NA, not applicable.

function of TORC1, the complex including mTOR and raptor (regulatory associated protein of TOR), and have less activity against TORC2, the complex including mTOR and rictor (rapamycin insensitive companion of TOR). Although the clinical activity of mTOR inhibitors in RCC was largely discovered empirically, the ability of the rapalogues to attenuate HIF-1α gene expression by reducing both mRNA and protein stabilization has long been proposed as a potential mechanism of action of these agents in RCC.[59,60] This situation may be particularly true in the clear cell variant, most of which possess biallelic alterations in the VHL gene,[61,62] resulting in the accumulation of HIF-1 and HIF-2 and the subsequent activation of their target genes, including VEGF, PDGF, TGF-α, and CXCR4.[63–65] However, although HIF-1α and HIF-2α are known to have overlapping effects on gene expression, HIF-2α has been argued by many to be the more relevant HIF with respect to the development and progression of RCC.[66,67] It has recently been shown that a substantial fraction of VHL−/− RCC express HIF-2α only.[48] Recent studies have also suggested that the translation of HIF-2α is more dependent on the activity of TORC2 and largely independent of the TORC1 activity.[68,69] Together these findings highlight the potential therapeutic value of simultaneously inhibiting both TORC1 and TORC2 in RCC.

A new generation of mTOR inhibitors is under development that are not allosteric inhibitors of mTOR but rather bind directly to the adenosine triphosphate-binding domain of mTOR, thereby inhibiting the function of both TORC1 and TORC2. The aforementioned ability to suppress HIF-2α expression would not be the only theoretic advantage of such agents in RCC. One of the primary activities of TORC1 inhibitors is believed to be the dephosphorylation and activation of eukaryotic translation initiation factor (eIF4E)-binding proteins (4EBPs), which function to sequester and block eIF4E from performing cap-dependent translation of certain difficult-to-translate mRNAs such as those of VEGF, cyclin D, c-Myc, and survivin.[69,70] However, the phosphorylation of 4E-BP1 has long been recognized to be less responsive to rapalogues than that of the S6 ribosomal protein and the suppression of 4E-BP1 phosphorylation by rapamycin is reversed within a few hours of drug exposure.[71] The active site inhibitors of mTOR would therefore also have the added advantage of achieving more effective suppression of 4E-BP1 phosphorylation and therefore attenuation of cap-dependent translation. Whether these theoretic advantages will translate into superior clinical activity will be an area of active investigation in the coming years.

Novel Immunotherapy Approaches

As discussed earlier, immunotherapy with HD IL-2 maintains the advantage over other therapies of offering a higher percentage of durable responses for patients with advanced RCC. However, the possibility of achieving these durable responses must be balanced with the potential toxicity of HD IL-2. Nonetheless, it must be conceded that at least a subset of RCC remain responsive to immune-stimulating agents. Novel immunotherapy approaches will seek to further exploit the immune-responsiveness of RCC and avoid the well-described toxicities of HD IL-2. Although this topic is covered in more detail in the article by Rosenblatt and McDermott elsewhere in this issue, a few novel immune targets are worthy of special mention.

Although the exact mechanism by which HD IL-2 exerts its antitumor activity remains unknown, it is widely believed that immune-stimulating agents result in the generation, activation, or expansion of a population of T lymphocytes that recognize antigens expressed by RCC. Improved understanding of various mechanisms by which T-cell activation can be positively or negatively regulated has led to the development of agents that can activate the immune system by modulating costimulatory signals on T cells. These novel immune therapies include antibodies against CTLA-4 and PD-1.

CTLA-4 is a costimulatory receptor expressed on the surface of activated T lymphocytes that, when activated, prevents further lymphocyte proliferation. Preventing engagement of this inhibitory signal has emerged as a strategy to augment or release an antitumor immune response. Currently approved by the FDA for the treatment of patients with metastatic melanoma, ipilimumab, an antibody directed against CTLA-4, has seen a limited evaluation in patients with metastatic RCC. In a phase II trial run by the National Cancer Institute Surgery Branch, 2 cohorts of patients with advanced RCC received 2 different dosing schedules of ipilimumab: a 3-mg/kg loading dose followed by either 1-mg/kg or 3-mg/kg maintenance doses every 3 weeks.[72] Of the 21 patients receiving the 1-mg/kg maintenance dose, 1 patient (4.7%) experienced a partial response. Of 40 patients treated with the 3-mg/kg maintenance dose, 5 (12.5%) experienced partial responses. Responses were observed in patients who had failed previous HD IL-2, suggesting that there is no clear cross-resistance. Given its recent FDA approval for melanoma, ipilimumab will likely see further evaluation in RCC in the near future.

PD-1 is another costimulatory receptor that is expressed on activated T lymphocytes and when activated downmodulates T-cell function. A major ligand for PD-1, B7-H1 (PD-L1), was shown to be overexpressed in many RCC, and greater expression was associated with worse prognosis.[73] It has been suggested that expression of B7-H1 by RCC is a strategy to evade immune detection and activation. Efforts are under way to block PD-1 activation as a means of reactivating an antitumor immune response. MDX-1106 is a monoclonal antibody directed against PD-1 that was recently assessed in a phase I trial including many patients with advanced RCC.[74] MDX-1106 was administered in doses of 1, 3, and 10 mg/kg given every 2 weeks. Of 16 patients with RCC treated at various doses, 5 patients (31%) achieved objective responses, including 1 complete response. This promising activity coupled with a mild toxicity profile has prompted the rapid assessment of MDX-1106 in multiple phase II trials in patients with advanced RCC. Over the next several years, agents such as ipilimumab and MDX-1106 will likely be assessed, along with HD IL-2, in various sequences and combinations with the goal of achieving higher rates of durable responses than what is possible with currently available therapies.

Therapeutic Targets Identified by Resistance Mechanisms

Elucidating the mechanism by which RCC develops resistance to VEGF-targeted therapies is perhaps the most critical priority for RCC research. Because complete responses to these antiangiogenic agents remain rare, it is clear that most RCC possess the intrinsic ability to survive the immediate insult of hypoxia and nutrient deprivation induced by the reduction in tumor vasculature and are able to eventually activate escape pathways to restore tumor perfusion. It is hoped that the identification of critical signaling pathways that mediate both the intrinsic resistance to antiangiogenic agents and the delayed restoration of microvasculature angiogenic escape will identify novel therapeutic targets in RCC. Efforts directed toward this end have already identified several such targets.

Angiopoietins

The angiopoietins (Angs) are ligands for the endothelial-specific tyrosine kinase receptors Tie-1 and Tie-2 and are believed to play a critical role in vessel maturation and the maintenance of vessel integrity. Ang-1 and Ang-2 are the most frequently implicated Angs in tumor angiogenesis and are specific ligands for Tie-2. Ang-2 is highly expressed by the endothelial cells of many tumors and is believed to act in tandem with VEGF to promote tumor-mediated angiogenesis. Activation of the Ang/Tie-2 axis had been implicated in both basal angiogenesis in response to hypoxia in RCC and in vascular survival in the setting of VEGF blockade.[75,76] AMG-386 is an antiangiopoietin peptibody (an Ang-recognizing peptide fused to the Fc region of an antibody) that can inhibit the interaction between Ang-1 and Ang-2 with Tie-2. Given the possible synergistic relationship between VEGF and Ang-2 in promoting angiogenesis, the combination of AMG-386 with VEGF-targeted agents has emerged as a therapeutic strategy in RCC. Although a randomized phase II trial in patients with advanced RCC failed to show a prolongation in the PFS in patients treated with sorafenib in combination with 2 different doses of AMG-386 compared with placebo, a higher objective response rate was noted in the AMG-386–containing arms.[77] A single-arm phase II trial combining sunitinib with AMG-386 in patients with treatment-naive or cytokine-refractory metastatic RCC is ongoing and results are expected soon.

IL-8

IL-8 is a member of the CXC family of chemokines and is known to be a potent proangiogenic factor. Angiogenesis mediated by IL-8 may occur in a VEGF-independent manner as suggested by Mikukami and colleagues[78] in a colon cancer xenograft model in which VEGF signaling was opposed. It was recently shown in multiple RCC xenograft models that IL-8 secretion was upregulated in tumors treated with sunitinib coincident with restoration of microvasculature heralding treatment resistance.[79] Concurrent treatment of the same xenograft models with sunitinib and a neutralizing antibody against IL-8 resulted in the restoration of sensitivity of the tumors to sunitinib. In patients with clear cell RCC resistant to sunitinib, expression of IL-8 was found to be increased in their archived tumor specimens, suggesting that IL-8 may play a role in upfront resistance to VEGF-targeted agents in addition to a role in delayed resistance. Efforts to develop therapeutic strategies to inhibit IL-8–mediated signaling are under way and there will be great interest in examining the additive effects of these agents in combination with VEGF-targeted therapies in RCC in the years to come.

FGF

FGF is a soluble growth factor produced by both tumors and tumor microenvironment, which are also potent angiogenic factors signaling through tyrosine kinase receptors. FGF-2 was initially found to be upregulated by Casanovas and colleagues[80] in an islet cell tumor model of acquired resistance to VEGF-targeted therapy. Welti and colleagues[81] recently showed that FGF-2 can oppose the antiangiogenic effect of sunitinib by directly stimulating a proangiogenic signal in endothelial cells. This effect was opposed by concurrent treatment with an inhibitor of the FGF receptor tyrosine kinase. Furthermore, greater than 50% of human RCC specimens were found to strongly express FGF-2 in both the tumor cell and tumor endothelium. Taken together, these findings suggest that there may be some value to the simultaneous targeting of both FGF and VEGF signaling. There are now several multitargeted TKIs in various stages of clinical development with broad activity against VEGFR-1, VEGFR-2, PDGFR-β, and FGF receptor 1. Many of these agents, such as E7080 (Eisai Pharmaceuticals, Tokyo, Japan) and Dovitinib (TKI258, Novartis Pharmaceuticals, Basel, Switzerland) are in active clinical study in RCC, and the results of these studies will inform the value of this therapeutic approach.

Emerging Novel Therapeutic Targets

In addition to the therapeutic targets identified by studies into resistance to VEGF-targeted therapy, several other molecular targets will likely be actively investigated in RCC in the upcoming years. Those targets closest to therapeutic investigation in the near future are discussed in the following sections.

Phosphoinositide 3-kinase/Akt

The aforementioned clinical activity of the rapalogues in RCC has highlighted the potential relevance of the mTOR pathway to RCC pathogenesis and progression. The kinase activity of mTOR is regulated by a complex system of upstream and downstream elements including phosphoinositide 3-kinase (PI3-K), Akt, and the tumor suppressor PTEN homolog. The PI3-K/Akt pathway regulates the function of a broad array of proteins involved in cell growth, proliferation, motility, adhesion, neovascularization, and cell death.[82] One of the potential mechanisms of resistance to RCC to TORC1 inhibitors is through the feedback activation of the PI3-K/Akt. Treatment with TORC1 inhibitors has been shown in some cases to result in the activation of PI3-K through a feedback loop involving the insulinlike growth factor 1 receptor.[83] TORC1 inhibitors also can activate Akt directly through the derepression of TORC2, which results in TORC2-mediated phosphorylation of Akt on Ser^{473}.[84] PI3-K/Akt signaling activates an array of kinases, transcription factors, and other proteins besides mTOR that promote cell growth and survival.[85] This prosurvival effect is primarily executed by Akt through a variety of pathways including the negative regulation of factors promoting the expression of death genes (eg, inactivation of forkhead family proteins), positive regulation of prosurvival genes (eg, activation of NF-κB), direct phosphorylation of proapoptotic proteins (eg, inactivation of BAD), and regulation of the cell cycle. Disruption of any of these prosurvival signals may have therapeutic benefits that complement the effects of mTOR inhibition and enhance antitumor activity, a notion that has been supported in preclinical studies both in vitro and in vivo.[86]

Inhibitors of PI3-K and Akt are now entering active clinical development in RCC. Because the catalytic domain of mTOR and p110α subunit of PI3-K are structurally related, multiple agents are also in development that have dual inhibitory activity against PI3-K and mTOR. In addition to being inhibitors of PI3-K, these agents have the added benefit of directly inhibiting mTOR kinase activity, thereby inhibiting the function of both TORC1 and TORC2. Preclinical studies have also supported the efficacy of these dual inhibitors in RCC.[87] Should these agents prove superior to allosteric inhibitors of TORC1 in clinical studies, it is possible that they may replace the rapalogues in the therapeutic landscape of RCC within the next several years.

Hepatocyte growth factor/c-MET

Directly involved through germline mutation in hereditary papillary RCC, c-MET is a tyrosine kinase and protooncogene the activation of which is believed to promote tumor invasiveness. Activation of c-MET in RCC has been linked to VHL loss as well as hypoxia and may play an important role in malignant progression.[88,89] Higher expression of c-MET in RCC tumor specimens has been associated with higher tumor grade and clinical stage and was also found to be an independent predictor of poor OS.[90] Similar to many of the molecular targets mentioned earlier, c-MET has also been implicated in the development of resistance to VEGF-targeted therapy through maintenance of an alternate angiogenic pathway.[91] Treatment of RCC xenografts resistant to sunitinib with the combination of sunitinib and a selective c-MET inhibitor resulted in significantly greater inhibition of tumor growth than treatment with either agent alone.

Inhibition of c-MET signaling is being explored clinically either through direct inhibitors of c-MET receptor tyrosine kinase activity or through disruption of the interaction of c-MET with its ligand hepatocyte growth factor (HGF) (ie, HGF antibody). These agents are now likely to be explored both as single agents and in combination with VEGF-targeted therapy in patients with advanced RCC. XL184 (Exelixis Pharmaceuticals), a potent small molecule inhibitor of both c-MET and VEGFR2, is being investigated in a phase I drug interaction study in RCC and may develop as an attractive agent for patients who have failed previous VEGF-targeted therapy.

HIF-2α

As discussed earlier, it is now largely accepted that HIF-2α is the more relevant HIF in RCC with respect to malignant transformation and progression. As the upregulation of HIF levels as a result of loss of VHL function that characterizes most clear cell RCC results in the activation of many other genes that may drive tumor survival and proliferation besides *VEGF* and *PDGF* (eg, TGFα, CXCR4), successful inhibition of HIF-2α may have broader therapeutic effects than currently available VEGF-targeted agents. However, although HIF-2α is clearly an attractive therapeutic target in RCC, there are no direct inhibitors of HIF-2α in active clinical assessment in RCC. Efforts are under way to develop such agents, and successful evaluation of these agents in RCC may represent a major therapeutic advancement in the next several years.

SUMMARY

Although significant strides have been made in RCC treatment in the last several years, physicians and researches must still face many challenges to further improve therapeutic outcomes for patients. With so many agents now approved by the FDA for the treatment of patients with advanced RCC, to maximize the therapeutic benefits of these agents, physicians must determine optimal dosing strategies, sequences, or combinations by which to administer them. Furthermore, with multiple agents that have potentially distinct mechanisms of action, it will be even more critical to identify and develop patient selection strategies to direct the most appropriate therapies to individual patients. The next several years will see a multitude of novel agents assessed in RCC. Although the efficacy of many of these agents has yet to be established, should this situation be the case, clinicians will face the difficult task of integrating these new therapies into the already complicated therapeutic landscape in RCC.

REFERENCES

1. Jemal A, Siegel R, Xu J, et al. Cancer statistics. CA Cancer J Clin 2010;60(5): 277–300.
2. Motzer RJ, Mazumdar M, Bacik J, et al. Survival and prognostic stratification of 670 patients with advanced renal cell carcinoma. J Clin Oncol 1999;17(8):2530–40.
3. Heng DY, Xie W, Regan MM, et al. Prognostic factors for overall survival in patients with metastatic renal cell carcinoma treated with vascular endothelial growth factor-targeted agents: results from a large, multicenter study. J Clin Oncol 2009;27(34):5794–9.
4. Escudier B, Szczylik C, Hutson TE, et al. Randomized phase II trial of first-line treatment with sorafenib versus interferon Alfa-2a in patients with metastatic renal cell carcinoma. J Clin Oncol 2009;27(8):1280–9.
5. Amato RJ, Harris P, Dalton M, et al. A phase II trial of intra-patient dose-escalated sorafenib in patients (pts) with metastatic renal cell cancer (MRCC). J Clin Oncol 2007;25:18S [abstract: 5026].
6. Houk BE, Bello CL, Poland B, et al. Relationship between exposure to sunitinib and efficacy and tolerability endpoints in patients with cancer: results of

a pharmacokinetic/pharmacodynamic meta-analysis. Cancer Chemother Pharmacol 2010;66(2):357–71.

7. Rini BI. Biomarkers: hypertension following anti-angiogenesis therapy. Clin Adv Hematol Oncol 2010;8(6):415–6.

8. Motzer RJ, Hutson TE, Olsen MR, et al. Randomized phase II multicenter study of the efficacy and safety of sunitinib on the 4/2 versus continuous dosing schedule as first-line therapy of metastatic renal cell carcinoma: renal EFFECT trial. J Clin Oncol 2011;29(Suppl 7) [abstract: #LBA308].

9. Motzer RJ, Michaelson MD, Rosenberg J, et al. Sunitinib efficacy against advanced renal cell carcinoma. J Urol 2007;178(5):1883–7.

10. Escudier B, Bellmunt J, Negrier S, et al. Phase III trial of bevacizumab plus interferon alfa-2a in patients with metastatic renal cell carcinoma (AVOREN): final analysis of overall survival. J Clin Oncol 2010;28(13):2144–50.

11. Atkins MB, Hidalgo M, Stadler WM, et al. Randomized phase II study of multiple dose levels of CCI-779, a novel mammalian target of rapamycin kinase inhibitor, in patients with advanced refractory renal cell carcinoma. J Clin Oncol 2004;22(5):909–18.

12. Motzer RJ, Escudier B, Oudard S, et al. Efficacy of everolimus in advanced renal cell carcinoma: a double-blind, randomised, placebo-controlled phase III trial. Lancet 2008;372(9637):449–56.

13. Cho DC, Puzanov I, Regan MM, et al. Retrospective analysis of the safety and efficacy of interleukin-2 after prior VEGF-targeted therapy in patients with advanced renal cell carcinoma. J Immunother 2009;32(2):181–5.

14. Rini BI, Michaelson MD, Rosenberg JE, et al. Antitumor activity and biomarker analysis of sunitinib in patients with bevacizumab-refractory metastatic renal cell carcinoma. J Clin Oncol 2008;26(22):3743–8.

15. Rini BI, Wilding G, Hudes G, et al. Phase II study of axitinib in sorafenib-refractory metastatic renal cell carcinoma. J Clin Oncol 2009;27(27):4462–8.

16. Heng DY, MacKenzie MJ, Vaishampayan UN, et al. Primary anti-VEGF refractory metastatic renal cell carcinoma (mRCC): clinical characteristics, risk factors and subsequent therapy. J Clin Oncol 2011;29:7S [abstract: 305].

17. Sosman JA, Atkins MB, McDermott DF, et al. Updated results of phase I trial of sorafenib (s) and bevacizumab (B) in patients with metastatic renal cell cancer (mRCC). J Clin Oncol 2008;26(15S):252s [abstract: 5011].

18. Feldman DR, Baum MS, Ginsberg MS, et al. Phase I trial of bevacizumab plus escalated doses of sunitinib in patients with metastatic renal cell carcinoma. J Clin Oncol 2009;27(9):1432–9.

19. Levine RJ, Maynard SE, Qian C, et al. Circulating angiogenic factors and the risk of preeclampsia. N Engl J Med 2004;350(7):672–83.

20. Bukowski RM, Kabbinavar FF, Figlin RA, et al. Randomized phase II study of erlotinib combined with bevacizumab compared with bevacizumab alone in metastatic renal cell cancer. J Clin Oncol 2007;25(29):4536–41.

21. Hainsworth JD, Spigel DR, Burris HA 3rd, et al. Phase II trial of bevacizumab and everolimus in patients with advanced renal cell carcinoma. J Clin Oncol 2010;28(13):2131–6.

22. Merchan JR, Liu G, Fitch T, et al. Phase I/II trial of CCI-779 and bevacizumab in stage IV renal cell carcinoma: phase I safety and activity results. J Clin Oncol 2007;25:18S [abstract: 5034].

23. Escudier B, Negrier S, Gravis G, et al. Can the combination of temsirolimus and bevacizumab improve the treatment of metastatic renal cell carcinoma (MRCC)? Results of the randomized TORAVA phase II trial. J Clin Oncol 2010;28:15S [abstract: 4516].

24. Rini BI, Halabi S, Rosenberg JE, et al. Bevacizumab plus interferon alfa compared with interferon alfa monotherapy in patients with metastatic renal cell carcinoma: CALGB 90206. J Clin Oncol 2008;26(33):5422–8.

25. Dandamudi UB, Ghebremichael MS, Sosman JA, et al. A phase II study of bevacizumab (B) and high-dose aldesleukin (IL-2) in patients (p) with metastatic renal carcinoma (mRCC): a Cytokine Working Group Study (CWGS). J Clin Oncol 2010;28:15S [abstract: 4530].

26. Hudes G, Carducci M, Tomczak P, et al. Temsirolimus, interferon alfa, or both for advanced renal-cell carcinoma. N Engl J Med 2007;356(22):2271–81.

27. Motzer RJ, Hutson TE, Tomczak P, et al. Sunitinib versus interferon alfa in metastatic renal-cell carcinoma. N Engl J Med 2007;356(2):115–24.

28. McDermott DF, Regan MM, Clark JI, et al. Randomized phase III trial of high-dose interleukin-2 versus subcutaneous interleukin-2 and interferon in patients with metastatic renal cell carcinoma. J Clin Oncol 2005;23(1):133–41.

29. Yang JC, Sherry RM, Stienberg SM, et al. A three-arm randomized comparison of high and low dose intravenous and subcutaneous interleukin-2 in the treatment of metastatic renal cancer. J Clin Oncol 2003;21:3127.

30. Mcdermott DF, Ghebremichael M, Signoretti S, et al. The high-dose aldesleukin (HD IL-2) "Select" trial in patients with metastatic renal cell carcinoma (mRCC). J Clin Oncol 2010;28:15S [abstract: 4514].

31. Upton MP, Parker RA, Youmans A, et al. Histologic predictors of renal cell carcinoma response to interleukin-2-based therapy. J Immunother 2005;28(5):488–95.

32. Motzer RJ, Bacik J, Mariani T, et al. Treatment outcome and survival associated with metastatic renal cell carcinoma of non-clear-cell histology. J Clin Oncol 2002;20(9):2376–81.

33. Atkins M, Regan M, McDermott D, et al. Carbonic anhydrase IX expression predicts outcome of interleukin 2 therapy for renal cancer. Clin Cancer Res 2005;11(10):3714–21.

34. Bui MH, Seligson D, Han KR, et al. Carbonic anhydrase IX is an independent predictor of survival in advanced renal clear cell carcinoma: implications for prognosis and therapy. Clin Cancer Res 2003;9(2):802–11.

35. Jaeger E, Waldman R, Roydasgupta R, et al. Array-based comparative genomic analysis of interleukin-2 complete responders in patients with metastatic renal cell carcinoma. J Clin Oncol 2008;26:15S [abstract: 5043].

36. Delgado DC, Hank JA, Kolesar J, et al. Genotypes of NK cell KIR receptors, their ligands, and Fcgamma receptors in the response of neuroblastoma patients to Hu14.18-IL2 immunotherapy. Cancer Res 2010;70(23):9554–61.

37. Gajewski TF, Louahed J, Brichard VG. Gene signature in melanoma associated with clinical activity: a potential clue to unlock cancer immunotherapy. Cancer J 2010;16(4):399–403.

38. Sullivan RJ, Hoshida Y, Brunet J, et al. A single center experience with high-dose (HD) IL-2 treatment for patients with advanced melanoma and pilot investigation of a novel gene expression signature as a predictor of response. J Clin Oncol 2009;27:15S [abstract: 9003].

39. Libermann TA, Bhasin M, Joseph MG, et al. Gene expression profiling signatures associated with RCC response to IL-2 therapy. J Immunother 2008;31(9):958.

40. Dutcher JP, de Souza P, McDermott D, et al. Effect of temsirolimus versus interferon-alpha on outcome of patients with advanced renal cell carcinoma of different tumor histologies. Med Oncol 2009;26(2):202–9.

41. Choueiri TK, Plantade A, Elson P, et al. Efficacy of sunitinib and sorafenib in metastatic papillary and chromophobe renal cell carcinoma. J Clin Oncol 2008;26(1):127–31.

42. Cho D, Signoretti S, Dabora S, et al. Potential histologic and molecular predictors of response to temsirolimus in patients with advanced renal cell carcinoma. Clin Genitourin Cancer 2007;5(6):379–85.

43. Figlin RA, de Souza P, McDermott D, et al. Analysis of PTEN and HIF-1alpha and correlation with efficacy in patients with advanced renal cell carcinoma treated with temsirolimus versus interferon-alpha. Cancer 2009;115(16):3651–60.

44. De Benedetti A, Graff JR. eIF-4E expression and its role in malignancies and metastases. Oncogene 2004;23(18):3189–99.

45. Urano J, Sato T, Matsuo T, et al. Point mutations in TOR confer Rheb-independent growth in fission yeast and nutrient-independent mammalian TOR signaling in mammalian cells. Proc Natl Acad Sci U S A 2007;104(9):3514–9.

46. Escudier B, Eisen T, Stadler WM, et al. Sorafenib for treatment of renal cell carcinoma: final efficacy and safety results of the phase III treatment approaches in renal cancer global evaluation trial. J Clin Oncol 2009;27(20):3312–8.

47. Patel PH, Chadalavada RS, Ishill NM, et al. Hypoxia-inducible factor (HIF)1a and 2a in cell lines and human tumor predicts response to sunitinib in renal cell carcinoma (RCC). J Clin Oncol 2008;26 [abstract: 5008].

48. Gordan JD, Lal P, Dondeti VR, et al. HIF-alpha effects on c-Myc distinguish two subtypes of sporadic VHL-deficient clear cell renal carcinoma. Cancer Cell 2008;14(6):435–46.

49. Choueiri TK, Vaziri SA, Jaeger E, et al. von Hippel-Lindau gene status and response to vascular endothelial growth factor targeted therapy for metastatic clear cell renal cell carcinoma. J Urol 2008;180(3):860–5 [discussion: 865–6].

50. Gad S, Sultan-Amar V, Meric J, et al. Somatic von Hippel-Lindau (VHL) gene analysis and clinical outcome under antiangiogenic treatment in metastatic renal cell carcinoma: preliminary results. Target Oncol 2007;2:3–6.

51. Hutson TE, Davis ID, Macheils JH, et al. Biomarker analysis and final efficacy and safety results of a phase II renal cell carcinoma trial with pazopanib (GW786034), a multi-kinase angiogenesis inhibitor. J Clin Oncol 2008;26:15S [abstract: 5046].

52. Beroukhim R, Brunet JP, Di Napoli A, et al. Patterns of gene expression and copy-number alterations in von-Hippel Lindau disease-associated and sporadic clear cell carcinoma of the kidney. Cancer Res 2009;69(11):4674–81.

53. Keefe SM, Moyneur E, Meyers S, et al. Dose reductions and delays in patients (pts) with renal cell carcinoma (RCC) treated with sorafenib (SR) or sunitinib (SU): retrospective analysis of two large U.S. health care claims databases. J Clin Oncol 2008;28:15 [abstract: 6090].

54. Eskens F, De Jonge MJ, Esteves B, et al. Updated results from a phase I study of AV-951 (KRN951), a potent and selective VEGFR-1, -2 and -3 tyrosine kinase inhibitor, in patients with advanced solid tumors. Proc Annu Meet Am Assoc Cancer Res 2008;49:LB201.

55. Chow LQ, Eckhardt SG. Sunitinib: from rational design to clinical efficacy. J Clin Oncol 2007;25(7):884–96.

56. Bhargava P, Esteves B, Al-Adhami M, et al. Activity of tovozanib (AV-951) in patients with renal cell carcinoma (RCC): subgroup analysis from a phase II randomized discontinuation trial (RDT). J Clin Oncol 2010 ASCO Annual Meetings Proceedings 2010;28(15S):366S.

57. Rixe O, Bukowski RM, Michaelson MD, et al. Axitinib treatment in patients with cytokine-refractory metastatic renal-cell cancer: a phase II study. Lancet Oncol 2007;8(11):975–84.

58. Rini BI, Wilding GT, Hudes G, et al. Axitinib (AG-013736) in patients with metastatic renal cell cancer refractory to sorafenib. J Clin Oncol 2007. ASCO Annual Meetings Proceedings 2007;25:18S [abstract: 5032].
59. Hudson CC, Liu M, Chiang GG, et al. Regulation of hypoxia-inducible factor 1alpha expression and function by the mammalian target of rapamycin. Mol Cell Biol 2002;22(20):7004–14.
60. Turner KJ, Moore JW, Jones A, et al. Expression of hypoxia-inducible factors in human renal cancer: relationship to angiogenesis and to the von Hippel-Lindau gene mutation. Cancer Res 2002;62(10):2957–61.
61. Kenck C, Wilhelm M, Bugert P, et al. Mutation of the VHL gene is associated exclusively with the development of non-papillary renal cell carcinomas. J Pathol 1996;179(2):157–61.
62. Foster K, Prowse A, van den Berg A, et al. Somatic mutations of the von Hippel-Lindau disease tumour suppressor gene in non-familial clear cell renal carcinoma. Hum Mol Genet 1994;3(12):2169–73.
63. Jaakkola P, Mole DR, Tian YM, et al. Targeting of HIF-alpha to the von Hippel-Lindau ubiquitylation complex by O2-regulated prolyl hydroxylation. Science 2001;292(5516):468–72.
64. Iliopoulos O, Kibel A, Gray S, et al. Tumour suppression by the human von Hippel-Lindau gene product. Nat Med 1995;1(8):822–6.
65. de Paulsen N, Brychzy A, Fournier MC, et al. Role of transforming growth factor-alpha in von Hippel–Lindau (VHL)(–/–) clear cell renal carcinoma cell proliferation: a possible mechanism coupling VHL tumor suppressor inactivation and tumorigenesis. Proc Natl Acad Sci U S A 2001;98(4):1387–92.
66. Kondo K, Klco J, Nakamura E, et al. Inhibition of HIF is necessary for tumor suppression by the von Hippel-Lindau protein. Cancer Cell 2002;1(3):237–46.
67. Kondo K, Kim WY, Lechpammer M, et al. Inhibition of HIF2alpha is sufficient to suppress pVHL-defective tumor growth. PLoS Biol 2003;1(3):E83.
68. Toschi A, Lee E, Gadir N, et al. Differential dependence of hypoxia-inducible factors 1 alpha and 2 alpha on mTORC1 and mTORC2. J Biol Chem 2008;283(50):34495–9.
69. Ma XM, Blenis J. Molecular mechanisms of mTOR-mediated translational control. Nat Rev Mol Cell Biol 2009;10(5):307–18.
70. Graff JR, Konicek BW, Carter JH, et al. Targeting the eukaryotic translation initiation factor 4E for cancer therapy. Cancer Res 2008;68(3):631–4.
71. Choo AY, Yoon SO, Kim SG, et al. Rapamycin differentially inhibits S6Ks and 4E-BP1 to mediate cell-type-specific repression of mRNA translation. Proc Natl Acad Sci U S A 2008;105(45):17414–9.
72. Yang JC, Hughes M, Kammula U, et al. Ipilimumab (anti-CTLA4 antibody) causes regression of metastatic renal cell cancer associated with enteritis and hypophysitis. J Immunother 2007;30(8):825–30.
73. Thompson RH, Dong H, Kwon ED. Implications of B7-H1 expression in clear cell carcinoma of the kidney for prognostication and therapy. Clin Cancer Res 2007; 13(2 Pt 2):709s–15s.
74. Sznol MPJ, Smith DC, Brahmer JR, et al. Safety and antitumor activity of biweekly MDX-1106 (Anti-PD-1, BMS936558/ONO-4538) in patients with advanced refractory malignancies. J Clin Oncol 2010;28(15S):205s.
75. Yamakawa M, Liu LX, Belanger AJ, et al. Expression of angiopoietins in renal epithelial and clear cell carcinoma cells: regulation by hypoxia and participation in angiogenesis. Am J Physiol Renal Physiol 2004;287(4):F649–57.
76. Huang J, Bae JO, Tsai JP, et al. Angiopoietin-1/Tie-2 activation contributes to vascular survival and tumor growth during VEGF blockade. Int J Oncol 2009;34(1):79–87.

77. Rini BI, Szczylik C, Tanner NM, et al. AMG 386 in combination with sorafenib in patients (pts) with metatstatic renal cell cancer (mRCC): a randomized, double-blind, placebo controlled, phase II study. J Clin Oncol 2011;29(Suppl 7) [abstract: 309].

78. Mizukami Y, Jo WS, Duerr EM, et al. Induction of interleukin-8 preserves the angiogenic response in HIF-1alpha-deficient colon cancer cells. Nat Med 2005; 11(9):992–7.

79. Huang D, Ding Y, Zhou M, et al. Interleukin-8 mediates resistance to antiangiogenic agent sunitinib in renal cell carcinoma. Cancer Res 2010;70(3):1063–71.

80. Casanovas O, Hicklin DJ, Bergers G, et al. Drug resistance by evasion of antiangiogenic targeting of VEGF signaling in late-stage pancreatic islet tumors. Cancer Cell 2005;8(4):299–309.

81. Welti JC, Gourlaouen M, Powles T, et al. Fibroblast growth factor 2 regulates endothelial cell sensitivity to sunitinib. Oncogene 2011;30(10):1183–93.

82. Nicholson KM, Anderson NG. The protein kinase B/Akt signalling pathway in human malignancy. Cell Signal 2002;14(5):381–95.

83. Wan X, Harkavy B, Shen N, et al. Rapamycin induces feedback activation of Akt signaling through an IGF-1R-dependent mechanism. Oncogene 2007;26(13): 1932–40.

84. Sarbassov DD, Guertin DA, Ali SM, et al. Phosphorylation and regulation of Akt/PKB by the rictor-mTOR complex. Science 2005;307(5712):1098–101.

85. Cantley LC. The phosphoinositide 3-kinase pathway. Science 2002;296(5573): 1655–7.

86. Sourbier C, Lindner V, Lang H, et al. The phosphoinositide 3-kinase/Akt pathway: a new target in human renal cell carcinoma therapy. Cancer Res 2006;66(10): 5130–42.

87. Cho DC, Cohen MB, Panka DJ, et al. The efficacy of the novel dual PI3-kinase/mTOR inhibitor NVP-BEZ235 compared with rapamycin in renal cell carcinoma. Clin Cancer Res 2010;16(14):3628–38.

88. Pennacchietti S, Michieli P, Galluzzo M, et al. Hypoxia promotes invasive growth by transcriptional activation of the met protooncogene. Cancer Cell 2003;3(4): 347–61.

89. Koochekpour S, Jeffers M, Wang PH, et al. The von Hippel-Lindau tumor suppressor gene inhibits hepatocyte growth factor/scatter factor-induced invasion and branching morphogenesis in renal carcinoma cells. Mol Cell Biol 1999;19(9):5902–12.

90. Gibney G, Conrad P, Aziz SA, et al. C-met as a therapeutic target using ARQ197 in renal cell carcinoma. J Clin Oncol 2011;29(Suppl 7) [abstract: 360].

91. Shojaei F, Lee JH, Simmons BH, et al. HGF/c-Met acts as an alternative angiogenic pathway in sunitinib-resistant tumors. Cancer Res 2010;70(24):10090–100.

Index

Note: Page numbers of article titles are in **boldface** type.

Hematol Oncol Clin N Am 25 (2011) 937–950
doi:10.1016/S0889-8588(11)00080-3
0889-8588/11/$ – see front matter © 2011 Elsevier Inc. All rights reserved.

hemonc.theclinics.com

Moving?

Make sure your subscription moves with you!

To notify us of your new address, find your **Clinics Account Number** (located on your mailing label above your name), and contact customer service at:

Email: journalscustomerservice-usa@elsevier.com

800-654-2452 (subscribers in the U.S. & Canada)
314-447-8871 (subscribers outside of the U.S. & Canada)

Fax number: 314-447-8029

Elsevier Health Sciences Division
Subscription Customer Service
3251 Riverport Lane
Maryland Heights, MO 63043

*To ensure uninterrupted delivery of your subscription, please notify us at least 4 weeks in advance of move.

Printed and bound by CPI Group (UK) Ltd, Croydon, CR0 4YY

03/10/2024

01040446-0011